The 3P's for Advanced Healthcare Providers

Pathophysiology, Physical Assessment, and Pharmacology

Julia L. Rogers, DNP, APRN, CNS, FNP-BC, FAANP
Associate Professor, DNP Program Coordinator
College of Nursing
Purdue University Northwest
Hammond, Indiana
Nurse Practitioner
Medical Staff
Northwest Medical Group Pulmonary and Critical Care Medicine
Valparaiso, Indiana
Hospitalist Nurse Practitioner
Medical Staff
TeamHealth
Valparaiso, Indiana

Jodi A. Allen, DNP, RN, FNP-C
Assistant Professor and FNP Program Coordinator
College of Nursing
Purdue University Northwest
Hammond, Indiana

ELSEVIER

Elsevier
3251 Riverport Lane
St. Louis, Missouri 63043

THE 3P'S FOR ADVANCED HEALTHCARE
PROVIDERS

ISBN: 978-0-323-93726-9

Publisher's note: Elsevier takes a neutral position with respect to territorial disputes or
jurisdictional claims in its published content, including in maps and institutional affiliations.

Notice

Practitioners and researchers must always rely on their own experience and knowledge
in evaluating and using any information, methods, compounds, or experiments
described herein. Because of rapid advances in the medical sciences in particular,
independent verification of diagnoses and drug dosages should be made. To the
fullest extent of the law, no responsibility is assumed by Elsevier, authors, editors,
or contributors for any injury and/or damage to persons or property as a matter
of products liability, negligence or otherwise, or from any use or operation of any
methods, products, instructions, or ideas contained in the material herein.

Content Strategist: Heather Bays-Petrovic, Grace Onderlinde
Senior Content Development Manager: Lisa Newton
Senior Content Development Specialist: Laura Goodrich
Publishing Services Manager: Deepthi Unni
Senior Project Manager: Manchu Mohan
Design Direction: Patrick Ferguson

Printed in India

Last digit is the print number: 9 8 7 6 5 4 3 2 1

Working together
to grow libraries in
developing countries

www.elsevier.com • www.bookaid.org

This book is dedicated to the students who motivate us to be better educators and practitioners. We encourage you to continue to carry the torch that will enlighten future nurses.

Julia's:

To my husband, Dwayne; my son, Zachery, and his wife, Emily; and my daughter, Shane. Thanks for always standing by my side. Each of you bring joy and laughter into my life each and every day. I am proud to be part of such an amazing ohana. Ohana means family, and family means nobody is ever left behind or forgotten. To my sisters and brothers: Darla, Theresa, David, Martha, James, John, Robert, and Michael; and in memory of my sisters Vera, Teena, and Loretta and my brother Joseph. Each of you were a part of who I am today, and I appreciate you more than you know.

Jodi's:

To my husband, Daniel, who provides me with endless love and support. You truly are the banks to my river. Thank you for being my partner in every adventure. To my family, who encourage me in all I do. I could not do anything without each of you cheering me on. To my mom, who modeled the art of listening and quiet confidence; you remain a part of all I do.

Jodi Allen, DNP, RN, FNP-C
Assistant Professor and FNP Program
  Coordinator
College of Nursing
Purdue University Northwest
Hammond, Indiana

Corrine M. Djuric, DNP, RN, FNP-C, CWOCN
Assistant Clinical Professor
College of Nursing
Purdue University Northwest
Hammond, Indiana
Family Nurse Practitioner
Wound Ostomy Clinic
Community Hospital
Munster, Indiana

Felipe Oria, Nursing Student
Research Assistant
College of Nursing
Purdue University Northwest
Hammond, Indiana

Julia L. Rogers, DNP, APRN, CNS, FNP-BC, FAANP
Associate Professor, DNP Program
  Coordinator
College of Nursing
Purdue University Northwest
Hammond, Indiana
Nurse Practitioner
Medical Staff
Northwest Medical Group Pulmonary and
  Critical Care Medicine
Valparaiso, Indiana
Hospitalist Nurse Practitioner
Medical Staff
TeamHealth
Valparaiso, Indiana

Marianne Schallmo, DNP, RN, APRN, ANP-BC
Associate Dean Undergraduate Nursing
College of Nursing
Purdue University Northwest
Hammond, Indiana

Susan Feeney, DNP, FNP-C, FNP-BC, FAANP
Associate Professor of Nursing and Associate
    Dean for Advanced Practice Programs
Tan Chingfen Graduate School of Nursing
    at UMass Chan Medical School
Worcester, Massachusetts

Jill Olmstead, DNP, ANP-BC, FAANP
Nurse
Department of Gastroenterology
Providence St. Joseph Health
Fullerton, California

The intent of *The 3P's for Advanced Healthcare Providers* is to illustrate the three principles of higher education in nursing—pathophysiology, physical assessment, and pharmacology—with clarity and accuracy while demonstrating their interconnectedness.

Interdisciplinary research has led to significant advancements in understanding the individual differences in disease risk, physical and biologic markers, diagnostic strategies, and individualized treatment. Importantly, the forward movement of the three P's continues to advance knowledge within the context of social, economic, educational, environmental, and political processes that determine how disease is defined, experienced, assessed, and treated.

There is a synergistic relationship among the three P's. *Pathophysiology* is the study of abnormal physiologic processes associated with the causes, consequences, or concomitants of disease or injury. *Physical assessment* is the organized systemic process of collecting subjective and objective data based up a health history and examination. Physical assessment is performed to determine the physiologic measurements and physical clues to a potential pathology that may reflect the pathophysiologic process of a specific disease. *Pharmacology* is directly related to the pathophysiology of a disease by providing the body with counteractive means to reset the body back to homeostasis through medication. The physical assessment will have abnormal results based on the pathophysiologic process of a disease; however, after effective pharmacotherapy, the assessment should return to normal or back to baseline.

Interweaving the three P's has created excitement. However, it has also created the problem of how students, professors, and clinicians can bring all three together in one succinct format, instead of creating three separate courses that build on each other. Attempting to translate and compress three main ideas into one interweaving idea for students and clinicians is challenging. The approach for this book was to streamline the content for all three P's and present the information in an organized and logical connective sequence using current evidence-based practice guidelines, literature, and research. The primary focus is on making the connection between the pathophysiology, physical examination findings, and pharmacotherapies for the top 40 diagnoses seen in practice.

The book was designed with the following goals:

- Organize the content in a logical and uniform format to facilitate the learning and teaching of all three concepts.
- Emphasize the readability of the material for improved comprehension of how all three P's are connected.
- Present information that considers diversity connections, the geriatric and pediatric populations, and acute care data.
- Provide the most current and relevant information on etiology, epidemiology, pathophysiology, clinical manifestations, and treatment for disease processes.
- Integrate health promotion and disease prevention by updating risk factors, explaining relationships between diversity and disease, and referencing screening recommendations.
- Deliver the most up-to-date information by providing links to the latest guidelines for each disease.

Organization and Content

The book is organized into units and chapters. Each unit focuses on a specific body system, which is then broken down into individual disease chapters. The discussion of each disease in the chapters is developed in a logical flow that begins with an introductory paragraph on the disease's etiology and epidemiology, followed by a section on its pathophysiology, then a section on its physical examination components (i.e., subjective, objective, and diagnostics), and finally a comprehensive plan section that includes pharmacology components (e.g., medications and vaccines); links to the most recent practice guidelines; education topics; health promotion and disease prevention; and follow-up recommendations. A summary of diversity, geriatric, pediatric, and acute care considerations is included in each chapter within boxes. Some disease processes have algorithms at the end of the chapter that present the three P's in a straightforward and reasonable context.

Pathophysiology Section

The pathophysiology section is set up to explain the essential components of the disease process and how those would specifically relate to the physical assessment findings and specific pharmacotherapies that would be prescribed to eliminate the cause of disease or at least attempt to reset the body back to homeostasis. Pathophysiology incorporates basic, translational, and clinical research to advance the understanding of disease and dysfunction.

Physical Examination Section

This section focuses on subjective and objective information that will inform the diagnosis in each chapter. The subjective information provided is not exhaustive; rather, it provides common subjective complaints and history components that are typical for the diagnosis in each chapter. The objective information highlights the abnormal physical examination findings for each diagnosis and also is not exhaustive. No specific vital signs have been included, as these are individualized for each person being examined. **Hallmark** physical examination findings are designated in **boldface**, and **red flag** physical examination findings are designated in **boldface** and are underlined. Some chapters demonstrate physical examination differences via different font colors to identify the diagnosis that may present with those specific physical examination findings.

The recommended diagnostic testing for each specific disease is also listed in this section.

Plan
Pharmacology Section

This section begins with links to the most recent practice guidelines for each of the 40 disease processes, followed by recommended pharmacology treatment. Medication classes are listed, along with specific dosages when possible. The recommended vaccines are also available.

The section also links to the most recent practice guidelines, provides specific education topics to be discussed with clients, and offers health promotion and disease prevention strategies and follow-up recommendations.

Features to Promote Learning

Ease of learning has been enhanced by designing a number of features that guide and support understanding, including the following:

- *Consistent headings* to underscore the path of each disease from the pathophysiology to the clinical manifestations, to the evaluation and pharmacotherapy treatment.
- More than 160 *boxes* dedicated to *diversity considerations*, *geriatric considerations*, *pediatric considerations*, and *acute care considerations*. Each box provides an overview of the most current research, clinical developments, and treatments of disease.

ACKNOWLEDGMENTS

To Tamara, thank you for understanding the importance of something that can make a profound impact on nursing practice. For your willingness to forge ahead with this adventure, we will be forever grateful.

To Heather, your guidance on this project has been stellar. Through all the ups and downs, you kept us joyful and were a stabilizing force for us. Thank you for supplying us with all of the material we needed to create this book.

To Laura, thank you for making so many last-minute (quick) changes to improve the book, for acquiring the art and tables, and for your continual administrative support. Thank goodness, you kept us on track.

To the Development and Production teams for creating some amazing art and making the book better than we had envisioned.

To Marianne and Corrine for your contributions to this body of work.

To Felipe for having such dedication to nursing and the advancement of knowledge. You created wonderful algorithms and gathered evidence-based practice information that will be beneficial to the readers of this book. Your help was invaluable to us.

To our colleagues at PNW's College of Nursing for continually supporting scholarly activities, promoting teaching excellence, and enhancing the student experience.

CONTENTS

SECTION 1 **Neurologic System**

1 Cerebrovascular Accident 2
Julia L. Rogers ▪ Felipe Oria

2 Primary Headache Syndromes 12
Julia L. Rogers ▪ Felipe Oria

3 Seizure 26
Julia L. Rogers ▪ Felipe Oria

4 Traumatic Brain Injury 37
Julia L. Rogers ▪ Felipe Oria

SECTION 2 **Psychiatric System**

5 Anxiety 47
Jodi Allen ▪ Corrine M. Djuric

6 Depression 54
Jodi Allen ▪ Corrine M. Djuric

7 Posttraumatic Stress Disorder 62
Jodi Allen ▪ Corrine M. Djuric

SECTION 3 **Musculoskeletal System**

8 Arthritis 70
Jodi Allen

9 Conditions of the Spine 80
Jodi Allen

10 Soft Tissue Disorders 89
Jodi Allen

SECTION 4 **Hematologic System**

11 Iron Deficiency Anemia 97
Jodi Allen ▪ Corrine M. Djuric

12 Pernicious Anemia 104
Jodi Allen

13 Leukocytosis 110
Jodi Allen ▪ Corrine M. Djuric

SECTION 5   **Endocrine System**

14   Diabetes Mellitus Type 2   116
Jodi Allen

15   Hypothyroidism   123
Jodi Allen

SECTION 6   **Cardiovascular System**

16   Angina   131
Julia L. Rogers

17   Dysrhythmias   140
Julia L. Rogers

18   Heart Failure   154
Julia L. Rogers

19   Hyperlipidemia   169
Julia L. Rogers ▪ Marianne Schallmo

20   Hypertension   181
Julia L. Rogers ▪ Marianne Schallmo

SECTION 7   **Respiratory System**

21   Pneumonia   193
Julia L. Rogers

22   Chronic Obstructive Pulmonary Disease   203
Julia L. Rogers

23   Restrictive Lung Disease   212
Julia L. Rogers

24   Pharyngitis   222
Julia L. Rogers

SECTION 8   **Gastrointestinal System**

25   Abdominal Pain   232
Julia L. Rogers

26   Gastroesophageal Reflux Disease   243
Julia L. Rogers

27   Abdominal Hernia   251
Julia L. Rogers

28   Inflammatory Bowel Disease   258
Julia L. Rogers

29 Irritable Bowel Syndrome   268
Julia L. Rogers

30 Cholelithiasis   277
Julia L. Rogers

SECTION 9   **Genitourinary System**

31 Nephrolithiasis   285
Julia L. Rogers

32 Urinary Tract Infection   294
Julia L. Rogers

SECTION 10   **Integumentary System**

33 Acne Vulgaris   304
Jodi Allen ■ Corrine M. Djuric

34 Contact Dermatitis   311
Jodi Allen ■ Corrine M. Djuric

35 Psoriasis   318
Jodi Allen

36 Malignant Skin Lesions   325
Jodi Allen ■ Corrine M. Djuric

37 Integumentary Infections   333
Jodi Allen

SECTION 11   **Reproductive System**

38 Benign Prostatic Hypertrophy   340
Jodi Allen

39 Dysmenorrhea   346
Jodi Allen

40 Sexually Transmitted Infections   353
Jodi Allen

Index   361

Neurologic System

SECTION OUTLINE

1 Cerebrovascular Accident

2 Primary Headache Syndromes

3 Seizure

4 Traumatic Brain Injury

CHAPTER 1

Cerebrovascular Accident

Julia L. Rogers   Felipe Oria

Ischemic and Hemorrhagic

Cerebrovascular Accident

A cerebrovascular accident (CVA), commonly called a stroke, is the fifth leading cause of death in the United States (Feske, 2021). CVAs are classified as ischemic or hemorrhagic. Ischemic strokes account for 87% of all strokes and 75% of those occur among adults aged 65 years and older (Kleindorfer et al., 2021). Hemorrhagic strokes account for the other 13% (Sheth, 2022; Tsao et al., 2022). The risk factors include age, race, gender, previous stroke, hypertension, smoking, diabetes mellitus, cardiovascular disease, hypercholesteralemia, and hypercoagulopathy. Studies have shown a 40% lower incidence of stroke with tight blood pressure (BP) control (<130 mm Hg) as compared with standard BP control (130–139 mm Hg) (Tsao et al., 2022). The Global Burden of Disease study showed that 90.5% of the global burden of stroke was attributable to modifiable risk factors. Targeting these risk factors with secondary preventative strategies such as aspirin, statins, and antihypertensive medications combined with diet modification, exercise, and smoking cessation can result in an 80% cumulative risk reduction in recurrent vascular events (Kleindorfer et al., 2021).

Pathophysiology

ISCHEMIC

Ischemic strokes are caused by cerebrovascular obstruction from a thrombus or embolus. Cardiovascular disease processes predispose an individual to clot or embolus formation. The embolus travels from the heart to the brain and becomes lodged in the cerebral arteries, causing inadequate blood supply and subsequently inadequate oxygen supply to cerebral tissue, leading to loss of function (Powers & Hubner, 2023). Cerebral thrombosis develops most often from a coagulopathy that causes clot formation (e.g., factor V leiden), atherosclerosis, or an inflammatory disease process that damages arterial walls. Atherosclerotic plaques may rupture or move, or fragments may break apart from the arterial vessel wall, obstructing the cerebrovascular structures. Other sources of embolism include fat, air, tumor, bacterial clumps, and foreign bodies (Powers & Hubner, 2023). If blood flow is restored quickly, neuronal function usually returns without infarction; this is commonly called a transient ischemic attack (TIA) (Feske, 2023). If loss of blood flow or low blood flow (<10 mL/min per 100 g; normal is 50 mL/min per 100 g) lasts long enough, irreversible tissue damage occurs.

HEMORRHAGIC

Hemorrhagic stroke is caused by a spontaneous hemorrhage in intracerebral, subarachnoid, or subdural spaces (Powers & Hubner, 2023). The primary cause of an intracerebral hemorrhagic stroke is chronic hypertension (Fig. 1.1). Other causes include traumatic brain injury, amyloid angiopathy, tumor, coagulopathy, or illicit drug use, particularly cocaine. Primary smaller arteries and arterioles become damaged by chronic hypertension, causing microaneurysms. As blood pressure rises, the aneurysms are under increased pressure, causing them to rupture in these smaller vessels and leading to extensive bleeding, which is a medical emergency (Powers & Hubner, 2023). Occasionally a slow bleed may occur caused by veins being pulled away from the dura, seen more commonly in the elderly. The bleeding may be subtle and not recognized right away because the brain atrophy that occurs with aging leaves room within the cranial vault for accumulating blood. As the hemorrhage continues to expand, there is increasing intracranial pressure, which compresses the brain tissue and causes edema, leading to the clinical manifestations (Powers & Hubner, 2023).

Physical Clinical Presentation

SUBJECTIVE

Documenting a thorough and detailed history of the patient's symptoms is extremely important (Box 1.1). The history of present illness for a patient with a CVA should always include the time of the initial onset of symptoms. Patients with hemorrhagic stroke generally report an abrupt but not an instantaneous onset, with complaints of focal neurologic signs over minutes to days. An ischemic stroke is reported as instantaneous (Sheth, 2022). Ask the patient how soon after symptoms began did they arrive at the hospital and whether they received thrombolysis (tissue plasminogen activator). Next, inquire about precipitaing factors leading up to the event, initial symptoms, and the location, intensity, and quality of manifestations. Ask how the symptoms progressed and

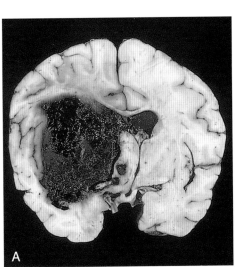
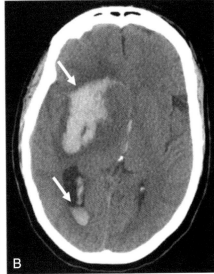

Fig. 1.1 Subdural hematoma and bridging veins. (A) Acute intracerebral hemorrhage. A fresh hematoma has disrupted and expanded the left cerebral hemisphere, causing the midline structures to shift to the right. Uncontrolled hypertension is an important cause of this catastrophic lesion. (B) Head computed tomography (CT) scan of intracerebral hemorrhage. Note that the acute hemorrhage appears hyperdense (*white*) on the CT scan. (From Kumar, V., Cotran, R. S., & Robbins, S. L. (2003). *Robbins basic pathology* (7th ed.). Saunders.)

> **BOX 1.1 ■ Pediatric Considerations**
>
> The pediatric population is not immune from having a cerebrovascular accident (CVA). The clinical manifestations are similar to those in adults and include weakness, numbness, and slurred speech. Ischemic strokes are the most common type in children and are associated with congenital heart disease, cerebral arteriovenous malformation, sickle cell disease, and infection. Because genetics play a role in CVAs, it is crucial to obtain a complete and thorough history on any individual who is starting family planning (Felling et al., 2023; Ferriero et al., 2019).

> **BOX 1.2 ■ Diversity Considerations**
>
> Identifying how genetics play a role in cerebrovascular accidents (CVA) is a rapidly developing field. The inheritance trait is produced from the cumulative effects of many genes, referred to as polygenic. In fact, about 38% of all ischemic strokes are caused by polygenic disorders. The advancements made in genomics have allowed for personalized prevention of CVA and novel individualized treatment possibilities. A comprehensive plan for primary stroke prevention might be possible with the use clinical information, the combined genetic risk scores, extended polygenic risk scores, and risk factor profiles. These can be combined to estimate the cumulative contribution of known genetic factors to a specific outcome of stroke. Currently, research is being conducted to determine new biomarkers for genetic causes of stroke and novel targets for gene therapy (Ekkert et al., 2021).

whether the patient has expereinced previous episodes, and if so, whether the symptoms were the same. Specifically ask about headache, nausea or vomiting, and a change in level of consciousness, as these can further differentiate hemorrhagic from ischemic stroke. Additionally, ask whether the patient had or still has weakness, sensory disturbances, visual disturbances, dysphagia, dysarthria, vertigo, or pain. If the response is yes, ask about localization or lateralization. Document the patient's dominant hand. Determine when the patient was hospitalized, for how long, and the course of treatment while hospitalized. Ask where the patient went for acute rehabilitation. Document allergies, medications, and medical, social, and family histories. Review the current medication list with the patient, documenting any changes. Is or was the patient taking oral contraception? When reviewing past medical history, it is important to ask about any potential risk factors (hypertension, atrial fibrillation, hyperlipidemia, hypertriglyceridemia, diabetes, previous TIA or CVA, hypercoagulable disease, carotid stenosis, prosthetic heart valves, or migraines with aura). Document any family history of stroke in first-degree relatives, hypercoagulable disorders (e.g., factor V), and genetic disorders (Box 1.2). Inquire about the current or past use of tobacco, alcohol, or drugs, and determine amount used and length of time. Finally, ask about social determinants of health.

OBJECTIVE*

Generalized: Weakness unilateral; <u>**slurred speech**</u>; fatigue

   Neurological: <u>**Confusion**</u>; aphasia; <u>**dysphagia**</u> (**receptive and/or expressive**); dysarthria; cranial nerve palsies; hemisensory loss; **unilateral body neglect**; overactive, asymmetric deep tendon reflexes (biceps, patellar, and Achilles); **hemiparesis; paresthesia unilateral**; *positive Romberg sign*; **pronator drift**; vertigo; **headache**; *complete cranial nerve assessment* should be completed

---

*Hallmark signs are bolded and <u>**Red flags are bolded and underlined**</u>. *Italics are for assessment techniques.*

HEENT: Blurred vision; downward and inward eye deviation; miotic pupils; pinpoint (but reactive) pupils; absent or impaired horizontal gaze (eye gaze preference is toward the side of the lesion); ocular bobbing (a sign in which the eyes rapidly and conjugately deviate downward and then slowly upward to midposition); facial weakness; **facial droop unilateral**; **tongue deviation**; **smile unequal**

Cardiovascular: Irregular rate and/or irregular rhythm; murmur

Genitourinary: Incontinence; hesitancy

Musculoskeletal: Weakness unilateral; **poor or hyperexcitable flexion or extension unilateral**; muscle stiffness

Psychiatric: Flat affect; gaze; depression; anxious; apathy; memory loss

(Ball et al., 2023; Dains et al., 2024; Powers & Hubner, 2023; Sheth, 2022)

Evaluation and Differential Diagnoses

DIAGNOSTICS

- Preventative
  - Blood pressure: Screen for hypertension.
  - Electrocardiogram: Screen for atrial fibrillation and other cardiac disease.
  - Carotid ultrasound: Screen for stenosis.
  - Polysomnogram: Screen for sleep apnea.
  - Swallow study: Screen for dysphagia.
  - Lipid panel: Screen for hyperlipidemia and hypertriglyceridemia.
  - Fasting glucose and HbA1C: Screen for diabetes.
  - Activated protein C: Screen for factor V.
- Acute hospital ischemic and hemorrhagic stroke management (Box 1.3)

(Kleindorfer et al., 2021; Powers & Hubner, 2023; Sheth, 2022)

BOX 1.3 ■ Acute Care Considerations

Acute hospital stroke management: The immediate objective of ischemic stroke treatment is to improve perfusion and prevent further tissue damage.
- Evaluate using National Institutes of Health Stroke Scale.
- Emergency brain imaging
- Acute ischemic stroke
  - Noncontrast head computed tomography (CT) scan: CT scan may be normal shortly after onset of acute ischemic stroke. Lack of hemorrhage or cause for focal deficit provides support for intravenous thrombolysis.
  - Magnetic resonance imaging scan: Sensitive for early identification
- Acute hemorrhagic stroke
  - Noncontrast head CT
  - Acute hemorrhage represents an absolute contraindication for intravenous thrombolytic therapy.
- Antithrombotic medications for acute ischemic stroke
  - Tissue plasminogen activator: Alteplase or tenecteplase (must meet criteria and have no contraindication)
  - Given within 3 hours of onset of symptoms
  - In-hospital infusion only

(Feske, 2021; Sheth, 2022; Warner et al., 2019; Wilson & Ashcraft, 2019)

DIFFERENTIAL DIAGNOSIS

- Seizure
- Brain tumor
- Toxic metabolic disorders (e.g., hyponatremia, hypoglycemia)
- Encephalitis

Plan

GUIDELINE RESOURCES

- AHA/ASA Guidelines. (n.d.). Guidelines for the early management of patients with acute ischemic stroke: 2019 update to the 2018 guidelines for the early management of acute ischemic stroke. https://www.heart.org/-/media/Files/Professional/Quality-Improvement/Get-With-the-Guidelines/Get-With-The-Guidelines-Stroke/2019UpdateAHAASAAIS GuidelineSlideDeckrevisedADL12919.pdf
- Hoh, B. L., Ko, N. U., Amin-Hanjani, S., Hsiang-Yi Chou, S., Cruz-Flores, S., Dangayach, N. S., Derdeyn, C. P., Du, R., Hänggi, D., Hetts, S. W., Ifejika, N. L., Johnson, R., Keigher, K. M., Leslie-Mazwi, T. M., Lucke-Wold, B., Rabinstein, A. A., Robicsek, S. A., Stapleton, C. J., Suarez, J. I., … Welch, B. G. (2023). 2023 guideline for the management of patients with aneurysmal subarachnoid hemorrhage: A guideline from the American Heart Association/American Stroke Association. *Stroke, 54*(7), e314–e370. https://doi.org/10.1161/str.0000000000000436
- Kleindorfer, D., Towfighi, A., Chaturvedi, S., Cockroft, K. M., Gutierrez, J., Lombardi-Hill, D., Kamel, H., Kernan, W. N., Kittner, S. J., Leira, E. C., Lennon, O., Meschia, J. F., Nguyen, T. N., Pollak, P. M., Santangeli, P., Sharrief, A. Z., Smith, S. C. Jr., Turan, T. N., & Williams, L. S. (2021). 2021 guideline for the prevention of stroke in patients with stroke and transient ischemic attack: A guideline from the American Heart Association/American Stroke Association. *Stroke, 52*(7), e364–e467. https://doi.org/10.1161/str.0000000000000375

Pharmacotherapy

- Acute care treatment for stroke (see Box 1.3)
- Medications for prevention
  - Antiplatelet (after TIA or ischemic stroke):
    - Aspirin 81–325 mg daily WITH
    - Clopidogrel 75 mg daily OR
    - Dipyridamole/aspirin 1 tablet daily for 2 weeks, then increase to 1 tablet twice daily
  - Anticoagulant:
    - Indicated for stroke prevention if:
      - Mechanical heart valve; atrial fibrillation – nonvalvular – estimate risk CHA2DS2-VASc score; intracardiac thrombus; hypercoagulable states; cerebral venous sinus thrombosis
    - Warfarin
    - Factor Xa inhibitors (apixaban, rivaroxaban, edoxaban)
    - Direct thrombin inhibitor (dabigatran)
  - Hypertension:
    - BP goal of <130/80 mm Hg antihypertensive based on comorbidities:
      - Thiazide diuretic

- Angiotensin-converting enzyme inhibitor
- Angiotensin II receptor blocker
- Hyperlipidemia: Goal LDL-C <100 mg/dL:
  - Atorvastatin 80 mg daily
  - Atherosclerotic disease: Goal LDL-C <70 mg/dL:
    - Statin
    - Ezetimibe (if needed with statin)
  - Very high risk (stroke + major atherosclerotic cardiovascular disease or stroke + high-risk comorbidities), already taking a statin and with ezetimibe with LDL-C >70 mg/dL:
    - Proprotein convertase subtilisin/kexin type 9
- Diabetes mellitus: Goal HbA1C ≤7%:
  - Glucose-lowering agent with cardiac benefit
- Smoking cessation aids should be offered to any person currently smoking tobacco.

(Kleindorfer et al., 2021; Kim et. al., 2023; Powers & Hubner, 2023; Sheth, 2022; Teasell et al., 2020)

NONPHARMACOTHERAPY

- Postacute discharge needs focus on poststroke complications and secondary stroke prevention (Box 1.4).
- Screen, evaluate, and address
  - Social determinants of health and health equity needs
  - Oral contraceptive use
  - Hormone replacement therapy
  - Factor V Leiden
  - Substance use
  - Activities of daily living
  - Fall risk
  - Depression

(Kleindorfer et al., 2021; Teasell et al., 2020)

- Educate
  - Medication compliance and importance of use in preventing future strokes
  - Modifiable risk factors
  - Prevention of poststroke complications
  - Home BP monitoring
  - Self-management
- Lifestyle and behavioral modifications
  - Weight reduction
  - Low-salt Mediterranean diet or Dietary Approaches to Stop Hypertension diet
  - Regular exercise and physical activity
  - Smoking cessation
  - Continue rehabilitation (see Box 1.4)

(Kleindorfer et al., 2021; Teasell et al., 2020)

- Complementary treatment
  - Psychosocial rehabilitation
  - Complementary and alternative therapies with natural medicines and supplements may interact with prescription medications. Obtain a complete medication history.
- Referral (identify and refer for treatment of comorbid conditions*)
  - Neurologist
  - Speech therapy

BOX 1.4 ■ Older Adult Considerations

A comprehensive geriatric assessment is key in initiating a holistic approach to rehabilitation for an elderly patient. Older patients who have suffered a stroke tend to have a longer stay in an acute care hospital and then continue treatment in an extended care facility (ECF) instead of an acute rehabilitation center. This approach may not work in favor of the patient. Generally, (ECF) rehabilitation is less aggressive in physical and occupational therapies. Many times the patient's primary care provider is not involved in the care. The best approach to a holistic rehabilitation program is to have an interdisciplinary treatment team including the provider, nurses, physiotherapists, occupational therapists, speech therapists, and social workers who have experience in and with the gerontology population and who work with rehabilitation plans that include individualized goals. (Achterberg, 2020).

- ■ Therapy: Physical and occupational
- ■ Dietitian
- ■ Cardiologist* (cardiovascular disease)
- ■ Hematologist* (factor V)
- ■ Pulmonologist* (sleep apnea)
- ■ Cardiovascular surgeon (*carotid artery stenosis; patent foramen ovale closure)
- ■ Follow-up
  - ■ Primary care provider office visit within 2 weeks of hospital discharge
  - ■ Neurologist within 1 month of hospital discharge
  - ■ Follow-up every 3 months

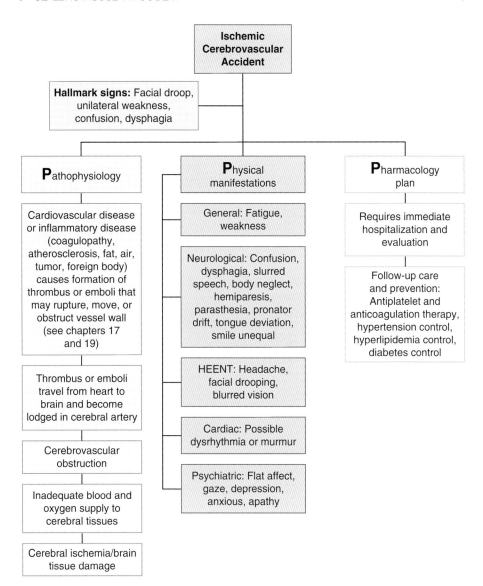

Algorithm 1.1 Ischemic Cerebrovascular Accident

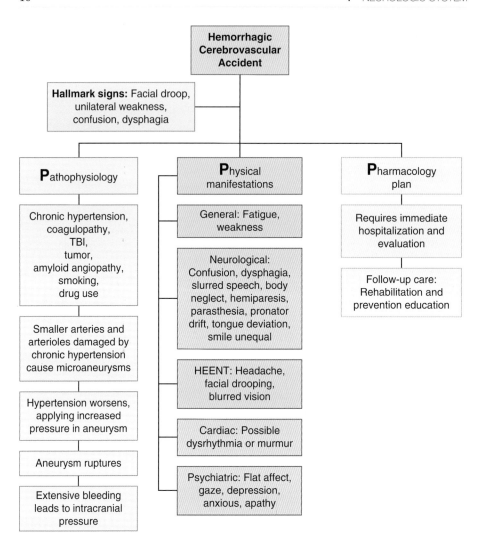

TBI = Traumatic brain injury

Algorithm 1.2   Hemorrhagic Cerebrovascular Accident

References

Achterberg, W. P. (2020). Geriatric assessment and rehabilitation in older stroke patients. *EClinicalMedicine, 24*, 100438.

Ball, J. W., Dains, J. E., Flynn, J. A., Solomon, B. S., & Stewart, R. W. (2023). *Seidel's guide to physical examination: An interprofessional approach* (9th ed). St. Louis: Elsevier.

Dains, J. E., Baumann, L. C., & Scheibel, P. (2024). *Advanced health assessment & clinical diagnosis in primary care* (7th ed). St. Louis: Elsevier.

Ekkert, A., Šliachtenko, A., Grigaitė, J., Burnytė, B., Utkus, A., & Jatužis, D. (2021). Ischemic stroke genetics: What is new and how to apply it in clinical practice? *Genes, 13*(1), 48. https://doi.org/10.3390/genes13010048.

Felling, R. J., Jordan, L. C., Mrakotsky, C., deVeber, G., Peterson, R. K., Mineyko, A., Feldman, S. J., Shapiro, K., Lo, W., & Beslow, L. A. (2023). Roadmap for the assessment and management of outcomes in pediatric stroke. *Pediatric Neurology, 141*(78), 93–100. doi:10.1016/j.pediatrneurol.2023.01.00836805967.

Ferriero, D. M., Fullerton, H. J., Bernard, T. J., Billinghurst, L., Daniels, S. R., DeBaun, M. R., deVeber, G., Ichord, R. N., Jordan, L. C., Massicotte, P., Meldau, J., Roach, E. S., Smith, E. R., & American Heart Association Stroke Council and Council on Cardiovascular and Stroke Nursing. (2019). Management of Stroke in Neonates and Children: A Scientific Statement From the American Heart Association/American Stroke Association. *Stroke, 50*(3), e51–e96. doi:10.1161/str.0000000000000183.

Feske, S. K. (2021). Ischemic stroke. *American Journal of Medicine, 134*(12), 1457–1464.

Kim, J., Lee, J. S., Kim, B. J., Kang, J., Lee, K., Park, J., Kang, K., Lee, S. J., Kim, J. G., Cha, J., Kim, D., Park, T. H., Lee, K., Lee, J., Hong, K., Cho, Y., Park, H., Lee, B., Yu, K., Oh, M. S., Kim, D., Ryu, W., Choi, J. C., Kwon, J., Kim, W., Shin, D., Yum, K. S., Sohn, S. I., Hong, J., Lee, S., Park, M., Choi, K., Lee, J., Park, K., & Bae, H. (2023). Statin Treatment in Patients With Stroke With Low-Density Lipoprotein Cholesterol Levels Below 70 mg/dL. *JAHA, 12*(276), 1. doi:10.1161/jaha.123.030738 37681519.

Kleindorfer, D. O., Towfighi, A., Chaturvedi, S., Cockroft, K. M., Gutierrez, J., Lombardi-Hill, D., Kamel, H., Kernan, W. N., Kittner, S. J., Leira, E. C., Lennon, O., Meschia, J. F., Nguyen, T. N., Pollak, P. M., Santangeli, P., Sharrief, A. Z., Smith, S. C., Jr., Turan, T. N., & Williams, L. S. (2021). 2021 guideline for the prevention of stroke in patients with stroke and transient ischemic attack: A guideline from the American Heart Association/American Stroke Association. *Stroke, 52*(7), e364–e467.

Powers, J., & Hubner, K. (2023). Alterations of the brain, spinal cord, and peripheral nerves. In J. L., Rogers (Ed.), *McCance & Huether's pathophysiology: The biological basis for disease in adults and children* (9th ed., pp. 570-613). Elsevier.

Sheth, K. N. (2022). Spontaneous intracerebral hemorrhage. *New England Journal of Medicine, 387*(17), 1589–1596. https://doi.org/10.1056/NEJMra2201449.

Teasell, R., Salbach, N. M., Foley, N., Mountain, A., Cameron, J. I., de Jong, A., Acerra, N. E., Bastasi, D., Carter, S. L., Fung, J., Halabi, M-L., Iruthayarajah, J., Harris, J., Kim, E., Noland, A., Pooyania, S., Rochette, A., Stack, B. D., Symcox, E., … Lindsay, M. P. (2020). Canadian stroke best practice recommendations: Rehabilitation, recovery, and community participation following stroke. Part one: Rehabilitation and recovery following stroke; 6th edition update 2019. *International Journal of Stroke,, 15*(7), 763–788. https://doi.org/10.1177/1747493019897843.

Tsao, C. W., Aday, A. W., Almarzooq, Z. I., Alonso, A., Beaton, A. Z., Bittencourt, M. S., Boehme, A. K, Buxton, A. E., Carson, A. P., Commodore-Mensah, Y., Elkind, M. S. V., Evenson, K. R., Eze-Nliam, C., Ferguson, J. F., Generoso, G., Ho, J. E., Kalani, R., Khan, S. S., Kissela, B. M., … Martin, S. S. (2022). Heart disease and stroke statistics—2022 update: A report from the American Heart Association. *Circulation, 145*(8), e153–e639.

Warner, J. J., Harrington, R. A., Sacco, R. L., & Elkind, M. S. (2019). Guidelines for the early management of patients with acute ischemic stroke: 2019 update to the 2018 guidelines for the early management of acute ischemic stroke. *Stroke, 50*(12), 3331–3332.

Wilson, S. E., & Ashcraft, S. (2019). Ischemic stroke: Management by the nurse practitioner. *Journal for Nurse Practitioners, 15*(1), 41–53.e2. https://doi.org/10.1016/j.nurpra.2018.07.019.

CHAPTER 2

Primary Headache Syndromes

Julia L. Rogers ▦ Felipe Oria

Migraine, Cluster, and Tension

Headache Syndrome

Primary headache disorders include migraine, tension-type, and trigeminal autonomic cephalgias, which include cluster headaches. Although usually benign, headaches can be a symptom of a more serious structural abnormality or systemic disease. Headaches caused by underlying medical conditions such as brain tumor, meningitis, sinusitis, giant cell arteritis, or cerebral vascular disease are considered secondary headaches (Headache Classification Committee of the International Headache Society [IHS], 2018; Rogers & Spain, 2020). Nearly 3 billion individuals globally are estimated to have a headache disorder. Tension headaches account for 1.89 billion cases and migraine for 1.04 billion cases (Stovner et al., 2018). According to the Centers for Disease Control and Prevention ([CDC], 2023), 4.3% of adults aged 18 years and older reported a headache or migraine within the past 3 months, with females (6.2%) being three times as likely as males (2.2%) to suffer from a headache syndrome. Headache disorders are a leading cause of disability worldwide and the third cause of disability in people younger than 50 years of age (Stovner et al., 2018).

Pathophysiology

MIGRAINE

Migraine involves dysfunction of brain stem pathways that exert a controlling influence on sensory input (see Algorithm 2.1). The key pathway for pain is the trigeminovascular input from the meningeal vessels, which pass through the trigeminal ganglion, and transmit electrical nerve impulses in the trigeminocervical complex. In turn, these neurons project through the trigemino-thalamic tract and form synapses with neurons in the thalamus (Goadsby et al., 2002) (Fig. 2.1). Migraine aura is associated with cortical spreading depression (CSD). CSD is a spontaneous self-propagating wave of glial and neuronal depolarization that starts in the occipital region of the brain and spreads across the cortex, resulting in hyperactivity. CSD initiates the release of excitatory neurotransmitters that activate the trigeminal vascular system (afferent projections from cranial nerve V) (Powers & Hubner, 2023) (see Fig. 2.1). This leads to vasodilation of dural blood vessels, activation and release of inflammatory mediators and neurotransmitters, (e.g., serotonin, glutamate, and dopamine), meningeal inflammation, hypersensitivity to pain, and activation of areas that modulate pain and prodromal symptoms in the brain stem and forebrain (Powers & Hubner, 2023). The pain associated with a migraine is thought to occur from a gradual depolarization or excitation of the nociceptors in the meninges and calcitonin gene–related peptide (CGRP), which is a neuropeptide in the central and peripheral nervous systems. During a migraine, CGRP is released, causing neurogenic inflammation and increasing headache pain (Goadsby et al., 2002; Wiemann et al., 2023; Williams, 2020). This is the basis for prescribing a class of medications that block or inhibit action of CGRP (Charles et al., 2024; Moriarty & Mallick-Searle, 2016).

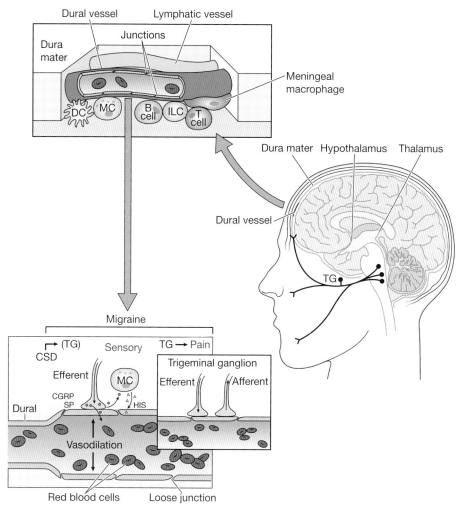

Fig. 2.1 Pathophysiology of headaches. *CSD*, cortical spreading depression; *CGRP*, calcitonin gene-related peptide; *HIS*, histamine; *MC*, mast cell; *SP*, substance P; *TG*, trigeminal ganglion.

CLUSTER

A cluster headache is thought to be initiated by activation of the posterior hypothalamus with secondary activation of the trigeminal autonomic reflex through the trigeminal-hypothalamic pathway (see Fig. 2.1). Trigeminovascular activation leads to the release of vasoactive neuropeptides and the formation of neurogenic inflammation, which initiates the pain cycle (see Algorithm 2.2) (Rogers & Spain, 2020). The severe unilateral pain that is associated with a cluster headache is mediated by activation of the first division of the trigeminal nerve (V1). Activation and outflow of the parasympathetic nervous system from the superior salivatory nucleus via the pterygopalatine (sphenopalatine) ganglion activates the trigeminal autonomic reflex. This leads to clinical manifestations such as lacrimation, nasal congestion, and rhinorrhea (Goadsby et al., 2002; Powers & Hubner, 2023).

TENSION

Tension-type headaches involve the central nervous system and the hypersensitivity of pain fibers originating from the trigeminal nerve. This leads to deficits in the descending inhibitory pain pathways located in the brain stem. A peripheral component also plays a role in the development of tension-type headaches as muscular sensitivity may be caused by the peripheral sensitization of myofascial sensory afferents (Rogers & Spain, 2020) (see Fig. 2.1 and Algorithm 2.3). Central mechanisms expressed as central sensitivities have also been implicated in chronic tension-type headaches. Other associative influences include psychological, environmental, and genetic factors. The genetic component has many possible sources, such as a circadian rhythm gene (PER3), orexin-B, and a receptor gene (pituitary adenylate cyclase–activating peptide) (Rogers & Spain, 2020).

Physical Clinical Presentation

SUBJECTIVE

Subjective findings help determine headache type. During the focused history, documentation should include the onset of symptoms; precipitating events; location, intensity, frequency, quality, and characteristics of pain; progression of symptoms; alleviating and exacerbating factors; previous episodes; and associated symptoms. Be alert to red flags such as "this is the worst headache I ever had in my life." Document allergies, ill contacts, autoimmune diseases, and medical, social, and family histories. (see Box 2.1)

The past medical history should include current and past medications or recent changes to medications by any provider. Document the dose and frequency of every medication, including supplements, vitamins, minerals, and over-the-counter medications. Assess medication overuse with anxiolytics, analgesics, and sedative hypnotics. List any comorbid conditions that could be contributory (hypertension, arrhythmia, hypercapnia, sleep apnea, anemia, hormonal changes), previous or recent head or neck trauma, and previous surgeries. Complete a review of body systems and include questions about jaw or neck symptoms, visual changes, dizziness, or dyspnea (US Department of Veterans Affairs, 2020; Williams, 2020).

During intake of social history, ask about any stress at home or work, history of posttraumatic stress, and any recent barometric changes. Individuals may complain of sensitivity to light or sound, nausea, and vomiting. Determine if there are any visual disturbances either before or during a migraine, known as auras, that may present as flashing lights (Walter, 2022). Be sure and inquire about exercise routine. Document electronic cigarette use or tobacco use, including cigarettes, cigars, and nicotine supplements, as well as exposure to secondhand smoke. Inquire about

---

BOX 2.1 ■ Diversity Considerations

A multitude of factors should be considered when caring for a patient with an acute or chronic headache. Research shows inequities in the treatment of individuals with a complaint of headache. Therefore health care providers need to consider any implicit bias when developing a plan of care for a patient with head pain. The factors include racism, socioeconomic status, insurance status, and geographical disparities contribute to treatment bias. However, multiple considerations can lead to equitable care. For example, health care providers can improve the screening process with questions to determine whether the patient has any unmet needs, advocate for improved insurance coverage for telemedicine, connect patients to community resources, and minimize assumptions about how much the patient and family understand the disease process, plan of care, and familiarity with the health care system (Kiarashi et al., 2021).

recreational marijuana use and illicit drug use. Obtain a 24-hour food diary and document how many glasses of water or other fluid is taken in during a 24-hour period to assess hydration status, specifically ask about coffee and caffeine intake, energy drinks, artificial sweeteners, and alcohol consumption. Ask how many hours of sleep per night is typical for the individual and if any naps are taken during the day (Table 2.1).

TABLE 2.1 ▪ **Primary Headache Differential Criteria**

Headache Type	Migraine	Cluster	Tension
Clinical Manifestations			
Onset	Gradual	Pain begins **quickly**, reaches a crescendo within minutes	Gradual
	May start with **prodromal period** for 1 hour to days before having a headache		
Location	Unilateral	Unilateral	**Bilateral**
	Often isolated to one side of the head	**Orbital**, supraorbital, and/or temporal	Often sensation like a **tight band** around the entire head
Duration	4–72 hours	15 minutes–3 hours	30 minutes–7 days
	Stages: Prodrome, aura, headache, postdrome		Episodic: Fewer than 15 days monthly, can be chronic; evolution from episodic version, more than 15 days monthly for at least 3 months
Frequency	Variable	1 every other day to 8 daily; often at same time each day; may have long periods of remission	Variable
Severity	Mild to severe	**Severe or very severe**	Mild to moderate
Quality	**Throbbing or pulsating**	**Stabbing**	**Tightening** pressure or tension
	Crescendo pattern	Pain is deep, continuous, excruciating, and explosive	Waxes and wanes
Aggravating factors	Aggravated by normal physical activity	Causes restlessness or agitation	**Triggered by stress**, sleep disorders; not aggravated by normal physical activity
Triggers		Normal or increased physical activity may improve symptoms	
Associated symptoms	Can be with or without **aura**; can have **nausea and/or vomiting**, fatigue, and dizziness	**Tearing and ptosis of the eye**, nasal congestion, referred pain to teeth	**Tenderness of pericranial muscles**
	Photophobia **and** phonophobia	May or may not have photophobia and/or phonophobia	No more than one photophobia **or** phonophobia
		May have nausea and/or vomiting	No nausea or vomiting
Age most common	Puberty–55 years	20–50 years	Teenage–50 years

Red flags to differentiate headache are **bolded and underlined**.
(Ford et al., 2021; Robbins et al., 2016; Powers & Hubner, 2023; Rogers & Spain, 2020; Walter, 2022; Williams, 2020; WHO, 2016)

OBJECTIVE*

The acronym **SNOOP(4)E** is for red flags: **S** = <u>**Systemic symptoms**</u>; **N** = <u>**Neurologicsymptoms**</u>; **O** = <u>**Onset abrupt or thunderclap**</u>; **O** = <u>**Older age at onset >50 years**</u> (see Box 2.3); **P(4)** = <u>**Progression/Pattern change, Precipitated by Valsalva, Postural aggravation, Papilledema**</u>; **E** = <u>**Exertion**</u>.

Generalized: *Weakness; fever; chills; night sweats;* <u>***severe headache pain (maximal intensity reached immediately)***</u>

Neurological: <u>***Confusion***</u>; <u>***impaired alertness/consciousness***</u>; <u>***change in behavior***</u>; CN II–XII may have irregularities; *decreased or no sensation to light touch or cold stimuli;* <u>***paresthesia***</u>; *tremor; speech changes; vertigo; positive Romberg sign; temporal arteritis; seizure*

(Note: *Damage to upper motor neuron[s] will show increased deep tendon reflexes, pronator drift, increased muscle tone, positive Babinski sign, and spastic paralysis with a clasp-knife reaction. Damage to lower motor neuron[s] will show decreased deep tendon reflexes, decreased muscle tone, negative Babinski sign, flaccid paralysis, muscle atrophy, and fasciculations.*)

HEENT: Headache; photophobia; <u>***papilledema***</u>; <u>***diplopia***</u>; <u>***ptosis***</u>; <u>***proptosis***</u>; <u>***pain with eye movements***</u>; rhinorrhea, nasal congestion, *fundoscopic exam with presence of low-amplitude nystagmus; vision changes; glaucoma; lymphadenopathy*

Neck: *Tenderness;* **neck stiffness**; *nuchal rigidity*

Cardiovascular: *Irregular rhythm; tachycardia; bounding pulse; murmur*

Pulmonary: *Inspection: Labored respirations; tachypnea; use of accessory muscles*
Auscultation: Wheezing; coarse rhonchi; rales

Musculoskeletal: <u>***Myalgias***</u>; examine cervical spine and surrounding musculature for *decreased range of motion; positive Spurling's test; unequal strength; poor or rigid flexion; poor or rigid extension*

Extremities: *Edema; cyanosis*

Psychiatric: *Memory loss; hallucinations; paranoia*

See Table 2.1 to differentiate headache type with objective findings. (See Algorithm 2.1, Algorithm 2.2, and Algorithm 2.3)

(Ball et al., 2023; Dains et al., 2024; Powers & Hubner, 2023; US Department of Veterans Affairs, 2020; Williams, 2020)

Evaluation and Differential Diagnoses

DIAGNOSTICS

- Diagnostic imaging
  - One or more red flags, then workup for a secondary headache disorder with either a magnetic resonance imaging, magnetic resonance angiography, magnetic resonance venography, or computed tomography scan of the head to rule out other structural conditions
- Craniocervical rotation test
- Estimated sedimentation rate elevated
- Lumbar puncture

(Ailani et al., 2021; Robbins et al., 2016; US Department of Veterans Affairs, 2020; Williams, 2020)

DIFFERENTIAL DIAGNOSIS

- Secondary headache as the result of another disease (e.g., brain tumor)
- Muscle contraction
- Allergies

*****Hallmark signs are bolded**, *Secondary causes of headache signs are italicized*, and <u>**Red flags are bolded and underlined**</u>.

Plan

GUIDELINE RESOURCES

- Ailani, J., Burch, R., & Robbins, M. S. (2021). The American Headache Society Consensus Statement: Update on integrating new migraine treatments into clinical practice. *Headache*, *61*(7), 1021–1039. https://doi.org/10.1111/head.14153
- Bendtsen, L., Evers, S., Linde, M., Mitsikostas, D. D., Sandrini, G., Schoenen, J., & EFNS. (2010). EFNS guideline on the treatment of tension-type headache—Report of an EFNS task force. *European Journal of Neurology*, *17*(11), 1318–1325. https://doi.org/10.1111/j.1468-1331.2010.03070.x
- Headache Classification Committee of the International Headache Society. The International Classification of Headache Disorders, 3rd edition. *Cephalalgia*, *38*(1), 1–211. https://doi.org/10.1177/0333102417738202
- Marmura, M. J., Silberstein, S. D., & Schwedt, T. J. (2015). The acute treatment of migraine in adults: The American Headache Society evidence assessment of migraine pharmacotherapies. *Headache*, *55*(1), 3–20. https://doi.org/10.1111/head.12499
- Management of Headache Guideline Summary. (2021). Guideline central. https://www.guidelinecentral.com/guideline/308835
- Robbins, M. S., Starling, A. J., Pringsheim, T., Becker, W. J., & Schwedt, T. J. (2016). Treatment of cluster headache: The American Headache Society evidence-based guidelines. *Headache*, *56*(7), 1093–1106. https://doi.org/10.1111/head.12866
- Silberstein, S. D., Holland, S., Freitag, F., Dodick, D. W., Argoff, C., Ashman, E., & Quality Standards Subcommittee of the American Academy of Neurology and the American Headache Society. (2012). Evidence-based guideline update: Pharmacologic treatment for episodic migraine prevention in adults: Report of the Quality Standards Subcommittee of the American Academy of Neurology and the American Headache Society. *Neurology*, *78*(17), 1337–1345. https://doi.org/10.1212/WNL.0b013e3182535d20
- US Department of Veterans Affairs. (2020). *VA/DoD clinical practice guidelines: Primary care management of headache.* https://www.healthquality.va.gov/guidelines/Pain/headacheVA/DoD
- See Box 2.2: Pediatric Considerations for Pediatric Guidelines

---

BOX 2.2 ■ Pediatric Considerations

The prevalence of headaches varies considerably in pediatric patients depending on diagnostic criteria and age. Migraine and tension-type headaches are the most predominant forms in school-age pediatric patients, with an average prevalence rate of 8% to 24%. Pediatric migraine is a disorder with substantial clinical differences compared to the adult form. Health care providers should follow the criteria of the International Headache Society to make a diagnosis of primary headache in pediatric patients and use the practice guidelines on acute and preventative treatments for migraine in children and adolescents published by the American Academy of Neurology to develop a plan of care. The use of calcitonin gene–related peptide receptor antagonists is recommended in adolescent patients with frequent migraine attacks (≥8 headache days/month), with moderate to severe disability associated with migraine, and who have failed ≥2 preventative therapies (i.e., propranolol, topiramate and cinnarizine, or amitriptyline plus cognitive behavioral therapy) (Iannone et al., 2022; IHS, 2018; Oskoui et al., 2019a, 2019b; Szperka et al., 2018).

Practice Guideline link:

- Practice guideline update summary: Acute treatment of migraine in children and adolescents: Report of the Guideline Development, Dissemination, and Implementation Subcommittee of the American Academy of Neurology and the American Headache Society. https://headache-journal.onlinelibrary.wiley.com/doi/full/10.1111/head.13628.

Pharmacotherapy

- Medications
  - Migraine: (see Algorithm 2.1)
    - Acute episodic or chronic treatment*:
      - Mild to moderate: Nonsteroidal antiinflammatory drugs (NSAIDs): aspirin, cele-coxib, diclofenac, ibuprofen, naproxen; caffeinated analgesic combinations
      - Moderate to severe: Triptans, ergotamine derivatives, gepants,** ditans,** selective serotonin receptor agonist, neuromodulation**
      - See Box 2.4 for acute care treatment of migraines
    - Preventative treatment*:
      - Oral: Candesartan, divalproex sodium, frovatriptan, metoprolol, propranolol, timo-lol, topiramate, valproate sodium
      - Parenteral: CGRP mAbs***—eptinezumab, erenumab, fremanezumab, galcanezumab
  - Cluster: (see Algorithm 2.2)
    - Acute episodic or chronic treatment*:
      - Sumatriptan subcutaneous injection (episodic or chronic)
      - Zolmitriptan nasal spray
      - Oxygen 6–12 L/min (episodic)
      - Sphenopalatine ganglion stimulation (chronic/dissatisfied with current treatment)
      - Galcanezumab
    - Prophylactic treatment*:
      - Suboccipital steroid injection
      - Civamide nasal spray
      - Lithium
      - Verapamil
      - Warfarin
      - Melatonin
  - Tension: (see Algorithm 2.3)
    - Acute episodic or chronic treatment*:
      - Aspirin or NSAIDs or acetaminophen
      - Ketoprofen
      - Diclofenac
      - Combination of simple analgesic or NSAID plus caffeine
    - Preventative treatment*:
      - Amitriptyline
      - Mirtazapine
      - Venlafaxine
- Smoking cessation aids should be offered to any person currently smoking tobacco.
(Ailani et al., 2021; Robbins et al., 2016; US Department of Veterans Affairs, 2020; Williams, 2020)

NONPHARMACOTHERAPY

- Educate
  - Eliminate triggers:
    - Food, additives, alcohol, environmental, occupational, irritants

---

*Medications with established efficacy are listed here. Medications with evidence of probable efficacy in acute migraine treatment are not listed here.

**Must meet criteria for initiating treatment with gepants, ditans, or neuromodulatory devices.

***Must meet criteria for initiating treatment with monoclonal antibodies to CGRP or its receptor.

BOX 2.3 ■ Older Adult Considerations

Proper treatment of headache in older adults requires the recognition of secondary causes, comorbid diseases, and drug-induced or medication-overuse headaches. A new-onset migraine is concerning and should be immediately evaluated for a secondary cause, because it is unusual after the age of 60 years. The most common secondary causes of headache in this age group are medication overuse, polypharmacy, altered drug pharmacokinetics, trauma to the head and/or neck, and comorbidities such as depression, obstructive sleep apnea, or cardiovascular disorders (Togha et al., 2022).

BOX 2.4 ■ Acute Care Considerations

Many individuals with a severe headache seek treatment in the emergency department (ED). In the United States, annual health care expenditures from ED visits just for migraine headaches are approximately $700 million. It can be difficult for a health care provider to narrow down the diagnosis of head pain in the ED without diagnostic testing, because occasionally, migraine with aura can mimic a transient ischemic attack or cerebral vascular accident (stroke). If concerned about a stroke, obtain a computed tomography scan. Migraine can be associated with acute complications that require urgent recognition and management, such as status migrainosus and migrainous infarction, which increase the risk for an ischemic stroke, and migraine aura–triggered seizure. The goals of treating migraine in the ED are to relieve pain, relieve migraine-associated symptoms, and return the patient to normal functioning. Medications used to treat acute pain from headaches in the ED are acetaminophen, nonsteroidal antiinflammatory drugs, and triptans. Opioids should be avoided. In cases of severe migraine, ketorolac intramuscular injection can be used (Cortel-LeBlanc et al., 2023; Marmura et al., 2015).

- Headache diary
- Self-management
- Disease progression

(Williams, 2020)

- Lifestyle and behavioral modifications
  - Smoking cessation
  - Dietary trigger avoidance
  - Regular exercise
  - Maintaining hydration
  - Eating regularly
  - Getting sufficient sleep

(Burch, 2019)

- Complementary treatment
  - Neuromodulation (Grimsrud & Halker Singh, 2018)—cluster:
    - External trigeminal nerve stimulation
    - Noninvasive vagus nerve stimulator
    - Single-pulse transcranial magnetic stimulation
  - Cognitive behavioral therapy
  - Physical therapy—tension type; yoga and tai chi; chiropractic manipulation, massage (Tick et al., 2018; Williams, 2020)
  - Aerobic exercise and strength training
  - Mindfulness
  - Acupuncture (Tick et al., 2018; Williams, 2020; Zang et al., 2020)
  - Magnesium, feverfew, vitamin B2 (riboflavin), and coenzyme Q10 are used in prevention of migraine (Burch, 2019).

- Complementary and alternative therapies with natural medicines and supplements may interact with prescription medications. Obtain a complete medication history.
- Referral (identify and refer for treatment of comorbid conditions or secondary causes*)
  - Neurologist
  - Psychiatrist or psychologist
  - Cardiologist*
  - Gastroenterologist*
- Follow-up
  - Immediately for headache that worsens after treatment, very severe headache ("worst headache in my life"), or vision and/or mental status changes
  - Monthly while medication is being titrated or adjusted
  - Regularly if controlled

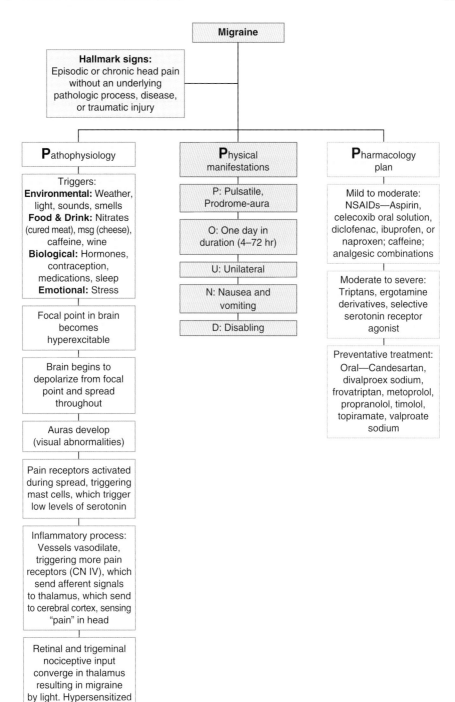

Migraine

Hallmark signs:
Episodic or chronic head pain without an underlying pathologic process, disease, or traumatic injury

Pathophysiology

Triggers:
Environmental: Weather, light, sounds, smells
Food & Drink: Nitrates (cured meat), msg (cheese), caffeine, wine
Biological: Hormones, contraception, medications, sleep
Emotional: Stress

Focal point in brain becomes hyperexcitable

Brain begins to depolarize from focal point and spread throughout

Auras develop (visual abnormalities)

Pain receptors activated during spread, triggering mast cells, which trigger low levels of serotonin

Inflammatory process: Vessels vasodilate, triggering more pain receptors (CN IV), which send afferent signals to thalamus, which send to cerebral cortex, sensing "pain" in head

Retinal and trigeminal nociceptive input converge in thalamus resulting in migraine by light. Hypersensitized visual cortex adds to photophobia.

Physical manifestations

P: Pulsatile, Prodrome-aura

O: One day in duration (4–72 hr)

U: Unilateral

N: Nausea and vomiting

D: Disabling

Pharmacology plan

Mild to moderate: NSAIDs—Aspirin, celecoxib oral solution, diclofenac, ibuprofen, or naproxen; caffeine; analgesic combinations

Moderate to severe: Triptans, ergotamine derivatives, selective serotonin receptor agonist

Preventative treatment: Oral—Candesartan, divalproex sodium, frovatriptan, metoprolol, propranolol, timolol, topiramate, valproate sodium

CN = cranial nerve
NSAIDs = nonsteroidal antiinflammatory drugs

Algorithm 2.1 Migraine headache

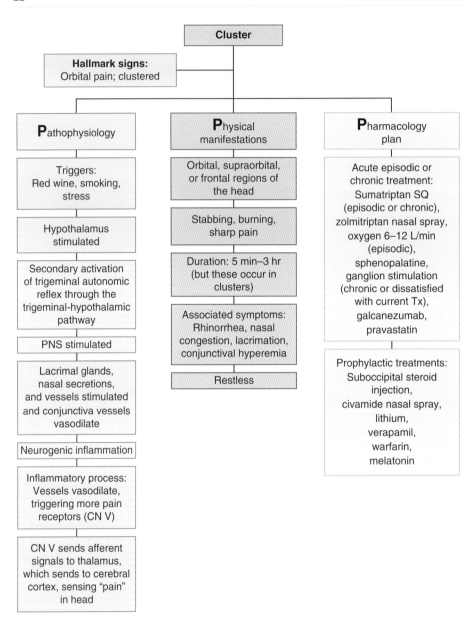

Cluster

Hallmark signs:
Orbital pain; clustered

Pathophysiology

Physical
manifestations

Pharmacology
plan

Triggers:
Red wine, smoking,
stress

Hypothalamus
stimulated

Secondary activation
of trigeminal autonomic
reflex through the
trigeminal-hypothalamic
pathway

PNS stimulated

Lacrimal glands,
nasal secretions,
and vessels stimulated
and conjunctiva vessels
vasodilate

Neurogenic inflammation

Inflammatory process:
Vessels vasodilate,
triggering more pain
receptors (CN V)

CN V sends afferent
signals to thalamus,
which sends to cerebral
cortex, sensing "pain"
in head

Orbital, supraorbital,
or frontal regions of
the head

Stabbing, burning,
sharp pain

Duration: 5 min–3 hr
(but these occur in
clusters)

Associated symptoms:
Rhinorrhea, nasal
congestion, lacrimation,
conjunctival hyperemia

Restless

Acute episodic or
chronic treatment:
Sumatriptan SQ
(episodic or chronic),
zolmitriptan nasal spray,
oxygen 6–12 L/min
(episodic),
sphenopalatine,
ganglion stimulation
(chronic or dissatisfied
with current Tx),
galcanezumab,
pravastatin

Prophylactic treatments:
Suboccipital steroid
injection,
civamide nasal spray,
lithium,
verapamil,
warfarin,
melatonin

PNS = parasympathetic nervous system part of the peripheral nervous system
CN = cranial nerve
Tx = treatment

Algorithm 2.2   Cluster headache

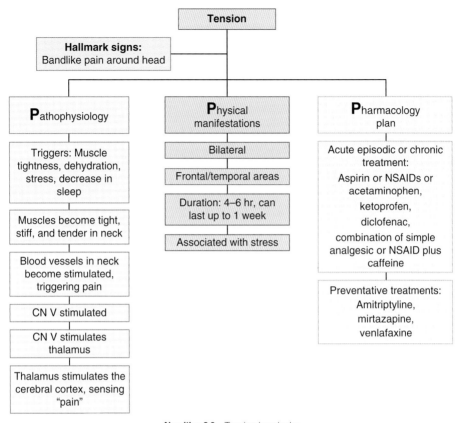

Algorithm 2.3 Tension headache

References

Ailani, J., Burch, R. C., Robbins, M. S., & Board of Directors of the American Headache Society. (2021). The American Headache Society consensus statement: Update on integrating new migraine treatments into clinical practice. *Headache, 61*(7), 1021–1039. https://doi.org/10.1111/head.14153.

Ball, J. W., Flynn, J. E., Solomon, B. S., & Stewart, R. W. (2023). *Seidel's guide to physical examination: An interprofessional approach* (9th Ed). St. Louis: Elsevier.

Burch, R. (2019). Migraine and tension-type headache: Diagnosis and treatment. *Medical Clinics of North America, 103*(2), 215–233. https://doi.org/10.1016/j.mcna.2018.10.003.

Centers for Disease Control and Prevention. (2023). QuickStats: Percentage of adults aged ≥18 years who have been bothered a lot by headache or migraine in the past 3 months, by sex and age group—National Health Interview Survey 2021. *Morbidity and Mortality Weekly Report, 72*(22), 611. http://doi.org/10.15585/mmwr.7222a6.

Charles, A. C., Digre, K. B., Goadsby, P. J., Robbins, M. S., & Hershey, A. (2024). Calcitonin gene-related peptide-targeting therapies are a first-line option for the prevention of migraine: An American Headache Society position statement update. *Headache, 64*(311), 333–341. doi:10.1111/head.14692.

Cortel-LeBlanc, M. A., Orr, S. L., Dunn, M., James, D., & Cortel-LeBlanc, A. (2023). Managing and preventing migraine in the emergency department: A review. *Annals of Emergency Medicine, 82*(6), 732–751. https://doi.org/10.1016/j.annemergmed.2023.05.024.

Dains, J. E., Baumann, L. C., & Scheibel, P. (2024). *Advanced health assessment & clinical diagnosis in primary care* (7th Ed). St. Louis: Elsevier.

Ford, B., Dore, M., & Harris, E. (2021). Outpatient primary care management of headaches: Guidelines from the VA/DoD. *American Family Physician, 104*(2), 316–320.

Goadsby, P. J., Lipton, R. B., & Ferrari, M. D. (2002). Migraine—Current understanding and treatment. *New England Journal of Medicine, 346*(4), 257–270.

Grimsrud, K. W., & Halker Singh, R. B. (2018). Emerging treatments in episodic migraine. *Current Pain Headache Report, 22*(61), 1–6. https://doi.org/10.1007/s11916-018-0716-2.

Headache Classification Committee of the International Headache Society. (2018). The International Classification of Headache Disorders, 3rd edition. *Cephalalgia, 38*(1), 1–211. https://doi.org/10.1177/0333102417738202.

Iannone, L. F., De Cesaris, F., & Geppetti, P. (2022). Emerging pharmacological treatments for migraine in the pediatric population. *Life, 12*(4), 536. https://doi.org/10.3390/life12040536.

Kiarashi, J., VanderPluym, J., Szperka, C. L., Turner, S., Minen, M. T., Broner, S., Ross, A. C., Wagstaff, A. E., Anto, M., Marzouk, M., Monteith, T. S., Rosen, N., Manrriquez, S. L., Seng, E., Finkel, A., & Charleston, L., 4th. (2021). Factors associated with, and mitigation strategies for, health care disparities faced by patients with headache disorders. *Neurology, 97*(6), 280–289.

Marmura, M. J., Silberstein, S. D., & Schwedt, T. J. (2015). The acute treatment of migraine in adults: The American Headache Society evidence assessment of migraine pharmacotherapies. *Headache, 55*(1), 3–20.

Moriarty, M., & Mallick-Searle, T. (2016). Diagnosis and treatment for chronic migraine. *Nurse Practitioner, 41*(6), 18–32. https://doi.org/10.1097/01.NPR.0000483078.55590.b3.

Oskoui, M., Pringsheim, T., Billinghurst, L., Potrebic, S., Gersz, E. M., Gloss, D., Holler-Managan, Y., Leininger, E., Licking, N., Mack, K., Powers, S. W., Sowell, M., Victorio, M. C., Yonker, M., Zanitsch, H., & Hershey, A. D. (2019a). Practice guideline update summary: Pharmacologic treatment for pediatric migraine prevention: Report of the Guideline Development, Dissemination, and Implementation Subcommittee of the American Academy of Neurology and the American Headache Society. *Neurology, 93*(11), 500–509.

Oskoui, M., Pringsheim, T., Holler-Managan, Y., Potrebic, S., Billinghurst, L., Gloss, D., Hershey, A. D., Licking, N., Sowell, M., Victorio, M. C., Gersz, E. M., Leininger, E., Zanitsch, H., Yonker, M., & Mack, K. (2019b). Practice guideline update summary: Acute treatment of migraine in children and adolescents: Report of the Guideline Development, Dissemination, and Implementation Subcommittee of the American Academy of Neurology and the American Headache Society. *Neurology, 93*(11), 487–499.

Powers, J., & Hubner, K. (2023). Alterations of the brain, spinal cord, and peripheral nerves. In J. L. Rogers (Ed.), *McCance & Huether's pathophysiology: The biological basis for disease in adults and children* (9th ed., pp. 597–599). Elsevier.

Robbins, M. S., Starling, A. J., Pringsheim, T. M., Becker, W. J., & Schwedt, T. J. (2016). Treatment of cluster headache: The American Headache Society evidence-based guidelines. *Headache, 56*(7), 1093–1106.

Rogers, J., & Spain, S. (2020). Understanding the most commonly billed diagnoses in primary care: Headache disorders. *Nurse Practitioner, 45*(10), 41–47.

Szperka, C. L., VanderPluym, J., Orr, S. L., Oakley, C. B., Qubty, W., Patniyot, I., Lagman-Bartolome, A. M., Morris, C., Gautreaux, J., Victorio, M. C., Hagler, S., Narula, S., Candee, M. S., Cleves-Bayon, C., Rao, R., Fryer, R. H., Bicknese, A. R., Yonker, M., Hershey, A. D., ... Gelfand, A. A. (2018). Recommendations on the use of anti-CGRP monoclonal antibodies in children and adolescents. *Headache, 58*(10), 1658–1669.

Stovner, L. J., Nichols, E., Steiner, T. J., Abd-Allah, F., Abdelalim, A., Al-Raddadi, R. M., Ansha, M. G., Barac, A., Bensenor, I. M., Doan, L. P., Edessa, D., Endres, M., Foreman, K. J., Gankpe, F. G., Gopalkrishna, G., Goulart, A. C., Gupta, R., Hankey, G. J., Hay, S. I., ... Murray, C. J. L. (2018). Global, regional, and national burden of migraine and tension-type headache, 1990–2016: A systematic analysis for the Global Burden of Disease study 2016. *Lancet Neurology, 17*(11), 954–976. https://doi.org/10.1016/S1474-4422(18)30322-3.

Tick, H., Nielsen, A., Pelletier, K. R., Bonakdar, R., Simmons, S., Glick, R., Ratner, E., Lemmon, R. L., Wayne, P., & Zador, V. (2018). Evidence-based non pharmacological strategies for comprehensive pain care: The consortium pain task force white paper. *Explore, 14*(3), 177–214. https://doi.org/10.1016/j.explore.2018.02.001.

Togha, M., Karimitafti, M. J., Ghorbani, Z., Farham, F., Naderi-Behdani, F., Nasergivehchi, S., Vahabi, Z., Ariyanfar, S., & Jafari, E. (2022). Characteristics and comorbidities of headache in patients over 50 years of age: A cross-sectional study. *BMC Geriatrics, 22*(1), 313. https://doi.org/10.1186/s12877-022-03027-1.

US Department of Veterans Affairs. (2020). VA/DoD clinical practice guidelines: Primary care management of headache. Retrieved July 21, 2023, from https://www.healthquality.va.gov/guidelines/Pain/headache.

Walter, K. (2022). What is migraine? *JAMA, 327*(1), 93.

Wiemann, M., Zimowski, N., Blendow, S., Enax-Krumova, E., Naegel, S., Fleischmann, R., & Strauss, S. (2023). Evidence for converging pathophysiology in complex regional pain-syndrome and primary headache disorders: results from a case–control study. *J Neurol, 271*(297), 1850–1860. doi:10.1007/s00415-023-12119-w.

Williams, K. A. (2020). Headache management in a veteran population: First considerations. *Journal of the American Association of Nurse Practitioners, 32*(11), 758–763. http://doi.org/10.1097/JXX.0000000000000539.

Zang, N., Houle, T., Hindyieh, N., & Aurora, S. K. (2020). Systematic review: Acupuncture vs standard pharmacological therapy for migraine prevention. *Headache, 60*(2), 309–317. https://doi.org/10.1111/head.13723.

CHAPTER 3

Seizure

Julia L. Rogers ■ Felipe Oria

Epilepsy

Seizure

Seizure is not a specific disease entity but rather represents a manifestation of disease. A seizure is a sudden transient disruption in brain electrical function caused by abnormal excessive discharges of cortical neurons. Any disorder that alters the neuronal environment may cause seizure activity (Powers & Hubner, 2023). There are several conditions associated with seizure disorders, including metabolic disorders, congenital malformations, genetic predisposition, perinatal injury, postnatal trauma, myoclonic syndromes, infection, brain tumor, vascular disease, drug or alcohol abuse, and toxins (Box 3.1) (Powers & Hubner, 2023). Febrile seizures are the most common type of seizure in pediatrics (Algorithm 3.1 and Box 3.2). Seizures are classified as generalized, affecting the brain bilaterally; or focal, located in one specific area of the brain.

Epilepsy

Epilepsy is a disease of the brain that causes seizures. Epilepsy is defined using the following criteria: (1) two unprovoked seizures occurring more than 24 hours apart; (2) one unprovoked seizure that has at least a 60% risk of recurrence after two unprovoked seizures, occurring over the next 10 years; and (3) diagnosis of an epilepsy syndrome (Powers & Hubner, 2023). Epilepsy affects approximately 3 million adults and 470,000 children in the United States (Centers for Disease Control and Prevention [CDC], 2020).

Pathophysiology

Epilepsy results from genetic mutations and environmental factors that disrupt normal neuronal function. The dysfunction may be caused from abnormalities in synaptic transmission, an imbalance in the brain's excitatory (Glutamate) and inhibitory (Gamma-Aminobutyric Acid [GABA]) neurotransmitters, alterations of receptors and ion channels activated by neurotransmitters, or the development of abnormal nerve connections or loss of nerves after injury. Antileptic medications target these mechanisms by stabilizing ion channels and neurotransmitters, which is the reason they are effective in treating seizures. The International League Against Epilepsy has proposed six groups for categorizing etiology of epilepsy: genetic, structural, metabolic, immune, infectious, and unknown (National Institute for Health and Care Excellence [NICE], 2022; Piccenna et al., 2023; Powers & Hubner, 2023).

A group of neurons may exhibit an involuntary depolarization, a change in the membrane potential that makes a neuron more likely to fire an action potential. The hyperexcitable neurons are easily activated by hyperthermia, hypoxia, hypoglycemia, electrolyte disturbances (hyponatremia

---

BOX 3.1 ■ Diversity Considerations

Seizures can be influenced by various factors including the inflammatory response, cortisol levels, and glutamate activity in the brain. Research has shown that estrogen may promote seizure activity by initiating excitatory glutamate receptors. Progesterone, and its metabolites (primarily allopregnanolone), has the opposite effect and has an inhibitory effect. It is this hormonal interplay that makes it difficult to manage seizures in women. In fact, some women with epilepsy experience seizure patterns that directly correlate with changes in estrogen and progesterone levels. In catamenial epilepsy, which affects up to 70% of females with epilepsy, is characterized by seizures clustering around cyclic phases of the menstrual cycle. Seizures tend to increase near menses, when estrogen levels are increased and progesterone levels are decreased. The decrease of estrogen during menopause tends to correlate with a decline in seizure activity, and the increased risk of osteoporosis, stroke, and coronary heart disease. The combination of estrogen and progesterone is often prescribed to ease the vasomotor and other symptoms of menopause related to low estrogen levels. However, a provider must be conscientious of the proconvulsant effect of estrogen, and monitor the patient closely for increased seizure activity. (Carvalho et al., 2023).

BOX 3.2 ■ Pediatric Considerations

Pediatric patients require special consideration. Aside from different physiology and age-specific medical conditions, antiepileptic medications must be carefully dosed based on weight.

Febrile seizures are common in young children, with a peak incidence between 12 months and 18 months of age, affecting 2% to 5% of children under 5 years of age in Western countries. Febrile seizures, generally benign, with rare long-term sequelae, are influenced by a genetic and environmental factors, including viruses and vaccines (Algorithm 3.1). Seasonal patterns exist with fall and winter peaks associated with respiratory infections such as influenza and RSV. Peaks of febrile seizures in summer months are generally linked to gastroenteritis (e.g., enteroviruses). Another virus associated with febrile seizures is human herpesvirus-6, also known as roseola infantum or sixth disease. It is crucial to understand the etiology, assessment, and management of febrile seizures, including immediate airway management, vital sign monitoring, and medication administration. Additionally, educating parents about seizure response and addressing their concerns is an essential part of patient care. See Algorithm 3.1. (Sawires et al., 2022; Kim et. al., 2019; Mikkonen et. al., 2015).

---

most common), repeated sensory stimulation, and certain sleep phases. When the intensity reaches a threshold point, cortical excitation spreads. It is the excitation of the subcortical, thalamic, and brain stem areas that corresponds to the tonic phase. Muscle contractions become intense with increased muscle tone (Fig. 3.1A) and can lead to loss of consciousness. The clonic phase is associated with alternating contraction and relaxation of muscles (Fig. 3.1B). Inhibitory neurons in the cortex, anterior thalamus, and basal nuclei react to the cortical excitation, which initiates the clonic phase. Eventually, the neuronal discharge is interrupted, allowing time for muscle contractions to gradually decrease (Fig. 3.1C) and finally cease as the epileptogenic neurons become exhausted (NICE, 2022; Powers & Hubner, 2023).

Another concern is the amount of oxygen consumption during seizure activity. Although cerebral blood flow increases, oxygen and glucose are rapidly depleted, and lactate accumulates in brain tissue. Continued severe seizure activity has the potential for progressive hypoxic brain injury and irreversible damage. In addition, if a seizure focus in the brain is active for a prolonged period, a mirror focus may develop in contralateral normal tissue and cause seizure activity, particularly with focal (i.e., temporal or frontal lobe) epilepsy (NICE, 2022; Powers & Hubner 2023).

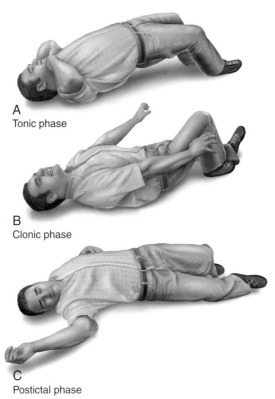

A
Tonic phase

B
Clonic phase

C
Postictal phase

Fig. 3.1 Tonic-clonic seizure activity. (A) Tonic phase. The patient's trunk is elevated with feet on the base and elbows are flexed with hands placed near the face. (B) Clonic phase. The patient is in supine position with one knee flexed and neck slightly above the ground. Arms are stretched straight. (C) Postictal phase. The patient is lying slightly sideways with one arm up and the other hand on one side of the chest. The upper knee is flexed. (From Black, J. M., & Hawks, J. H. (2009). *Medical-surgical nursing: Clinical management for positive outcomes* (8th ed.). Saunders.)

Physical Clinical Presentation

SUBJECTIVE

A thorough health history is a critical component in diagnosing epilepsy and establishing the cause and onset. Details of a seizure event should include a subjective report of sensations, altered consciousness, motor signs, behavioral changes, and environmental setting before and during the seizure. Note any potential triggers within the environment (e.g., flashing lights, loud noises). During the focused history, documentation should include the onset of symptoms precipitating events; location, intensity, and quality of pain; progression of symptoms; alleviating and aggravating factors; previous episodes; and associated symptoms. Document allergies, ill contacts, autoimmune diseases, and medical, social, and family histories (Goolsby & Grubbs, 2023; NICE, 2022; Powers & Hubner, 2023).

Two types of symptoms signal the preictal phase of a generalized tonic-clonic seizure: (1) a prodrome, which is characterized by early manifestations that occur hours to days before a seizure and may include anxiety, depression, or inability to think clearly; and (2) a focal seizure or aura that immediately precedes the onset of a generalized tonic-clonic seizure. Both may become familiar warning signs to the person experiencing recurrent generalized seizures that may enable the person to prevent injuries during the seizure. The ictus is the episode of the epileptic seizure with tonic-clonic activity. Relaxation of urinary and bowel sphincters may occur, leading to bladder and bowel incontinence. (Goolsby & Grubbs, 2023; NICE, 2022; Powers & Hubner, 2023).

OBJECTIVE*

Generalized: Malaise; weakness; fatigue; deep sleep

Neurological: Headache; generalized seizure or complex partial seizure that may take the form of a gustatory, visual, or auditory experience; a feeling of dizziness or numbness; **aura or just "a funny feeling"; seizure—tonic (muscle contraction with or just "a funny feeling"; seizure—tonic (muscle contraction with excessive muscle tone) and clonic (alternating contraction and relaxation of muscles)**; headache, **confusion**, aphasia, memory loss, and paralysis that may last hours or 1 to 2 days; **prolonged seizure activity (>5 minutes)**

HEENT: <u>Sclera conjunctiva with icterus</u>; **Blank stare; subtle eye blinking; pupillary response changes before and after seizure episode; lip smacking**; tongue biting

Cardiovascular: Tachycardia

Pulmonary: *Inspection:* Labored respirations; tachypnea; use of accessory muscles; **apnea** *Auscultation:* Wheezing; diminished

Genitourinary: Bladder and bowel **incontinence**

Musculoskeletal: Diminished strength; flexion; extension; **muscle contraction; rhythmic jerking movements**

Psychiatric: Sense of depression; anxious; memory loss

Phases: Preictal phase, occurs hours to a few days before the onset of a seizure; aura phase, immediately precedes the onset of a generalized tonic-clonic seizure; ictus phase, episode of the epileptic seizure with tonic-clonic activity; and postictal phase, follows an epileptic seizure with confusion and fatigue (Algorithm 3.2).

(Ball et al., 2023; Dains et al., 2024; Goolsby & Grubbs, 2023; NICE, 2022; Powers & Hubner, 2023)

Evaluation and Differential Diagnoses

DIAGNOSTICS

- Labs
  - Blood glucose, serum calcium, blood urea nitrogen, creatinine, and creatinine clearance
  - Cerebrospinal fluid examination
  - Genetic testing
  - Antibody testing with new-onset epilepsy if autoimmune encephalitis is suspected
- Urinalysis
  - Urine sodium
- Diagnostic imaging
  - Brain computed tomography or magnetic resonance imaging
  - Electroencephalogram
  - Combined electroencephalogram and functional magnetic resonance imaging
  - Electrocardiogram (12-lead)

(Krumholz et al., 2015; NICE, 2022; Powers & Hubner, 2023)

---

*Hallmark signs are bolded and <u>Red flags are bolded and underlined</u>.

DIFFERENTIAL DIAGNOSIS

- Convulsive concussion
- Drug intoxication or withdrawal
- Migraine with aura
- Psychogenic nonepileptic event
- Panic attack

Plan

GUIDELINE RESOURCES

- National Institute for Health and Care Excellence. (2022). *Epilepsies in children, young people and adults: Diagnosis and management. NICE guideline (NG217). Methods.* https://www.nice.org.uk/guidance/ng217
- Krumholz, A., Wiebe, S., Gronseth, G. S., Gloss, D., Sánchez, A. M., Arif, Liferidge, A. T., Martello, J., Kanner, A. M., Shinnar, S., Hopp, J. L., & French, J. A. (2015). Evidence-based guideline: Management of an unprovoked first seizure in adults: Report of the Guideline Development Subcommittee of the American Academy of Neurology and the American Epilepsy Society. *Neurology, 84*(16), 1705–1713. https://doi.org/10.1212/wnl.0000000000001487

Pharmacotherapy

Treatment options are linked to the pathophysiologic process of seizure activity, with the goal of correcting the offending agent. However, many times the underlying etiology is unknown, in which case medications, generally antiepileptic drugs, are used to reduce the rapid firing of neurons in the brain and thereby reduce calcium conduction.

- Medications (Algorithm 3.3)
  - Antiepileptic drug—individualized. Start treatment once the diagnosis of epilepsy is confirmed.
  - Monotherapy with antiepiletic medication (dependent on type of seizure—refer to guidelines)
    - If first-line monotherapy is unsuccessful, try monotherapy with another antiseizure medication, using caution during the changeover period:
      - Increase the dose of the second medicine slowly while maintaining the dose of the first medicine.
      - If the second medicine is successful, slowly taper off the dose of the first medicine.
      - If the second medicine is unsuccessful, slowly taper off the dose of the second medicine and consider an alternative.
  - If first- and second-line monotherapy medication is unsuccessful, consider trying an add-on treatment:
    - When starting an add-on treatment, carefully titrate the additional medicine and review treatment frequently, including monitoring for adverse effects such as sedation.
- Older adults require specialized treatment plans. See Box 3.3.
- Airway maintenance is a priority with seizure activity and needs to be ensured. (Box 3.4).

(Krumholz et al., 2015; NICE, 2022)

NONPHARMACOTHERAPY

- Individualized risk assessment for second seizure
  - Evaluate modifiable factors:

BOX 3.3 ■ Older Adult Considerations

Managing epilepsy in the elderly requires a comprehensive and individualized approach, involving a diverse team of healthcare professionals. This team typically includes epilepsy specialists, general neurologists, geriatricians, clinical pharmacists, primary care providers, and nurses with expertise in both neurology and geriatrics. The involvement of family members and caregivers is also crucial for optimal care delivery. Older adults with seizures present unique challenges due to age-related physiological changes and comorbidities. These factors necessitate careful consideration when selecting and administering antiseizure medications. Key concerns include altered drug metabolism, increased susceptibility to side effects (particularly cognitive impairment), and a higher risk of drug interactions due to polypharmacy. Providers should review the American Geriatrics Society's BEERS criteria for safe medication administration. Additionally, antiseizure medications can exacerbate or contribute to common geriatric issues such as osteoporosis, falls, and cardiovascular problems. The cognitive effects of some drugs may impair balance and reaction time, potentially increasing the risk of falls and accidents, including those involving motor vehicles. Therefore, treatment plans must balance seizure control with minimizing adverse effects and maintaining quality of life. Regular monitoring of drug levels, renal and hepatic function, bone density, and cognitive status is essential. Newer antiseizure medications with more favorable side effect profiles and fewer drug interactions are often preferred in this population. Patient and caregiver education about medication adherence, seizure recognition, and safety measures is also a critical component of effective epilepsy management in older adults. (Piccenna et al., 2023).

BOX 3.4 ■ Acute Care Considerations

A descriptive cross sectional study by Guterman et al., 2021, examined the clinical and economic burden of status epilepticus aiming to provide insight into the relationship between disease severity, outcomes, and healthcare costs. The research analyzed data from 43,988 U.S. hospitalizations between 2016 and 2018, categorizing patients based on their treatment complexity. The study classified status epilepticus cases into three groups: low, moderate, and high refractoriness, determined by the number and type of antiseizure medications administered. Key outcomes examined included mortality rates, hospital stay duration, and treatment costs. Results revealed that highly refractory status epilepticus cases, comprising 43.5% of the sample, had significantly worse outcomes. These patients experienced higher mortality rates, longer hospital stays, and substantially higher costs as compared to those with less refractory status epilepticus. The findings underscore the escalating burden of status epilepticus as it becomes more treatment-resistant. (Guterman et al., 2021).

- Mental health (e.g., depression, anxiety, psychosis, alcohol or substance misuse)
- Vascular risk factors (e.g., diabetes, hypertension, atrial fibrillation)
- Sepsis
- Educate
  - How to recognize a future seizure
  - First aid and initial safety guidance in case of another seizure
  - Risk reduction strategies
  - Contacts if they have a further seizure
  - Triggers that may provoke seizures
  - Medication adherence and potential side effects
  - Impact of epilepsy and treatment
  - Memory, attention, concentration, educational attainment, and work performance
  - Sudden Unexpected Death in Epilepsy (SUDEP)
  - Support and information on contraception and pregnancy for females and their partners to enable them to make informed decisions

- Lifestyle and behavioral modifications
  - Safety: Including activities that should be adapted or avoided; for example, showering rather than bathing, cooking safely, caring for babies and young children safely, and avoiding working at heights
  - Supervised swimming and water sports; no climbing above their height without supervision
  - Driving restrictions
- Complementary treatment
  - Psychosocial counseling
  - Complementary and alternative therapies with natural medicines and supplements may interact with prescription medications. Obtain a complete medication history.
- Referral
  - Neurologist
- Follow-up
  - Neurology specialist appointment within 2 weeks of a first suspected seizure or seizure recurrence after a period of remission for an assessment
  - Primary care office visit every 3 to 6 months

(NICE, 2022; Powers & Hubner, 2023)

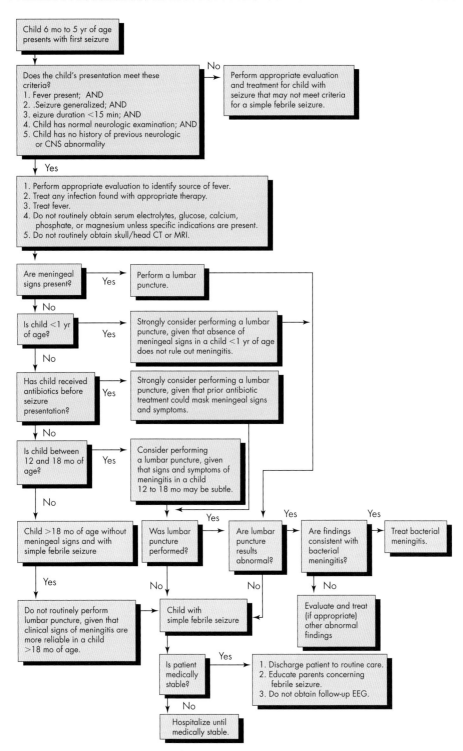

Algorithm 3.1 Febrile Seizures. (From Custer, J. W., & Rau, R. E. (2009). *The Harriet Lane handbook* (18th ed.). Mosby.)

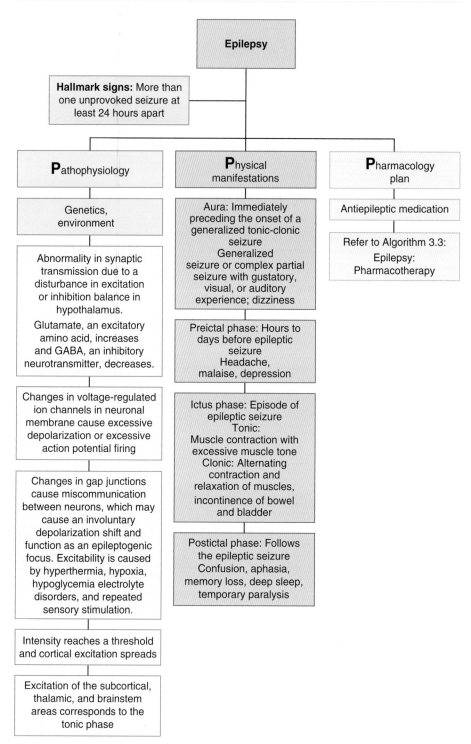

Epilepsy

Hallmark signs: More than one unprovoked seizure at least 24 hours apart

Pathophysiology

Genetics, environment

Abnormality in synaptic transmission due to a disturbance in excitation or inhibition balance in hypothalamus.
Glutamate, an excitatory amino acid, increases and GABA, an inhibitory neurotransmitter, decreases.

Changes in voltage-regulated ion channels in neuronal membrane cause excessive depolarization or excessive action potential firing

Changes in gap junctions cause miscommunication between neurons, which may cause an involuntary depolarization shift and function as an epileptogenic focus. Excitability is caused by hyperthermia, hypoxia, hypoglycemia electrolyte disorders, and repeated sensory stimulation.

Intensity reaches a threshold and cortical excitation spreads

Excitation of the subcortical, thalamic, and brainstem areas corresponds to the tonic phase

Physical manifestations

Aura: Immediately preceding the onset of a generalized tonic-clonic seizure
Generalized seizure or complex partial seizure with gustatory, visual, or auditory experience; dizziness

Preictal phase: Hours to days before epileptic seizure
Headache, malaise, depression

Ictus phase: Episode of epileptic seizure
Tonic:
Muscle contraction with excessive muscle tone
Clonic: Alternating contraction and relaxation of muscles, incontinence of bowel and bladder

Postictal phase: Follows the epileptic seizure
Confusion, aphasia, memory loss, deep sleep, temporary paralysis

Pharmacology plan

Antiepileptic medication

Refer to Algorithm 3.3:
Epilepsy:
Pharmacotherapy

Algorithm 3.2 Epilepsy

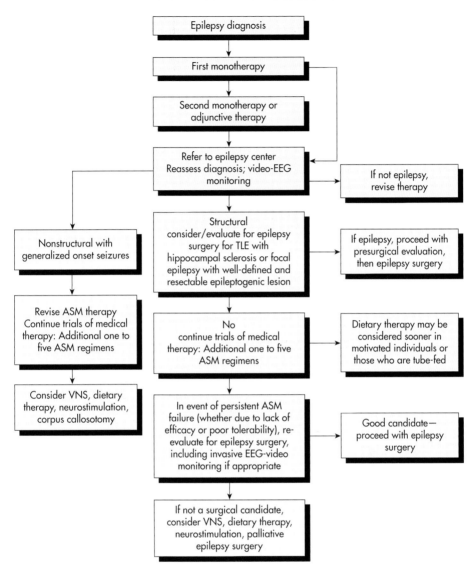

Algorithm 3.3 Epilepsy Pharmacotherapy. (From Jankovic, J., Mazziotta, J. C., & Pomeroy, S. L. (2022). In N. J. Newman (Ed.), *Bradley and Daroff's neurology in clinical practice* (8th ed.). Elsevier.)

References

Ball, J. W., Flynn, J. A., Solomon, B. S., & Stewart, R. W. (2023). *Seidel's guide to physical examination: An interprofessional approach* (9th ed). St. Louis: Elsevier.

Carvalho, V., Colonna, I., Curia, G., Ferretti, M. T., Arabia, G., Molnar, M. J., Lebedeva, E. R., Moro, E., de Visser, M., Bui, E., & Gender and Diversity Issues in Neurology Task Force of the European Academy of Neurology. (2023). Sex steroid hormones and epilepsy: Effects of hormonal replacement therapy on the seizures' frequency of postmenopausal women with epilepsy—A systematic review. *European Journal of Neurology, 30*(9), 2884–2898.

Centers for Disease Control and Prevention. (2024). Epilepsy fast facts. National Center for Chronic Disease Prevention and Health Promotion, Division of Population Health. https://www.cdc.gov/epilepsy/data-research/facts-stats/index.html#:~:text=Almost%203%20million%20U.S.%20adults,epilepsy%20are%20in%20the%20billions. Retrieved August 22, 2024.

Dains, J. E., Baumann, L. C., & Scheibel, P. (2024). *Advanced health assessment & clinical diagnosis in primary care* (7th ed). St. Louis: Elsevier.

Goolsby, M. J., & Grubbs, L. (2023). *Advanced Assessment: Interpreting Findings and Formulating Differential Diagnoses* (5th ed). Philadelphia: Elsevier, 9781719648301.

Guterman, E. L., Betjemann, J. P., Aimetti, A., Li, J. W., Wang, Z., Yin, D., Hulihan, J., Lyons, T., Miyasato, G., & Strzelczyk, A. (2021). Association between treatment progression, disease refractoriness, and burden of illness among hospitalized patients with status epilepticus. *JAMA Neurology, 78*(5), 588–595.

Kim, S. Y., Lee, N. M., Yi, D. Y., Yun, S. W., Lim, I. S., & Chae, S. A. (2019). Seasonal distribution of febrile seizure and the relationship with respiratory and enteric viruses in Korean children based on nationwide registry data. *Seizure, 73*, 9–13.

Krumholz, A., Wiebe, S., Gronseth, G. S., Gloss, D. S., Sanchez, A. M., Kabir, A. A., Liferidge, A. T., Martello, J. P., Kanner, A. M., Shinnar, S., Hopp, J. L., & French, J. A. (2015). Evidence-based guideline: Management of an unprovoked first seizure in adults: Report of the guideline development subcommittee of the American Academy of Neurology and the American Epilepsy Society: Evidence-based guideline. *Neurology, 84*(16), 1705–1713.

Mikkonen, K., Uhari, M., Pokka, T., & Rantala, H. (2015). Diurnal and seasonal occurrence of febrile seizures. *Pediatric neurology, 52*(4), 424–427.

National Institute for Health and Care Excellence (NICE). (2022). Epilepsies in children, young people and adults: Diagnosis and management. NICE guideline (NG217). Methods. https://www.nice.org.uk/guidance/ng217. Reviewed August 22, 2024.

Piccenna, L., O'Dwyer, R., Leppik, I., Beghi, E., Giussani, G., Costa, C., DiFrancesco, J. C., Dhakar, M. B., Akamatsu, N., Cretin, B., Krämer, G., Faught, E., & Kwan, P. (2023). Management of epilepsy in older adults: A critical review by the ILAE Task Force on Epilepsy in the Elderly. *Epilepsia, 64*(3), 567–585.

Powers, J., & Hubner, K. E. (2023). Alterations of the brain, spinal cord, and peripheral nerves. In J. L. Rogers (Ed.), *McCance & Huether's pathophysiology: The biological basis for disease in adults and children* (9th ed., pp. 570–617). Elsevier.

Sawires, R., Buttery, J., & Fahey, M. (2022). A review of febrile seizures: Recent advances in understanding of febrile seizure pathophysiology and commonly implicated viral triggers. *Frontiers in Pediatrics, 9*, 801321.

Wu, M. L., Chao, L. F., & Xiao, X. (2022). A pediatric seizure management virtual reality simulator for nursing students: A quasi-experimental design. *Nurse Education Today, 119*, 105550.

CHAPTER 4

Traumatic Brain Injury

Julia L. Rogers ▓ Felipe Oria

Concussion

Mild Traumatic Brain Injury: Concussion

A concussion is a mild traumatic brain injury (mTBI) caused by a direct or indirect biomechanical force transmitted to the head that leads to changes in physiologic and neurologic function affecting the physical, cognitive, emotional, and sleep domains. It is a predominantly functional rather than structural injury. The neurophysiologic event is related to sudden acceleration, deceleration (coup - counter coup), and rotational forces resulting from blunt impact to the head, neck, or body from a motor vehicle accident, sport or recreational injury, fall, or physical assault.

mTBI has an estimated annual incidence of 500 per 100,000 people in the United States (US) based on emergency room data. However, estimates are as high as 1153 per 100,000 people if community-based concussions are considered (Lithopoulos et al., 2022). In 2019, about 15% of all US high school students self-reported one or more sports- or recreation-related concussions within the preceding 12 months (Fig. 4.1; Box 4.1). People aged 75 years and older account for about 32% of hospitalizations related to traumatic brain injury (TBI) and 28% of TBI-related deaths (Jin, 2018) (Boxes 4.2 and 4.3). Males are almost twice as likely to be hospitalized with a TBI and have a mortality rate that is three times higher than that of females. When comparing mTBI rates by gender within the same sport (soccer, basketball, softball/baseball), females experience a higher rate of mTBI than their male counterparts at both the high school and collegiate levels (Jin, 2018). Unintentional fall is the leading mechanism of injury contributing to a nonfatal TBI (Jin, 2018).

Pathophysiology

The pathophysiologic process of mTBI involves a forceful direct impact to the head or face that may or may not involve a loss of consciousness. The brain is cushioned within the skull by cerebrospinal fluid, which protects the brain against penetrating trauma but is not always able to absorb the impact of a violent force. Therefore an abrupt blow to the head or even a rapid deceleration can cause the brain to contact the inner side of the skull and result in microscopic damage to brain cells, tearing of blood vessels, pulling of nerve fibers, and bruising of the brain without obvious structural damage visible on a computed tomography or magnetic resonance imaging scan (see Fig. 4.1) (Powers & Hubner, 2023). In severe cases, the brain tissue can swell and become compressed by the skull, leading to intracranial pressure (ICP) and limiting the flow of blood, which worsens the severity of the injury and can possibly lead to a cerebral vascular accident (CVA) (American Association of Neurological Surgeons, 2023).

There are two types of pathoanatomical lesions: focal and diffuse. Contact is the most common source of focal injuries and high rate of acceleration and deceleration or rotational forces are the

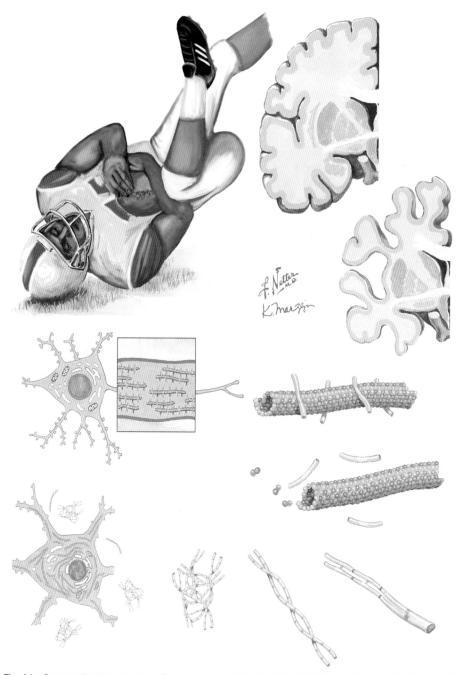

Fig. 4.1 Sports-related concussion. From top left clockwise: **Football Player Injury:** Sporting event causes concussion from coup - counter coup and rotation. **Normal Brain Anatomy:** A cross-sectional view of brain tissue showing normal anatomy. **Healthy Neuron:** An illustration of a normal neuron. **Damaged Neuron:** An illustration of a neuron with axonal damage due to concussion. **Intact Axons:** Axons in their normal, undamaged state. **Swelling Axons:** Axons undergoing swelling and disconnection. **Fragmented Axons:** Advanced neuronal damage post-concussion. (From Srinivasan, J., Chaves, C., Scott, B., & Small, J. E. (2020). *Netter's neurology* (3rd ed.). Elsevier.)

BOX 4.1 ■ Pediatric Considerations

There is a published guideline specifically for pediatric patients that includes 19 sets of recommendations on diagnosis, prognosis, and management/treatment of pediatric mild traumatic brain injury (mTBI). Recommendations include using validated clinical decision rules to identify children with mTBI at low risk for intracranial injury (ICI) in whom a computed tomography (CT) scan of the head is not indicated, as well as children who may be at higher risk for clinically important ICI and thus may warrant a CT scan of the head. The guidelines do not support routinely using magnetic resonance imaging (MRI) in the acute evaluation of suspected or diagnosed mTBI. It is important for health care providers to educate parents that recovery from pediatric mTBI is variable and that no single factor can predict symptom resolution or outcome. Be clear that symptoms generally resolve within 1 to 3 months after injury (Lumba-Brown et al., 2018). Refer to Guideline Resources in this chapter for URL to pediatric guidelines.

BOX 4.2 ■ Older Adult Considerations

Traumatic brain injury (TBI) presents a significant health concern, particularly among older adults. This demographic is particularly vulnerable due to added comorbidities such as hypertension, diabetes mellitus, and coronary heart disease, which can complicate treatment and recovery. Recent studies have shown that individuals aged 75 and above experience the highest rates of TBI-related hospitalizations. Interestingly, males show higher age-adjusted rates of fall-related TBI hospitalizations compared to females. This disparity might be explained by a combination of factors, including biological vulnerabilities, variations in healthcare-seeking behaviors, and differences in fall circumstances, such as a higher proportion of males experiencing falls from elevated positions like ladders, which are more likely to result in moderate to severe injuries, including TBI.

Unintentional falls are the primary cause of TBI-related hospitalizations within this same age group. The increasing use of anticoagulant therapies in older adults, while beneficial for managing chronic conditions such as atrial fibrillation, poses additional risks in the context of TBI from a sustained fall. These medications can increase the likelihood of intracranial hemorrhage, potentially exacerbating TBI complications. Healthcare providers should be vigilant in assessing older patients for TBI symptoms following falls or fall-related injuries, including seemingly unrelated incidents such as hip fractures. The clinical manifestations of periods of forgetfulness and other decreased cognitive abilities can be overlooked as just being part of aging, especially if the person does not remeber the fall or does not want to report the fall in fear of losing independence. The CDC (2023) provides an assessment tool, "The Stopping Elderly Accidents, Deaths, and Injuries" (STEADI) which provides a streamlined approach for healthcare providers to implement the American and British Geriatrics Societies' clinical practice guideline for fall prevention. (CDC, 2023, April 13; Peterson & Thomas, 2021; American Association of Neurological Surgeons, 2024).

most common cause of diffuse injuries. Injury is transferred from the outer to the inner regions of the brain, causing a breakdown of cellular homeostasis, neuroinflammation, diffuse bruising, apoptosis, oxidative stress, and neurodegeneration, which causes a decrease in plasticity and memory. The extent of rotationally induced diffuse brain injury is dependent on kinematics such as angular acceleration, rotational speed, and acceleration duration (Naumenko et al., 2023). The injured brain cells and tissue cause clinical manifestations such as headache, nausea, vomiting, impaired ability to concentrate, and difficulty sleeping. There is also mechanically induced brain injury, which initiates ionic, metabolic, inflammatory, and neurovascular changes in the central nervous system and can lead to acute, subacute, and chronic neurological consequences (Naumenko et al., 2023) (Algorithm 4.1).

BOX 4.3 ■ Diversity Considerations

Certain groups have a higher chance of sustaining a traumatic brain injury (TBI). Adults aged 75 years and older account for about 32% of TBI-related hospitalizations and 28% of TBI-related deaths. American Indian/Alaska Native children and adults have higher rates of TBI-related hospitalizations and deaths than other racial or ethnic groups. Factors that contribute to this disparity include higher rates of motor vehicle crashes, substance use, and suicide as well as difficulties in accessing appropriate health care. Studies suggest that service members and veterans who have sustained a TBI may have ongoing symptoms, experience co-occurring health conditions such as posttraumatic stress disorder and depression, have difficulty accessing health care (particularly mental health services), and report thinking about or planning a suicide attempt. Research suggests almost 50% of incarcerated individuals have a history of TBI. Compared to the general population, people who experience homelessness are two to four times more likely to have a history of TBI and up to 10 times more likely to have a history of a moderate or severe TBI (CDC, 2024, April 29).

Physical Clinical Presentation

SUBJECTIVE

During the focused neurologic history, documentation should include the onset of symptoms; whether there was loss of consciousness and if so, for how many minutes; precipitating events; location, intensity, and quality of pain; progression of symptoms; alleviating and aggravating factors; previous episodes; and associated symptoms. Document allergies and past medical, social, and family histories. Complete the Acute Concussion Evaluation Physician/Clinician Office Version form (Gioia et al., 2008), an evidence-based initial clinical evaluation tool for guiding the health care provider in the diagnosis of mTBI. Refer to Box 4.1 for information on assessing older adults for a TBI from a sustained fall.

mTBI is characterized by immediate but transitory clinical manifestations. There may be no loss of consciousness or there may be loss of consciousness for less than 30 minutes. An individual may be confused for several minutes after the injury or after regaining consciousness. Whether the person had a loss of consciousness or not, they may not remember what happened just prior to the injury (amnesia) (Powers & Hubner, 2023). It is important to ask witnesses of the injury if there was a period of loss or decreased consciousness and if so, the amount of time. A person with a concussion may not be able to recall memories of events immediately before or up to 24 hours after the event (Powers & Hubner, 2023). Common symptoms that are reported with concussion include physical, behavioral, and cognitive indicators. The individual or witness of the event may report altered level of consciousness and alteration in mental state with complaints of confusion, disorientation, and slowed thinking or processing of information, sometimes referred to as having brain fog or feeling dazed. Physical symptoms may include headache, weakness, loss of balance, change in vision, auditory sensitivity, and dizziness. The individual may also report difficulty falling asleep and mood swings (Powers & Hubner, 2023). It should raise a red flag if the individual reports a headache that continues to worsen or will not go away. The individual should be assessed in an acute care setting if there are reports of loss of consciousness, seizures, worsening symptoms, or symptoms that have not gone away after 10 to 14 days; history of multiple concussions; or inability to wake up. Behaviors and emotions may change and can include increased irritability, fatigue, anxiety, depression, and altered sleep patterns.

The mental status portion of the neurologic examination includes assessing a person's emotional responses; mood; ability to think, reason, and make judgments; and personality. It is important to identify the individual's strength and ability to interact with the environment. The diagnosis of concussion cannot be made on the basis of symptoms alone; rather, it must be made in the overall context of history, physical examination, and at times, additional clinical assessments.

OBJECTIVE*

Generalized: Lack of judgment; **impulsive**; **fatigue**

Neurological: Perform a complete neurologic exam. Cranial nerve examination must include reflexes, motor and sensory functioning, and coordination. **Confusion**; **memory loss**; **dizziness**; **difficulty concentrating**; sensitivity to light; loss of smell; loss of taste; <u>**slurred speech**</u>; <u>**weakness**</u>; <u>**paresthesia; decreased coordination**</u>; vertigo; **imbalance**; **abnormal deep tendon reflexes**

HEENT: Headache; **vision disturbances (double or blurry vision)**; strabismus; **ringing ears**; epistaxis

Cardiovascular: Regular rate rhythm; normal S1/S2

Pulmonary: Labored respirations; tachypnea; use of accessory muscles

Gastrointestinal: Nausea or vomiting; <u>**significant nausea or repeated vomiting**</u>

Genitourinary: Incontinence

Musculoskeletal: Strength, sensory, reflex, and coordination testing is usually normal but may reveal lack of muscle coordination.

Psychiatric: Memory loss; flat affect; depression; anxious

(Ball et al., 2023; Dains et al., 2024; Goolsby & Grubbs, 2019; Powers & Hubner, 2023)

Evaluation and Differential Diagnoses

DIAGNOSTICS

- Glasgow Coma Scale to assess mental status (mTBI Glasgow Coma Scale score is 13 to 15)
- Computed tomography (CT) or magnetic resonance imaging (MRI) scan of the head often presents normally as concussion is metabolic and microscopic in nature. The purpose of neuroimaging is to assess for other etiologies or injuries, such as hemorrhage or contusion, that may cause similar symptoms but require different management.

DIFFERENTIAL DIAGNOSIS

- Headache disorders (migraines, cluster, tension)
- Mental health diagnoses (anxiety, depression, or posttraumatic stress disorder)
- Attention deficit hyperactivity disorder
- Sleep dysfunction

Plan

GUIDELINE RESOURCES

- Ontario Neurotrauma Foundation. (2023). *Living concussion guidelines: Guideline for concussion & prolonged symptoms for adults 18 years of age or older*. https://concussionsontario.org
- Lumba-Brown, A., Yeates, K. O., Sarmiento, K., Breiding, M. J., Haegerich, T. M., Gioia, G. A., Turner, M., Benzel, E. C., Suskauer, S. J., Giza, C. C., Joseph, M., Broomand, C., Weissman, B., Gordon, W., Wright, D. W., Moser, R. S., McAvoy, K., Ewing-Cobbs, L., Duhaime, A. C., … Timmons, S. D. (2018). Centers for Disease Control and Prevention guideline on

---

*Hallmark signs are bolded and <u>**Red flags are bolded and underlined**</u>.

BOX 4.4 ■ Acute Care Considerations

The rapid transfer of traumatic brain injury (TBI) patients to trauma centers and the avoidance of secondary insults such as hypotension and hypoxia are paramount. The acute management of TBI focuses on the prevention of secondary injury through the avoidance of hypotension and hypoxia and maintenance of appropriate cerebral perfusion pressure and cerebral blood flow. Elevated intracranial pressure (ICP) can be managed in an intensive care unit with a combination of hyperosmolar therapy, cerebrospinal fluid drainage, pentobarbital coma, and decompressive craniectomy. It is important to include venous thromboembolism, stress ulcer, and seizure prophylaxis as well as nutrition and metabolic optimization in TBI patients (Vella et al., 2017).

---

the diagnosis and management of mild traumatic brain injury among children. *JAMA Pediatrics*, *172*(11), e182853–e182853. https://doi.org/10.1001/jamapediatrics.2018.2853
■ American College of Emergency Physicians. (2023). *Mild traumatic brain injury*. https://www.acep.org/patient-care/clinical-policies/mild-traumatic-brain-injury2
■ The Management of Concussion—Mild Traumatic Brain Injury Working Group. (2016). *VA/DoD clinical practice guideline for the management of concussion—Mild traumatic brain injury*. https://www.va.gov/covidtraining/docs/mTBICPGFullCPG50821816.pdf

Pharmacotherapy

■ Medications (Refer to guideline resources for specific dosages)
  ■ Posttraumatic headache:
    ▫ Analgesics (nonsteroidal antiinflammatory drugs)
  ■ Sleep disturbance:
    ▫ Gabapentin
    ▫ Amitriptyline
    ▫ Nortriptyline
    ▫ Melatonin
    ▫ Trazadone
  ■ Depression:
    ▫ Selective serotonin reuptake inhibitors (SSRIs)
    ▫ Serotonin and norepinephrine reuptake inhibitors (SNRIs)
    ▫ Tricyclic antidepressants
  ■ See Box 4.4.
(Stillman et al., 2017)

NONPHARMACOTHERAPY

■ Physical and cognitive rest 3 to 5 days after injury, followed by a gradual resumption of both physical and cognitive activities as tolerated, remaining below the level at which symptoms are exacerbated
■ Dizziness or vertigo
  ■ Dix-Hallpike maneuver and Epley maneuver
■ Sleep hygiene education
  ■ Minimize electronic screen time 1 hour before going to bed.
  ■ Go to bed and wake up at the same time each day.
  ■ Minimize or avoid caffeine, nicotine, and alcohol.
■ Educate on head injury prevention

- Remove hazards in the home that may contribute to falls. Secure rugs and loose electrical cords, put away toys, use safety gates, and install window guards. Install grab bars and handrails for the frail or elderly.
- Obey all traffic signals and be aware of drivers when cycling or skateboarding.
- Wear a seat belt every time, whether driving or riding in a motor vehicle.
- Never drive while under the influence of drugs or alcohol or ride as a passenger with anybody who is under the influence.
- Use helmets or protective headgear approved by the American Society for Testing and Materials for specific sports.
- Wear appropriate protective clothing for the sport.
- Do not participate in sports when ill or very tired.
- Keep unloaded firearms in a locked cabinet or safe, and store ammunition in a separate, secure location.

(CDC & National Center for Injury Prevention and Control, 2023; CDC, 2023, April 6)

- Complementary treatment
  - Counseling or neuropsychotherapy
- Referral
  - Neurologist
  - Physical therapy
  - Cognitive therapy
- Follow-up
  - Frequent monitoring of all head injuries is important.
  - Communicate with patient or family members within 4 to 12 hours after the injury and then periodically depending on the condition of the patient.

(Stillman et al., 2017)

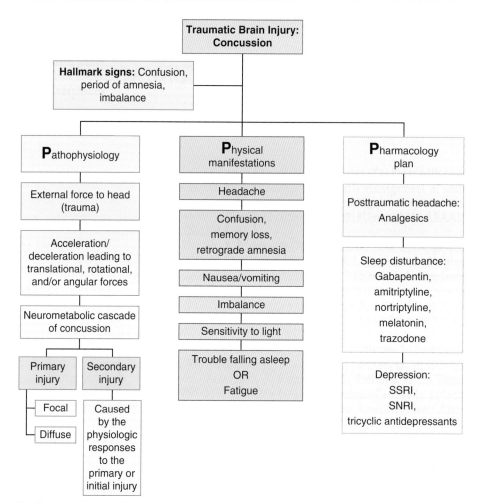

Algorithm 4.1 Traumatic Brain Injury: Concussion. *SNRI,* Serotonin and norepinephrine reuptake inhibitor; *SSRI,* Selective serotonin reuptake inhibitor.

References

American Association of Neurological Surgeons. (2024). Concussion. Retrieved [September 6, 2024], from https://www.aans.org/patients/conditions-treatments/concussion/

Ball, J. W., Dains, J. E., Flynn, J. A., Solomon, B. S., & Stewart, R. W. (2023). *Seidel's guide to physical examination* (10th ed.). Elsevier.

Centers for Disease Control and Prevention. (2023, April 6). Traumatic brain injury & concussion. Accessed September 6, 2024. https://www.cdc.gov/traumatic-brain-injury/

Centers for Disease Control and Prevention. (2023, April 13). About STEADI. Accessed September 6, 2024. https://www.cdc.gov/steadi/about/index.html

Centers for Disease Control and Prevention. (2024, April 29). *Traumatic brain injury and concussion: Health disparities and TBI.* Accessed September 6, 2024. https://www.cdc.gov/traumatic-brain-injury/health-equity/?CDC_AAref_Val=https://www.cdc.gov/traumaticbraininjury/health-disparities-tbi.html

Dains, J. E., Baumann, L. C., & Scheibel, P. (2024). *Advanced health assessment & clinical diagnosis in primary care* (7th ed.). Elsevier.

Gioia, G. A., Collins, M., & Isquith, P. K. (2008). Improving identification and diagnosis of mild traumatic brain injury with evidence: Psychometric support for the acute concussion evaluation. *Journal of Head Trauma Rehabilitation, 23*(4), 230–242.

Goolsby, M. J., & Grubbs, G. L. (2019). *Advanced assessment interpreting findings and formulating differential diagnoses* (4th ed.). F. A. Davis Company.

Jin, J (2018). Prevention of falls in older adults. *JAMA, 319*(16), 1734. https://doi.org/10.1001/jama.2018.43 96externalicon.

Lithopoulos, A., Bayley, M., Curran, D., Fischer, L., Knee, C., Lauzon, J., Nevison, M., Velikonja, D., & Marshall, S. (2022). Protocol for a living systematic review for the management of concussion in adults. *BMJ Open, 12*(7), e061282. https://doi.org/10.1136/bmjopen-2022-061282.

Lumba-Brown, A., Yeates, K. O., Sarmiento, K., Breiding, M. J., Haegerich, T. M., Gioia, G. A., Turner, M., Benzel, E. C., Suskauer, S. J., Giza, C. C., Joseph, M., Broomand, C., Weissman, B., Gordon, W., Wright, D. W., Moser, R. S., McAvoy, K., Ewing-Cobbs, L., Duhaime, A. C., … Timmons, S. D. (2018). Centers for Disease Control and Prevention guideline on the diagnosis and management of mild traumatic brain injury among children. *JAMA Pediatrics, 172*(11), e182853. https://doi.org/10.1001/jamapediatrics.2018.2853.

Marshall, S., Bayley, M., McCullagh, S., Berrigan, L., Fischer, L., Ouchterlony, D., & Velikonja, D. (2022). *Guideline for concussion/mild traumatic brain injury and persistent symptoms: (for Adults 18+ years of age).* Toronto, ON: Ontario Neurotrauma Foundation, 2018.

Naumenko, Y., Yuryshinetz, I., Zabenko, Y., & Pivneva, T. (2023). Mild traumatic brain injury as a pathological process. *Heliyon, 9*(7), e18342. https://doi.org/10.1016/j.heliyon.2023.e18342.

Peterson, A. B., & Thomas, K. E. (2021). Incidence of nonfatal traumatic brain injury–related hospitalizations—United States, 2018. *Morbidity and Mortality Weekly Report, 70*(48), 1664–1668. http://doi.org/10.15585/mmwr.mm7048a3.

Powers, J., & Hubner, K. (2023). Alterations of the brain, spinal cord, and peripheral nerves. In J. L. Rogers, (Ed.), *McCance & Huether's pathophysiology: The biological basis for disease in adults and children* (9th ed., pp. 570–578). Elsevier.

Stillman, A., Alexander, M., Mannix, R., Madigan, N., Pascual-Leone, A., & Meehan, W. P. (2017). Concussion: Evaluation and management. *Cleveland Clinic Journal of Medicine, 84*(8), 623–630.

Vella, M. A., Crandall, M. L., & Patel, M. B. (2017). Acute management of traumatic brain injury. *Surgical Clinics of North America, 97*(5), 1015–1030. https://doi.org/10.1016/j.suc.2017.06.003.

Psychiatric System

SECTION OUTLINE

5 Anxiety

6 Depression

7 Posttraumatic Stress Disorder

CHAPTER 5

Anxiety

Jodi Allen ▪ Corrine M. Djuric

Generalized Anxiety Disorder

Generalized Anxiety Disorder

Generalized anxiety disorder (GAD) is one of the most common mental health disorders in the United States. Prior to the COVID-19 pandemic, an estimated 3.1% of US adults aged 18 years and older had experienced GAD (National Institute of Mental Health, 2022). New literature suggests that the COVID-19 pandemic has created an environment that negatively affected and increased the prevalence of mental health conditions such as GAD (COVID-19 Mental Disorders Collaborators, 2021). Young adults (ages 18–24) are more likely to report symptoms of anxiety since the pandemic (Kaiser Family Foundation, 2023). Females have twice the risk of developing GAD than males (National Institute of Mental Health, 2022). GAD typically arises when a person is in their early 20s but can occur in childhood (Box 5.1) (Takahashi, 2023). Risk for anxiety is a complicated interplay between genetic, epigenetic, and environmental factors (Penninx et al., 2021). Like so many other psychiatric disorders, comorbid psychopathology increases the risk of developing GAD, with the strongest association between GAD and major depressive disorder (MDD) (Takahashi, 2023). An unfortunate complication of GAD is substance use disorder, which often results from self-medication with alcohol and illicit drugs to improve symptoms of GAD (Takahashi, 2023).

Pathophysiology

The pathophysiology of GAD is not fully understood, but abnormalities in three neurotransmitters—norepinephrine, serotonin, and gamma-aminobutyric acid—and their effects on the amygdala have been identified. The amygdala is the portion of the brain and limbic system that processes fear, stress, and/or threatening stimuli and can be overstimulated by these neurotransmitters. Magnetic resonance imaging studies of persons with GAD have identified elevated cingulate cortex activity, which is another portion of the limbic system. If overstimulation of either of these limbic system structures occurs, a large amount of stress hormone is released (see Algorithm 5.1). This causes an exaggerated stress response to manifest and possible development of GAD (Takahashi, 2023).

Physical Clinical Presentation

SUBJECTIVE

Excessive and persistent worries are the hallmark signs of GAD (Box 5.2) (Takahashi, 2023). These worries are often related to life events, health, job performance, or money. The worry experienced can seem out of proportion to the situation, frequently leading to physical symptoms

---

BOX 5.1 ■ Pediatric Considerations

Generalized anxiety disorder (GAD) is most often diagnosed in the pediatric population between the ages of 9 and 18 years. GAD is one of the most prevalent psychiatric disorders in pediatrics and is the second most common pediatric anxiety disorder; however, only 22% of adolescents who meet DSM-5 diagnostic criteria are diagnosed with GAD by their primary care provider. It is imperative to pay attention to cues that point to a traumatic experience as the cause of GAD in children. Nonpharmacologic management is the mainstay of treatment in children with GAD, focusing on behavioral interventions for the child and family. Cognitive behavioral therapy has shown the greatest treatment response in children, though mindfulness and psychodynamic therapy have shown benefit as well. It is recommended to refer an older child or adolescent to a pediatric mental health professional for determination of treatment plan (Garzon et al., 2020).

BOX 5.2 ■ Diversity Considerations

Culture impacts the ways in which behavior, emotion, and thought are expressed, including the way anxiety is expressed. A person from one culture may be comfortable expressing their anxieties while a person from another culture may find this challenging or even inexpressible. Health literacy plays a role in the ability to express the emotional aspects of anxiety; therefore persons with less knowledge about health systems may present with more physical symptoms related to generalized anxiety disorder (GAD) and an inability or uncertainty of how to address the emotional component. Health care providers should focus on providing compassionate, culturally appropriate care to gain the trust of persons with GAD. This allows for open dialogue and person-centered treatment plans for persons with GAD (Martinez, 2019).

BOX 5.3 ■ Acute Care Considerations

While panic attacks are less likely to occur in persons with generalized anxiety disorder (GAD), intense feelings of panic or worry along with other physical symptoms of anxiety can mimic signs and symptoms of a myocardial infarction (MI). Females, who are more likely to be diagnosed with GAD, also present with atypical symptoms of cardiovascular disease and MI. Astute health care providers will first rule out potential organic causes of anxiety related to GAD, but ruling out MI should be prioritized. GAD itself is associated with cardiovascular disease and can negatively impact cardiac health. Screening for cardiac disease indicators and educating persons with GAD on healthy behaviors to decrease the risk of cardiac disease is imperative to improve morbidity and mortality (American Heart Association, 2022; Centers for Disease Control and Prevention, 2020).

---

such as muscle tension, nausea, diarrhea, shortness of breath, restlessness, fatigue, irritability, and difficulty concentrating and sleeping (Takahashi, 2023). During the focused history, documentation should include the onset of symptoms; precipitating events; location, intensity, and quality of pain (if any); progression of symptoms; alleviating and aggravating factors; previous episodes; and associated symptoms. Severity of symptoms can fluctuate and is often linked to changes in stress levels experienced (Takahashi, 2023). Social history should be reviewed with a focus on substance use to ensure self-medication with illicit substances is not occurring. Review of family history can identify a genetic predisposition to GAD. Medication review, including prescription, over-the-counter, herbal, and illicit drug use, is imperative to ensure that one or more medications are not an organic cause of GAD. Consider asking about caffeine consumption as well. Cardiovascular disease is strongly associated with GAD, so careful review of this system and health promotion activities is paramount for prevention of comorbid complications (Box 5.3). Many disease processes, among them thyroid disease, arrhythmia, vitamin deficiencies, and asthma, can cause symptoms of anxiety and must be ruled out.

TABLE 5.1 ■ The Generalized Anxiety Disorder 7-item (GAD-7) Scale

Over the last 2 weeks, how often have you been bothered by the following problems	Not at all	Several days	More than half the days	Nearly every day
1. Feeling nervous, anxious or on edge	0	1	2	3
2. Not being able to stop or control worrying	0	1	2	3
3. Worrying too much about different things	0	1	2	3
4. Trouble relaxing	0	1	2	3
5. Being so restless that it is hard to sit still	0	1	2	3
6. Becoming easily annoyed or irritable	0	1	2	3
7. Feeling afraid as if something awful might happen	0	1	2	3
GAD-7 score obtained by adding score for each question (total points).				
A score of 8 points or higher is the cut-off for needing further identifying evaluation to determine presence and type of anxiety disorder				
The following cut-offs correlate with level of anxiety severity:				
Score 0–4:	Minimal Anxiety			
Score 5–9:	Mild Anxiety			
Score 10–14:	Moderate Anxiety			
Score 15 or greater:	Severe Anxiety			

From Sapra, A., Bhandari, P., Sharma, S., Chanpura, T., & Lopp, L. (2020). Using generalized anxiety disorder-2 (GAD-2) and GAD-7 in a primary care setting. *Cureus*, *12*(5), e8224. doi:10.7759/cureus.8224.

OBJECTIVE*

Generalized: Malaise; weight loss

    Neurological: Loss of focus during examination; inability to concentrate

    Cardiovascular/peripheral vascular: Tachycardia; palpitations

    Pulmonary: Tachypnea

    Gastrointestinal: Epigastric pain

    Musculoskeletal: Generalized muscle tension upon palpation

    Psychiatric: Excessive worry verbalized; irritability; **<u>suicidal ideations</u>** (the GAD-7 screening tool can assist in objective identification of symptoms consistent with GAD but is not diagnostic for GAD [Table 5.1]) (see Algorithm 5.1)

    (National Institute of Mental Health, 2022; Takahashi, 2023)

Evaluation and Differential Diagnoses

DIAGNOSTICS

There are no diagnostic tests indicated to detect GAD; however, they may be useful if there is a clinical suspicion that the anxiety is secondary to an underlying medical condition or substance.

- DSM-5 criteria for GAD (American Psychiatric Association, 2022)
  - Excessive anxiety and worry occurring more days than not for at least 6 months
  - Difficulty controlling the worry

---

*Hallmark signs are bolded and <u>Red flags are bolded and underlined</u>.

- Anxiety and worry associated with at least three of the following symptoms (with at least some symptoms having been present for more days than not for the past 6 months):
  - Restlessness or feeling on edge
  - Being easily fatigued
  - Difficulty concentrating or mind going blank
  - Irritability
  - Muscle tension
  - Sleep disturbance (difficulty falling or staying asleep or restless, unsatisfying sleep)
- Anxiety, worry, or physical symptoms causing clinically significant distress or impairment in social, occupational, or other important areas of functioning
- Disturbance not attributable to physiologic effects of a substance (drug, medication) or another medical condition
- Disturbance not better explained by another mental disorder

DIFFERENTIAL DIAGNOSES

- Organic disease processes: Cardiovascular disease, endocrine dysfunction (e.g., thyroid disease), and asthma are a few diseases that can mimic symptoms of GAD and must be ruled out (see Box 5.3).
- MDD: The characteristic of worry is distinctly different in MDD. Persons with MDD generally worry about past events whereas persons with GAD focus on future events (Box 5.4).
- Panic disorder: Persons with panic disorder will experience disabling paroxysmal panic attacks whereas patients with GAD generally will not.
(Takahashi, 2023)

Plan

GUIDELINE RESOURCES

- National Institute for Health and Care Excellence. (2020). Generalised anxiety disorder and panic disorder in adults: Management. https://www.nice.org.uk/guidance/cg113/chapter/Recommendations

Pharmacotherapy

- First-line treatment
  - Selective serotonin reuptake inhibitors (SSRIs) (e.g., citalopram, escitalopram, sertraline, paroxetine, fluoxetine, fluvoxamine), rather than other classes of medications, are suggested

as initial treatment. There is no evidence of superior agents within the class. Selection of SSRI should be individualized and include cost-effectiveness (see Algorithm 5.1).

- Select serotonin and norepinephrine reuptake inhibitors (SNRIs) (e.g., venlafaxine XR, duloxetine) are an alternative to SSRIs.
- If a person cannot tolerate SSRIs or SNRIs, consider pregabalin, but evaluate the person carefully for history of drug abuse and observe them for development of signs of abuse and dependence.
- Benzodiazepines should *not* be offered unless as a short-term measure during crisis and can be useful for agitation and insomnia symptoms in patients with no history of substance abuse. Duration should be short as they have a high abuse and dependence potential.

(National Institute for Health and Care Excellence [NICE], 2020)

NONPHARMACOTHERAPY

- Educate
  - Person and their family about the diagnosis of GAD, treatments, possible side effects of treatment, importance of adherence to both pharmacologic and nonpharmacologic therapy, and impact of overusing medications such as benzodiazepines
  - Family about danger signs related to self-harm, what to do if identified, and need for close follow-up
- Lifestyle
  - Smoking cessation
  - Regular physical activity (150 minutes/week)
  - Quality nutrition
  - Importance of self-care that promotes relaxation and stress reduction (including meditation and yoga)
- Referral
  - Cognitive behavior therapy: Duration is typically 12 to 15 sessions with evidence to support monthly "booster" sessions.
  - Psychiatry or psych-mental health nurse practitioner: If there is significant diagnostic uncertainty, complicating comorbidity (substance use disorder or MDD), suicidal ideation, poor response to standard treatment, or at any point when the treatment modality exceeds the experience of the clinician. Children should always be referred to a pediatric mental health professional.
- Follow-up:
  - Every 2 to 4 weeks for evaluation of pharmacotherapy effectiveness during the first 3 months of treatment or until stable
  - Every 3 months thereafter

(NICE, 2020)

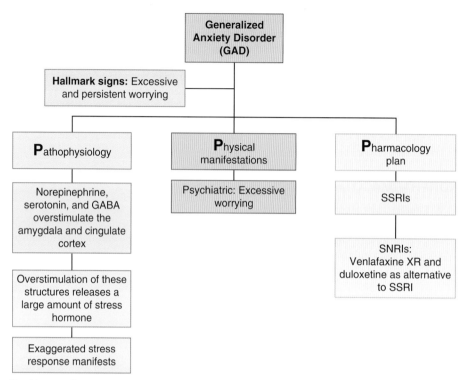

Algorithm 5.1   Generalized Anxiety Disorder (GAD). *GABA*, Gamma-aminobutyric acid; *SNRIs*, serotonin and norepinephrine reuptake inhibitors; *SSRIs*, selective serotonin reuptake inhibitors.

References

American Heart Association. (2022). How to tell the difference between a heart attack and panic attack. https://www.heart.org/en/news/2022/07/13/how-to-tell-the-difference-between-a-heart-attack-and-panic-attack.

American Psychiatric Association. (2022). Anxiety disorders. In *Diagnostic and statistical manual of mental disorders* (5th ed., text rev.). https://doi.org/10.1176/appi.books.9780890425787.

Centers for Disease Control and Prevention. (2020). Heart disease and mental health disorders. https://www.cdc.gov/heartdisease/mentalhealth.htm.

COVID-19 Mental Disorders Collaborators. (2021). Global prevalence and burden of depressive and anxiety disorders in 204 countries and territories in 2020 due to the COVID-19 pandemic. *Lancet, 398*(10312), 1700–1712. https://doi.org/10.1016/S0140-6736(21)02143-7.

Garzon, D. L., Starr, N. B., & Chauvin, J. (2020). Neurodevelopmental, behavioral, and mental health disorders. In D. L. Maaks, N. Starr, M. A. Brady, N. M. Gaylord, M. Driessnack, & K. G. Duderrstadt (Eds.), *Burns' pediatric primary care* (7th ed., pp. 424–425). Elsevier.

Kaiser Family Foundation. (2023). Latest federal data show that young people are more likely than older adults to be experiencing symptoms of anxiety. https://www.kff.org/coronavirus-covid-19/press-release/latest-federal-data-show-that-young-people-are-more-likely-than-older-adults-to-be-experiencing-symptoms-of-anxiety-or-depression.

King, B. M., Touhy, T. A., & Wilson, T. (2020). Mental health. In T. A. Touhy & K. Jett (Eds.), *Ebersole & Hess' Toward healthy aging: Human needs & nursing response* (10th ed., p. 349). Elsevier.

Martinez, K. G. (2019). Influences of cultural differences in the diagnosis and treatment of anxiety and depression. *Anxiety & Depression Association of America.* https://adaa.org/learn-from-us/from-the-experts/blog-posts/consumer/influences-cultural-differences-diagnosis-and.

National Institute for Health and Care Excellence. (2020). Generalised anxiety disorder and panic disorder in adults: Management. https://www.nice.org.uk/guidance/cg113/chapter/Recommendations.

National Institute of Mental Health. (2022, April). Mental health information: Anxiety disorders.https://www.nimh.nih.gov/health/topics/anxiety-disorders.

Penninx, B. W., Pine, D. S., Holmes, E. A., & Reif, A. (2021). Anxiety disorders. *Lancet, 397*(10277), 914–927. https://doi.org/10.1016/S0140-6736(21)00359-7.

Takahashi, L. K. (2023). Neurobiology of schizophrenia, mood disorders, anxiety disorders, posttraumatic stress disorder, and obsessive-compulsive disorder. In J. L. Rogers (Ed.), *McCance and Huether's pathophysiology: The biologic basis for disease in adults and children* (9th ed., pp. 630–633). Mosby-Elsevier.

CHAPTER 6

Depression

Jodi Allen ■ Corrine M. Djuric

Major Depressive Disorder

Major Depressive Disorder

Major depressive disorder (MDD) is one of the most common mental health disorders in the United States and is associated with functional disability and mortality. An estimated 21 million US adults (8.3%) have had at least one major depressive episode (MDE) (National Institute of Mental Health, 2023). Prevalence is higher among adult females (10.3%) compared to males (6.2%); in individuals aged 18 to 25 years (18.6%); those who report two or more races (13.9%) (Box 6.1); those with lower socioeconomic status; and those who are divorced, separated, or widowed. Prevalence is highest in those with Native American ethnicity (National Institute of Mental Health, 2023). While genetic components of MDD exist, developmental and environmental factors are equally important contributors to MDD (Takahashi, 2023). Numerous psychiatric disorders (69% have comorbid psychopathology) and nearly all chronic and disabling medical conditions increase the risk of developing MDD (American Psychiatric Association, 2022). MDD is an independent risk factor for increased morbidity and mortality from cardiac disease (National Institute of Mental Health, 2023). In 2020, only 66% of US adults aged 18 and older diagnosed with MDD received treatment (National Institute of Mental Health, 2023). The undertreatment of MDD can lead to poor outcomes, including suicide or self-harm.

Pathophysiology

MDD is a unipolar depression that correlates with a hypersecretion of cortisol and various neuroendocrine dysregulatory processes. The overproduction of corticotropin-releasing hormone causes hyperactivity of the hypothalamic-pituitary-adrenal cortex, which plays an essential role in a person's ability to cope with stress (Takahashi, 2023). Prolonged exposure to the released glucocorticoids is thought to suppress neurogenesis and cause hippocampal atrophy and a diminished ability to cope (Takahashi, 2023). Monoamine neurotransmitter imbalance in the brain has also been linked to unipolar depression, with serotonin (5-HT), dopamine (DA), and norepinephrine contributing. A decrease in norepinephrine has been associated with loss of alertness, attention, interest in pleasurable activities, and energy. Dopamine reduction has been associated with loss of pleasure, reward, and motivation. A decrease in serotonin has been linked to increased anxiety, compulsions, and obsessions (Takahashi, 2023). In recent studies, inflammation has been noted to trigger depression onset, and persons studied with MDD demonstrate an elevated level of C-reactive protein, a well-established inflammatory marker (Takahashi, 2023).

Physical Clinical Presentation

SUBJECTIVE

MDD presents with heterogeneous symptom(s); that is, no two adult persons may experience the same symptomatology, adding to the challenge of diagnosis. Symptomology in the pediatric population can be even more varied (Box 6.2). The key identifiers of MDD are unabating feelings of sadness and despair (see Algorithm 6.1). The dysphoric mood is frequently paired with other symptoms such as insomnia and diminished interest in pleasurable activities and relationships (Takahashi, 2023). Sleep disturbances can vacillate between difficulty falling asleep to difficulty staying asleep, which exacerbates fatigue common in MDD. Feelings of worthlessness and guilt as well as pessimism are common in persons with MDD (Takahashi, 2023). During the focused history, documentation should include the onset of symptoms; precipitating events; location, intensity, and quality of pain (if any); progression of symptoms; alleviating and aggravating factors; previous episodes; and associated symptoms. Depressive episodes may ebb and flow, though often occurring suddenly (Takahashi, 2023). Social history should be reviewed, with a focus on substance use as concurrent substance use disorder is common with MDD (Substance Abuse and Mental Health Services Administration, 2021). Review of family history can identify a genetic predisposition to mood disorders and substance abuse. Medication review, including prescription, over-the-counter, herbal, and illicit drug use, is imperative to ensure that one or more medications are not an organic cause of MDD. Suicide risk increases in depression, and any person presenting with depressive symptoms should be asked about suicidal ideations.

OBJECTIVE*

Abnormal findings may be absent in patients with MDD; however, a comprehensive physical and psychiatric assessment should be completed to rule out other organic causes of depressive symptoms.

Generalized: Weight gain or loss; unkempt appearance; tearful; poor eye contact

Neurological: Mental status changes; psychomotor agitation or slowing; diminished ability to concentrate; diminished attention span; diminished immediate memory recall

HEENT: Speech may be low in volume.

Psychiatric: Flat affect; **feelings of sadness and despair verbalized** (the PHQ-9 screening tool can assist in objective identification of symptoms consistent with MDD but is not diagnostic for MDD [Fig. 6.1]) (see Algorithm 6.1).

(National Institute of Mental Health, 2023; Takahashi, 2023)

Over the last 2 weeks, how often have you been bothered by any of the following problems? (Use "✔" to indicate your answer)	Not at all	Several days	More than half the days	Nearly every day
1. Little interest or pleasure in doing things	0	1	2	3
2. Feeling down, depressed, or hopeless	0	1	2	3
3. Trouble falling or staying asleep, or sleeping too much	0	1	2	3
4. Feeling tired or having little energy	0	1	2	3
5. Poor appetite or overeating	0	1	2	3
6. Feeling bad about yourself — or that you are a failure or have let yourself or your family down	0	1	2	3
7. Trouble concentrating on things, such as reading the newspaper or watching television	0	1	2	3
8. Moving or speaking so slowly that other people could have noticed? Or the opposite — being so fidgety or restless that you have been moving around a lot more than usual	0	1	2	3
9. Thoughts that you would be better off dead or of hurting yourself in some way	0	1	2	3

FOR OFFICE CODING ___0___ + _____ + _____ + _____

=Total Score: _____

If you checked off any problems, how **difficult** have these problems made it for you to do your work, take care of things at home, or get along with other people?

Not difficult at all ☐	Somewhat difficult ☐	Very difficult ☐	Extremely difficult ☐

*Hallmark signs are bolded and <u>**Red flags are bolded and underlined**</u>.

Interpretation

PHQ-9 Score	Depression Severity	Proposed Treatment Actions
0 – 4	None-minimal	None
5 – 9	Mild	Watchful waiting; repeat PHQ-9 at follow-up
10 – 14	Moderate	Treatment plan, considering counseling, follow-up and/or pharmacotherapy
15 – 19	Moderately Severe	Active treatment with pharmacotherapy and/or psychotherapy

Fig. 6.1 PHQ-9 screening tool with interpretation. This tool provides a way to *screen* persons with symptoms consistent with major depressive disorder (MDD) (recall that the only diagnostic confirmation is via the DSM-5 MDD criteria). The PHQ-9 tool has a sensitivity of 88% and a specificity of 88%, making it an effective screening tool. (Information Adapted From and Image Found American Psychological Association. (2019). Patient Health Questionnaire-9 (PHQ-9). https://www.psychiatry.org/getmedia/a3986be5-94af-42e7-afce-19234c2f4998/APA-DSM5TR-SeverityMeasureForDepressionAdult.pdf.)

Evaluation and Differential Diagnoses

DIAGNOSTICS

There are no diagnostic tests indicated to detect MDD; however, they may be useful if there is a clinical suspicion that the depression is secondary to an underlying medical condition or substance.

- DSM-5 criteria for MDD (American Psychiatric Association, 2022)
  - Five or more of the following symptoms need to have been present during the same 2-week period *along with* either (1) depressed mood or (2) loss of interest or pleasure:
    - Depressed mood most of the day, nearly every day, observable by others
    - Markedly diminished interest or pleasure in all or almost all activities most days or every day, observable by others
    - Significant unintentional weight loss or weight gain (more than 5% of body weight in 1 month) or a decrease or increase in appetite nearly every day
    - Insomnia or hypersomnia
    - Psychomotor changes (agitation or retardation) severe enough to be observable by others
    - Fatigue, low energy, or decreased efficiency in completing routine tasks
    - Feelings of worthlessness or excessive or inappropriate guilt nearly every day
    - Diminished ability to think or concentrate or indecisiveness nearly every day, observable by others
    - Recurrent thoughts of death, suicidal ideation, or suicide attempts
  - The symptoms cause clinically significant distress or impairment in social, occupational, or other important areas of functioning.
  - The symptoms are not attributable to the direct physiologic effects of a substance or to another medical condition.
  - There has never been a manic or hypomanic episode.
  - MDE is not better explained by schizophrenia spectrum or other psychotic disorders.

BOX 6.3 ■ Older Adult Considerations

Treatment of major depressive disorder (MDD) in the older adult can be difficult secondary to co-morbid conditions and the side effects of polypharmacy. Previously medications such as nortriptyline were recommended as first-line therapy for MDD, but best available evidence has changed to promote cognitive behavioral therapy first with concomitant use of selective serotonin reuptake inhibitors (SS-RIs) or serotonin and norepinephrine reuptake inhibitors (SNRIs). Keep in mind that antidepressants also have side effects that are often more prominent in older adults and tend to be dose dependent. The advice of "start low and go slow" with older adults applies to the prescribing of medications for MDD (American Psychological Association, 2019).

DIFFERENTIAL DIAGNOSES

- Organic disease processes: Many disease processes can mimic symptoms of MDD, such as hypothyroidism, mononucleosis, obstructive sleep apnea, systemic lupus erythematosus, vitamin D deficiency, and vitamin B12 deficiency, which must be ruled out.
- Bipolar depression: Bipolar depression is differentiated by the presence of periods of mania (feelings of euphoria or grandiosity) in addition to depression. The manic behavior is often identified by friends or family.
- Substance use disorder: Illicit substance use often precipitates feels of sadness and despair which can cause/exacerbate depressive symptoms. Assessing for substance use is imperative in all patients with suspected MDD.

(National Institute of Mental Health, 2023; Takahashi, 2023)

Plan

GUIDELINE RESOURCES

- American Psychological Association. (2019). Clinical practice guideline for the treatment of depression across three age cohorts. https://www.apa.org/depression-guideline/guide-line.pdf

Pharmacotherapy

Once a diagnosis of MDD is established, a combination of psychotherapy and pharmacologic therapy should start as soon as possible. Pharmacotherapy and psychotherapy alone are reasonable alternatives to combination therapy, but they are less effective.

- Selective serotonin reuptake inhibitors (SSRIs), serotonin and norepinephrine reuptake inhibitors, or norepinephrine and dopamine reuptake inhibitors are all first-line pharmacotherapy for MDD. Choice of medication and dosage should be based on a person-centered plan of care, taking symptoms, age, side effects, safety, cost, and convenience into consideration (see Algorithm 6.1) (Box 6.3).

(American Psychological Association, 2019; Takahashi, 2023)

NONPHARMACOTHERAPY

- Educate
  - Person and their family about the diagnosis of MDD, treatments, possible side effects of treatment (Box 6.4), and importance of adherence to both pharmacologic and nonpharmacologic therapy

> **BOX 6.4 ■ Acute Care Considerations**
>
> Serotonin syndrome is a potentially life-threatening condition associated with increased serotonergic activity in the central nervous system. Selective serotonin reuptake inhibitors (SSRIs) are the most commonly involved agents in the activation of serotonin syndrome. While serotonin syndrome frequently occurs due to a combination of at least two drugs that increase serotonin activity, it can occur from a single drug, particularly in susceptible persons such as older and younger adults. An estimated 15% of SSRI overdoses lead to mild or moderate serotonin toxicity. The classic serotonin syndrome triad involves altered mental status (ranging from anxiety to hyperactive delirium), autonomic abnormalities (tachycardia, hypertension, hyperthermia), and neuromuscular findings (tremor, hyperreflexia, clonus, and bilateral Babinski signs). While symptoms of serotonin syndrome often resolve within 24 hours of discontinuing SSRIs, severe cases require intensive medical care (Garel et al., 2021).

  - Family about danger signs related to self-harm, what to do if identified, and need for close follow-up
- Lifestyle
  - Smoking cessation
  - Regular physical activity (150 minutes/week)
  - Quality nutrition
  - Importance of self-care (including bright light therapy and/or yoga)
- Referral
  - Behavioral therapy, cognitive therapy, cognitive behavioral therapy, mindfulness-based cognitive therapy, interpersonal psychotherapy, psychodynamic therapies, or supportive therapy. If using an antidepressant medication, the use of cognitive behavioral therapy or interpersonal psychotherapy in combination demonstrates higher treatment efficacy.
  - Refer to psychiatry or psych-mental health nurse practitioner if there is significant diagnostic uncertainty, complicating comorbidity (substance use disorder or generalized anxiety disorder), suicidal ideation, poor response to standard treatment, or at any point when the treatment modality exceeds the experience of the clinician. Children should always be referred to a pediatric mental health professional.
- Follow-up
  - Every 1 to 2 weeks during the first month of pharmacotherapy to ascertain effectiveness and side effects (if any), then at least once in the following 4 to 8 weeks until stable and every 3 to 6 months thereafter. Improvement of symptoms can be identified by repeating the PHQ-9 screening tool and comparing to previous results (see Fig. 6.1).
  - Weekly for psychotherapy

(American Psychological Association, 2019)

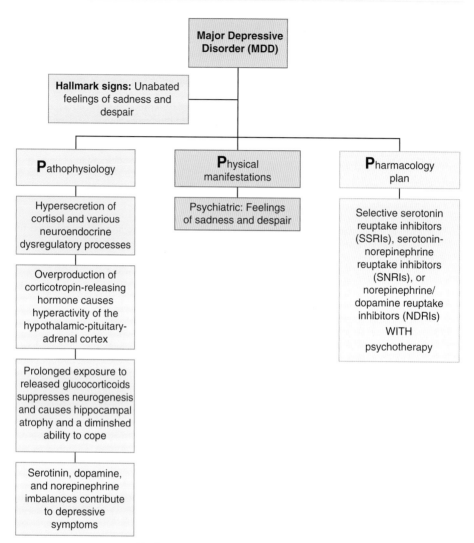

Algorithm 6.1 Major Depressive Disorder (MDD)

References

American Psychiatric Association. (2022). Depressive disorders. In *Diagnostic and statistical manual of mental disorders* (5th ed.). American Psychiatric Publishing. https://doi.org/10.1176/appi.books.9780890425787.

American Psychological Association. (2019). Clinical practice guideline for the treatment of depression across three age cohorts. https://www.apa.org/depression-guideline/guideline.pdf.

Bailey, R. K., Mokonogho, J., & Kumar, A. (2019). Racial and ethnic differences in depression: Current perspectives. *Neuropsychiatric Disease and Treatment, 15*, 603–609. https://doi.org/10.2147/NDT.S128584.

Garel, N., Greenway, K. T., Tabbane, K., & Joober, R. (2021). Serotonin syndrome: SSRIs are not the only culprit. *Journal of Psychiatry and Neuroscience, 46*(3), E369–E370. https://doi.org/10.1503/jpn.210001.

Garzon, D. L., Starr, N. B., & Chauvin, J. (2020). Neurodevelopmental, behavioral, and mental health disorders. In D. L.,Maaks, N.,Starr, M. A., Brady, N. M., Gaylord, M., Driessnack, & K. G., Duderrstadt. (Eds.), *Burns' pediatric primary care* (7th ed., pp. 428–432). Elsevier.

National Institute of Mental Health. (2023). Major depression. https://www.nimh.nih.gov/health/statistics/major-depression#part_2562.

Substance Abuse and Mental Health Services Administration. (2021). National survey of drug use and health. https://www.samhsa.gov/data/release/2021-national-survey-drug-use-and-health-nsduh-releases#annual-national-report.

Takahashi, L. K. (2023). Neurobiology of schizophrenia, mood disorders, anxiety disorders, posttraumatic stress disorder, and obsessive-compulsive disorder. In J. L., Rogers. (Ed.), *McCance and Huether's pathophysiology: The biologic basis for disease in adults and children* (9th ed., pp. 623–630). Mosby-Elsevier.

CHAPTER 7

Posttraumatic Stress Disorder

Jodi Allen ▪ Corrine M. Djuric

Posttraumatic Stress Disorder

Posttraumatic stress disorder (PTSD) is the only mental health disorder for which an event can be linked to an organic response. This response can develop within hours of the traumatic experience, after several months, or even after several years (Takahashi, 2023). Lifetime prevalence of PTSD ranges from 7% to 8% in the general US population (Takahashi, 2023). Higher rates of PTSD have been found in subgroups such as female, White, Native American, younger, previously married, those with less than a high school education, those in a lower socioeconomic bracket, and those living in rural areas (Box 7.1). Lower prevalence rates have been found outside North America (Goldstein et al., 2016). Apart from the groups with higher prevalence, risk factors for the likelihood of developing PTSD include poor social support, physical injury, childhood adversity (Box 7.2), increased duration of trauma, characteristics of the individual, and inciting event, particularly if the event is related to combat, sexual assault, or any event that caused a traumatic brain injury (Cyr et al., 2021; Takahashi, 2023). Family and/or personal history of substance abuse as well as other neuropsychiatric and psychiatric comorbid conditions (e.g., various forms of dementia, anxiety, depression, suicide, substance use disorder) can increase risk for PTSD (Box 7.3) (Goldstein et al., 2016).

Pathophysiology

The primary etiology of PTSD is exposure to a traumatic, terrifying, life-threatening event that induces pathophysiologic alterations in many neural structures and neurotransmitter systems. The amygdala, prefrontal cortex (PFC), and hippocampus play important roles in how fearful memories are stored, retrieved, and extinguished. The amygdala is a major player in processing fearful and threatening stimuli as well as modulating associative emotion or conditioned fear while the PFC plays a central role in cognitive control functions. Dopamine in the PFC influences impulse inhibition, prospective memory, and cognitive flexibility. In other words, the PFC is essential to fear processing, fear acquisition, avoidance behavior, and strategies to regulate fear response. In the presence of trauma-related stimuli, increased activity in the amygdala is identified while the PFC experiences diminished activity (see Algorithm 7.1). Continual dysregulation of fear-based memory can underline chronic PTSD where the PFC fails to control amygdala-induced activation of fear, which further compromises removal of fear memory. PTSD is linked to neurodegeneration caused by cellular aging and cortical thinning in areas of the brain associated with regulation of emotions and threats (Takahashi, 2023).

Physical Clinical Presentation

SUBJECTIVE

The principal feature of PTSD is one or more traumatic events causing painful, intrusive reexperiencing of the event(s) along with avoidance and emotional numbing behaviors. There are four

BOX 7.1 ■ Diversity Considerations

Trauma exposure is common across populations but particularly among lesbian, gay, bisexual, transgender, queer, and questioning (LGBTQ+) persons. LGBTQ+ persons experience higher rates of discrimination and victimization, which often complicates posttraumatic stress disorder (PTSD) treatment. Current best practice interventions for PTSD do not consider the pervasive stress experienced by LGBTQ+ persons and how the ongoing threat to safety they often experience can negatively affect typical PTSD interventions. Effective Skills to Empower Effective Men (aka ESTEEM) is a 10-session treatment that enhances emotion regulation skills, reduces avoidance patterns, and improves motivation and self-efficacy for behavior change. In a pilot trial among 63 gay and bisexual males, improved depression, alcohol use, and sexual risk-taking outcomes were identified. This is a promising endeavor that provides culturally appropriate evidence-based trauma treatment for a portion of LGBTQ+ persons with PTSD (Livingston et al., 2020).

BOX 7.2 ■ Pediatric Considerations

Posttraumatic stress disorder assessment in children is challenging, requiring careful interviewing with both the child and caregiver(s). If the traumatic event involves a caregiver, the nonoffending caregiver or other caretaker should be included in the interview. It is recommended *not* to use leading or prompting questions with children but to ask them directly if their privacy was invaded, how it happened, and how the injuries (if any) occurred. Referral to a pediatric behavioral health specialist is imperative and reporting to social services agencies is crucial for children under the age of 18 who have witnessed or experienced violence. Referencing the National Child Traumatic Stress Network (https://www.nctsn.org) can be helpful for health care providers who may care for children who experience trauma (Garzon et al., 2020).

BOX 7.3 ■ Older Adult Considerations

Evidence suggests that stressors associated with aging can exacerbate posttraumatic stress disorder (PTSD) symptoms in older adults. Functional and role changes that occur with aging, including increased physical issues that decrease independence, decreased social support, retirement, and bereavement, may be associated with increases in PTSD symptoms. Older adults may present for care related to physical symptoms associated with PTSD versus mental health, so careful screening should be undertaken to ensure proper diagnosis of PTSD and/or appropriate treatment for PTSD exacerbations. Evaluating for cognitive changes is necessary as PTSD is an independent risk factor in the development of dementia (Kaiser et al., 2019).

behavioral symptom diagnostic cluster categories (Fig. 7.1): (1) intrusive memories of the trauma (nightmares, flashbacks, sudden intrusive memories of the event); (2) avoidance (avoid any situation or activity that might revive the memory of the traumatic event); (3) negative thought pattern and mood (distorted sense of blame of self or others, isolation, diminished interest in activities); and (4) hyperarousal (on edge, unprovoked anger, aggressive or reckless behavior, sleep disturbance, hypervigilance) (American Psychiatric Association, 2022). During the focused history, documentation should include the onset of symptoms; precipitating events; location, intensity, and quality of pain (if any); progression of symptoms; alleviating and aggravating factors; previous episodes; and associated symptoms. Hyperarousal symptoms and how persons reexperience traumatic events can be different for each individual experiencing PTSD, so careful and supportive history taking is imperative (Marx et al., 2022). Physical manifestations of PTSD can present with headaches, palpitations, abdominal pain, and nausea and vomiting, and an organic cause for these symptoms must be ruled out (see Algorithm 7.1) (Marx et al., 2022). While most persons exhibit symptoms within a few months of the traumatic event, many can experience a delayed onset. Persons experiencing PTSD can self-report as feeling "normal" for an extended period of

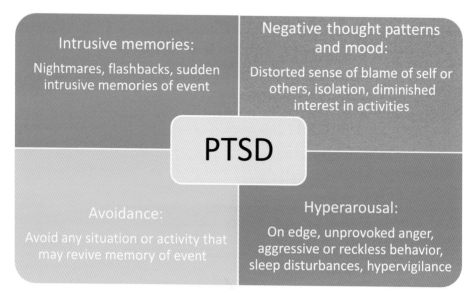

Fig. 7.1 Behavioral symptom diagnostic clusters of posttraumatic stress disorder. *PTSD,* Posttraumatic stress disorder. (Adapted from American Psychiatric Association. (2022). *Diagnostic and statistical manual of mental disorders* (5th ed.). American Psychiatric Publishing. https://doi.org/10.1176/appi.books.978089-425787).

time, but reexperiences of the traumatic event can be accelerated in times of stress (American Psychological Association [APA], 2017). Careful medication review should be done to ensure that the symptoms are not related to medication side effects (APA, 2017). All persons with subjective signs of PTSD should be screened for suicidal ideations (Box 7.4) (APA, 2017).

OBJECTIVE*

- Generalized: Malaise; **avoidance**
- Neurological: <u>**Mental status changes**</u>
- Cardiovascular/peripheral vascular: Palpitations; tachycardia; hypertension
- Gastrointestinal: Abdominal pain; vomiting
- Integumentary: Compulsive excoriations
- Psychiatric: Flat affect; **hyperarousal**; **anxiousness**; **nervousness**; <u>**suicidal ideations**</u>

(APA, 2017; US Department of Veterans Affairs, 2023)

Evaluation and Differential Diagnoses

DIAGNOSTICS

- The Clinician-Administered PTSD Scale for DSM-5, the gold standard in PTSD assessment, is a 30-item questionnaire corresponding to the DSM-5 diagnostic criteria for PTSD. There are three versions corresponding to different time periods: symptoms over the past week, past month (for current PTSD), and/or worst month (for lifetime PTSD). The questionnaire takes 45 to 60 minutes to complete (Marx et al., 2022).

---

*Hallmark signs are bolded and <u>Red flags are bolded and underlined</u>.

> **BOX 7.4 ■ Acute Care Considerations**
>
> A strong relationship exists between posttraumatic stress disorder (PTSD) and suicide. When controlling for comorbid disorders and physical illness, research has identified that persons with PTSD are at higher risk for suicide attempts. Alterations in coping mechanisms, intrusive memories/thoughts, anger, and impulsivity increase the risk of suicide attempts for persons with PTSD. Combat-related guilt in veterans appears to be the most significant predictor of suicide attempts and preoccupation with suicide. Education of family members in proper identification of suicidal ideations should be included in the usual care of persons with PTSD and their family. Health care providers can use the Ask Suicide-Screening Questions tool for persons 8 years of age and older to aid in clinical identification of suicidal ideations. This tool provides next steps to ensure that safety is maintained and acute clinical care can be provided as needed (Hudenko et al., 2022; National Institute of Mental Health, 2020).

- DSM-5 Criteria for PTSD (US Department of Veterans Affairs, 2023): https://www.ptsd.va.gov/professional/treat/essentials/dsm5_ptsd.asp#one.

DIFFERENTIAL DIAGNOSES

- Acute stress disorder (ASD): Symptoms associated with ASD are very similar to PTSD. However, ASD is the diagnosis for the first 30 days following the traumatic event. Persons who remain symptomatic after 30 days should be reevaluated using the DSM-5 criteria for PTSD.
- Substance-induced anxiety: This form of anxiety is related to the effect of medication(s) or toxin(s) exposure.
- General anxiety disorder: This can mimic symptoms of PTSD, but the person will meet DSM-5 criteria for general anxiety disorder.

(American Psychiatric Association, 2022)

Plan

GUIDELINE LINKS

- American Psychological Association. (2017). *Clinical practice guideline for the treatment of PTSD*. https://www.apa.org/ptsd-guideline/ptsd.pdf.

Pharmacotherapy

- Selective serotonin reuptake inhibitors: Specifically, sertraline (Zoloft) and paroxetine (Paxil) are approved by the US Food and Drug Administration for treatment of PTSD. Fluoxetine (Prozac) is considered off-label use for PTSD.
- Serotonin and norepinephrine reuptake inhibitors (SNRIs): Specifically, venlafaxine ER (Effexor) is considered off-label use for PTSD.
- Prazosin: This can be used for PTSD-associated nightmares and to improve quality of sleep.
- Benzodiazepines should be avoided as they are associated with increased risk of PTSD symptoms, aggression, depression, and substance use.

(APA, 2017; Takahashi, 2023)

NONPHARMACOTHERAPY

- Educate
  - Person and their family about the chronic nature of PTSD, treatments, possible side effects of treatment, and importance of adherence to both pharmacologic and nonpharmacologic therapy

- Family about danger signs related to self-harm, what to do if identified, and need for close follow-up (particularly for persons of any age prescribed SNRIs and for persons under the age of 30 prescribed either a selective serotonin reuptake inhibitor or an SNRI)
- Lifestyle
    - Smoking cessation
    - Regular physical activity (150 minutes/week)
    - Quality nutrition
    - Importance of self-care that promotes relaxation (including meditation)
- Referral
    - One of the following: Cognitive behavioral therapy, cognitive processing therapy, cognitive therapy, or prolonged exposure therapy is strongly recommended; brief eclectic psychotherapy, eye movement desensitization and reprocessing therapy, and narrative exposure therapy are additional options
    - Psychiatry or psych-mental health nurse practitioner: If there is significant diagnostic uncertainty, suicidal ideation, failure to respond to initial treatments, or at any point when the treatment modality exceeds the experience of the clinician
- Follow-up
    - Weekly for psychotherapy
    - Every 2 to 3 weeks for pharmacotherapy until stable

(APA, 2017)

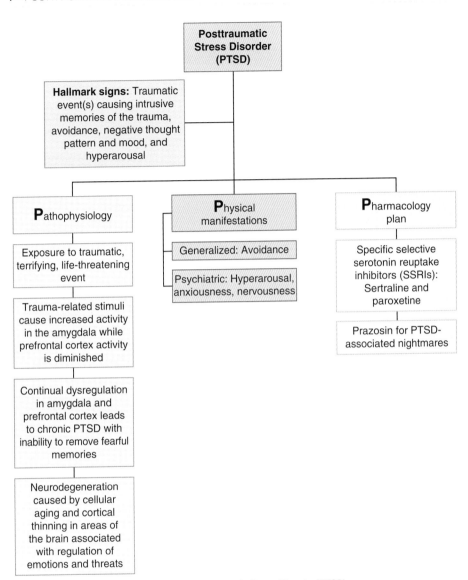

Posttraumatic Stress Disorder (PTSD)

Hallmark signs: Traumatic event(s) causing intrusive memories of the trauma, avoidance, negative thought pattern and mood, and hyperarousal

Pathophysiology

Exposure to traumatic, terrifying, life-threatening event

Trauma-related stimuli cause increased activity in the amygdala while prefrontal cortex activity is diminished

Continual dysregulation in amygdala and prefrontal cortex leads to chronic PTSD with inability to remove fearful memories

Neurodegeneration caused by cellular aging and cortical thinning in areas of the brain associated with regulation of emotions and threats

Physical manifestations

Generalized: Avoidance

Psychiatric: Hyperarousal, anxiousness, nervousness

Pharmacology plan

Specific selective serotonin reuptake inhibitors (SSRIs): Sertraline and paroxetine

Prazosin for PTSD-associated nightmares

Algorithm 7.1   Posttraumatic Stress Disorder (PTSD)

References

American Psychiatric Association. (2022). Trauma-and stressor-related disorders. In *Diagnostic and statistical manual of mental disorders* (5th ed.). American Psychiatric Publishing. https://doi.org/10.1176/appi.books.9780890425787.

American Psychological Association (2017). *Clinical practice guidelines for the treatment of PTSD*. https://www.apa.org/ptsd-guideline/ptsd.pdf.

Cyr, S., Guo, X., Marcil, M. J., Dupont, P., Jobidon, L., Benrimoh, D., Guertin, M. C., & Brouillette, J. (2021). Posttraumatic stress disorder prevalence in medical populations: A systematic review and meta-analysis. *General Hospital Psychiatry, 69*, 81–93. https://doi.org/10.1016/j.genhosppsych.2021.01.010.

Garzon, D. L., Starr, N. B., & Chauvin, J. (2020). Neurodevelopmental, behavioral, and mental health disorders. In D. L. Maaks, N. Starr, M. A. Brady, N. M. Gaylord, M. Driessnack, & K. G. Duderrstadt (Eds.), *Burns' pediatric primary care* (7th ed., pp. 427–428). Elsevier.

Goldstein, R. B., Smith, S. M., Chou, S. P., Saha, T. D., Jung, J., Zhang, H., Pickering, R. P., Ruan, W. J., Huang, B., & Grant, B. F. (2016). The epidemiology of DSM-5 posttraumatic stress disorder in the United States: Results from the National Epidemiologic Survey on Alcohol and Related Conditions-III. *Social Psychiatry and Psychiatric Epidemiology, 51*(8), 1137–1148. https://doi.org/10.1007/s00127-016-1208-5.

Hudenko, W., Homaifar, B., & Wortzel, H. (2022). *The relationship between PTSD and suicide*. US Department of Veterans Affairs. https://www.ptsd.va.gov/professional/treat/cooccurring/suicide_ptsd.asp.

Kaiser, A. P., Cook, J. M., Glick, D. M., & Moye, J. (2019). Posttraumatic stress disorder in older adults: A conceptual review. *Clinical Gerontology, 42*(4), 359–376. https://doi.org/10.1080/07317115.2018.1539801.

Livingston, N. A., Berke, D., Scholl, J., Ruben, M., & Shipherd, J. C. (2020). Addressing diversity in PTSD treatment: Clinical considerations and guidance for the treatment of PTSD in LGBTQ populations. *Current Treatment Options Psychiatry, 7*(2), 53–69. https://doi.org/10.1007/s40501-020-00204-0.

Marx, B. P., Lee, D. J., Norman, S. B., Bovin, M. J., Sloan, D. M., Weathers, F. W., Keane, T. M., & Schnurr, P. P. (2022). Reliable and clinically significant changes in the clinician-administered PTSD scale for DSM-5 and PTSD checklist for DSM-5 among male veterans. *Psychological Assessment, 34*(2), 197–203. https://doi.org/10.1037/pas0001098.

National Institute of Mental Health. (2020). *Ask suicide-screening questions (ASQ) toolkit*. https://www.nimh.nih.gov/sites/default/files/documents/research/research-conducted-at-nimh/asq-toolkit-materials/asq-tool/screening_tool_asq_nimh_toolkit.pdf.

Takahashi, L. K. (2023). Neurobiology of schizophrenia, mood disorders, anxiety disorders, posttraumatic stress disorder, and obsessive-compulsive disorder. In J. L. Rogers (Ed.), *McCance and Huether's pathophysiology: The biologic basis for disease in adults and children* (9th ed., pp. 633–634). Mosby-Elsevier.

US Department of Veterans Affairs (2023). *PTSD and DSM-5*. https://www.ptsd.va.gov/professional/treat/essentials/dsm5_ptsd.asp#one.

Musculoskeletal System

SECTION OUTLINE

8 Arthritis

9 Conditions of the Spine

10 Soft Tissue Disorders

CHAPTER 8

Arthritis

Jodi Allen

Osteoarthritis and Rheumatoid Arthritis

Arthritis

The two most commonly diagnosed forms of arthritis in the United States are osteoarthritis (OA) and rheumatoid arthritis (RA). OA affects approximately 80% of US adults over the age of 65, and globally it is found to be the cause of moderate to severe disability in 43 million people (Smallheer & Reeves, 2023). RA affects 1.3 million US adults (still a significant number) and 1% of the total world population (Xu & Wu, 2021). Each form varies in its pathophysiology, presentation, and pharmacologic management, but both share some characteristics and risk factors. Many of the same joints can be affected by both forms of arthritis; however, the etiology and mechanism of pain differ vastly between the two. Obesity is a major risk factor for both forms of arthritis, as is a family history of OA or RA (Mohammed et al., 2020). Both forms of arthritis create a financial burden on the economy due to loss of work, disability, and high treatment and management costs (Mohammed et al., 2020). The key distinction between OA and RA is found in the cause of the joint pain. OA is caused by mechanical wear and tear to the affected joint(s) while RA is caused by an autoimmune response and thus produces systemic symptoms (Smallheer & Reeves, 2023). Proper identification of the key indicators that differentiate OA from RA is imperative to ensure appropriate treatment and lessen the burden of pain and potential disability (Box 8.1).

Pathophysiology

OSTEOARTHRITIS

The etiology of OA is degeneration with eventual loss and inappropriate repair of articular cartilage. The chondrocytes of the articular cartilage are damaged as a result of biomechanical stress. These changes lead to increased chondrocyte injury, with alteration of chondrocyte signaling and extracellular matrix (Smallheer & Reeves, 2023). The destruction of the extracellular matrix, which provides critical elastic support to disperse pressure and stress with joint movement and is critical for biomechanical properties of cartilage, is progressive and a hallmark of OA (see Algorithm 8.1) (Smallheer & Reeves, 2023). Chondrocytes release matrix metalloproteases that degrade collagen. The affected collagen causes subchondral bone thickening and osteophyte formation, which in turn affects bone, synovium, ligament, muscle, and periarticular fat within the joint(s) (Smallheer & Reeves, 2023). Chronic inflammation contributes to disease progression, joint dysfunction, pain, stiffness, and functional limitation.

OA is classified into two categories: primary (idiopathic) and secondary. Primary OA is most commonly diagnosed when no predisposing trauma or disease is present yet risk factors are identified (Mohammed et al., 2020). Age (45 and older), female gender, obesity, genetics, and previous joint injury are risk factors for primary OA. Secondary OA is identified with preexisting joint abnormalities, including congenital joint disorders, inflammatory arthritis (including RA), avascular necrosis, infectious arthritis, Paget's disease, osteoporosis, osteochondritis dissecans, metabolic disorders, hemoglobinopathy, Ehlers-Danlos syndrome, or Marfan syndrome (Smallheer & Reeves, 2023).

RHEUMATOID ARTHRITIS

The etiology of RA is chronic and autoimmune in nature. CD4 helper T cells are initiated by the immune system and promote inflammation by producing cytokines that stimulate other inflammatory cells and foster tissue injury (Smallheer & Reeves, 2023). The most significant cytokines leading to the destructive nature of RA are interferon-gamma, which activates macrophages and synovial cells; IL-17, which stimulates neutrophils and monocytes; TNF and IL-1, which cause synovial cells to secrete proteases that are damaging to hyaline cartilage; and RANKL, which activates bone resorption and erosion (Smallheer & Reeves, 2023). Further protein structure and function are altered, chemokines attract T cells, and chronic inflammation results (Smallheer & Reeves, 2023). As part of the autoimmune response, normal antibodies become autoantibodies that attack self-antigens, or host tissues. These altered antibodies are known as rheumatoid factors (RFs) and are found in the serum of persons with RA (Smallheer & Reeves, 2023). B lymphocytes produce more RFs and T lymphocytes cause the release of enzymes that perpetuate the inflammatory response. With the release of multiple immunoregulatory cytokines and inflammatory enzymes, osteoclasts are eventually generated, causing bone destruction, the hallmark of RA (see Algorithm 8.2). Self-antigens perpetuate, leading to constant inflammation and formation of immune complexes that spread to articular cartilage, fibrous joint capsules, bone, and surrounding ligaments and tendons, causing pain, joint deformity, and functional loss (Smallheer & Reeves, 2023). The autoimmune nature of RA will produce systemic manifestations in other organs such as the skin, eyes, lungs, and heart.

Female gender, environmental factors (particularly silica and textile dust exposure), genetics/epigenetics, smoking, and periodontal disease are risk factors for developing RA (Xu & Wu, 2021).

Physical Clinical Presentation

SUBJECTIVE

The clinical manifestations of both OA and RA can occur subtly and insidiously, with pain that is often ignored initially. During the focused history, documentation should include the onset of symptoms; precipitating events; location, intensity, and quality of pain; progression of symptoms;

> ### BOX 8.2 ■ Pediatric Considerations
>
> Juvenile idiopathic arthritis (JIA), formerly known as juvenile rheumatoid arthritis, is a persistent arthritis lasting more than 6 weeks in children younger than 16 years of age. The pathophysiology is that of adult-onset rheumatoid arthritis, with the rate of JIA higher in females than in males. Oligoarticular (four or fewer joints involved) is the type diagnosed most often, with the most common presentation being a morning limp due to knee involvement. Systemic JIA presents with common symptoms such as fever (higher than in adults with rheumatoid arthritis) and drowsiness. JIA is a diagnosis of exclusion, and the child should be monitored to identify joint pain that persists for more than 6 weeks. Any child with suspected JIA should be referred to a pediatric rheumatologist (John & Brady, 2020).

---

alleviating and aggravating factors; previous episodes; and associated symptoms. Any musculoskeletal pain should prompt questions about functional decline and/or changes to activities of daily living caused by the pain (Rogers & Allen, 2021). The person's medical history should identify autoimmune disorders and other musculoskeletal disorders, environmental exposures (related to RA), occupational history of overuse of the joint(s), previous trauma and/or surgery to the joint(s), recreational activities and their effect on the joint(s), and family history of OA, RA, autoimmune, or other musculoskeletal disorders (Rogers & Allen, 2021). The classic triad of symptoms in OA includes joint pain that worsens with use and improves with rest, morning joint stiffness (for no more than 30 minutes after waking) or joint stiffness due to inactivity, and motor restriction (Smallheer & Reeves, 2023). Persons with OA report a grating or cracking sound from the affected joint(s), known as crepitus; muscle weakness; and balance issues (Smallheer & Reeves, 2023). The most commonly affected joints in OA are the hands, knees, hips, and spine, but any joint(s) can be affected, especially if weight bearing or used repetitively. OA often affects joints asymmetrically while RA affects joints symmetrically and bilaterally (Smallheer & Reeves, 2023). Persons with RA may complain of systemic symptoms initially, such as fatigue, weakness, lowgrade fever, weight loss, and generalized aches and stiffness (Box 8.2) (Smallheer & Reeves, 2023). The classic joint pain and stiffness noted in RA is felt in the morning, lasting for approximately 1 hour after awakening and subsiding as the day goes on (Smallheer & Reeves, 2023). The most commonly affected joints in RA are the hands, wrists, knees, and ankles.

OBJECTIVE*

It is imperative for the practitioner to examine joints symmetrically, without garments obscuring the exam and while still honoring the privacy of the person. When assessing the affected joint(s), the practitioner should examine the joint(s) above and below the painful joint(s), as well. During range-of-motion (ROM) testing, active range of motion (AROM) is preferred over passive range of motion (Rogers & Allen, 2021).

Generalized: **Fatigue** (RA); **weight loss** (RA); **low-grade fever** (RA)

Neurological: Decreased sensation to upper and/or lower extremities via monofilament and/or vibratory sensation assessment (RA); diminished reflexes (OA)

HEENT: Scleral injections (RA)

Cardiovascular/peripheral vascular: **Cardiac rub** (RA); ecchymosis on upper/lower extremities (RA)

Pulmonary: **Pleural friction rub** (RA); crackles (RA)

Musculoskeletal: Inspection: Little to minimal edema (OA)/minimal to moderate edema (RA) of affected joints; **bony deformities—bony joint enlargement** (OA); **Heberden's nodes**

---

*Hallmark signs are bolded and <u>Red flags are bolded and underlined</u>.

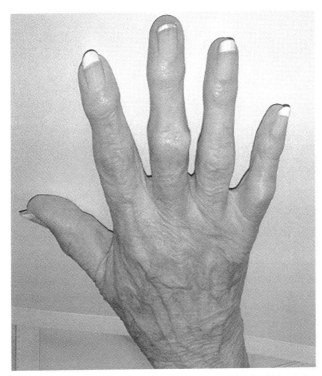

Fig. 8.1 Osteoarthritis (OA) of the hand. Note the Heberden's nodes at the distal interphalangeal joint and the Bouchard's nodes at the proximal interphalangeal joint. Both are prominent osteophytes (or bony outgrowths), which are typical features of OA. (From Stern, A. G., Moxley, G., Rao, T. P., Disler, D. G., McDowell, C. L., Park, M., & Schumacher, H. R. (2004). Utility of digital photographs of the hand for assessing the presence of hand. *Osteoarthritis and Cartilage, 12*(5), 360–365. https://doi.org/10.1016/j.joca.2004.01.003.)

in the distal interphalangeal **(DIP) joints** and Bouchard's nodes in the proximal interphalangeal **(PIP) joints** (OA; Fig. 8.1)/**boutonniere deformity** and/or **swan neck deformity** in affected joints (RA; Fig. 8.2); **rheumatoid nodules** over extensor surfaces of elbows and fingers (RA); gait abnormality such as a limp (OA). Palpation: **Tenderness to affected joint(s)** (OA/RA); **crepitus** (OA). ROM: **Limited and painful AROM** (OA)/**decreased and painful AROM** or **immobility** (RA) of affected joint(s) (see Algorithms 8.1 and 8.2).

Integumentary: Erythema and warmth to affected joint(s) (RA)
(Smallheer & Reeves, 2023)

Evaluation and Differential Diagnoses

DIAGNOSTICS

Osteoarthritis

- Diagnosis based on history and physical exam
- Plain radiograph(s) of affected joint(s) to confirm OA/rule out other diagnoses
- No laboratory testing required to diagnose OA, but to rule out conditions such as RA

(Smallheer & Reeves, 2023)

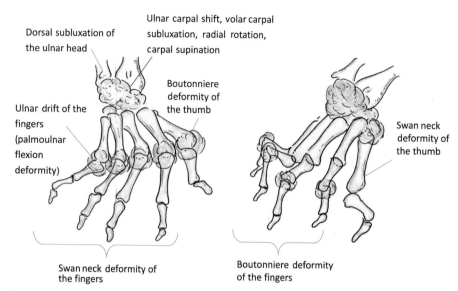

Fig. 8.2 Rheumatoid arthritis (RA) of the hand. Swan neck and boutonniere deformities are classic assessment findings in RA. (From Ishikawa, H. (2017). The latest treatment strategy for the rheumatoid hand deformity. *Journal of Orthopaedic Science, 22*(4), 583–592. https://doi.org/10.1016/j.jos.2017.02.007.)

Rheumatoid Arthritis

- Laboratory testing
  - RF: Alone, *not* diagnostic
  - Anticyclic citrullinated peptide antibody: More specific for RA
  - Complete blood count: Can diagnose anemia found commonly with RA
  - Erythrocyte sedimentation rate: Elevated in active RA; nonspecific indicator
  - C-reactive protein: Elevated in active RA; nonspecific indicator
- Radiography
  - Plain X-rays of affected joints are not reflective of RA in the early stages but can identify bone erosions after 1 to 2 years of symptoms, particularly in the hands and feet.
  - Magnetic resonance imaging can identify bone erosions in early disease, but cost versus benefit must be evaluated.

(Taylor, 2020)

DIFFERENTIAL DIAGNOSES

Differentiating between OA and RA is important, as each is a differential diagnosis for the other. Other OA differentials include gout, septic arthritis, and bursitis. Other RA differentials include systemic lupus erythematosus, Sjogren's syndrome, and chronic Lyme disease.

Plan

GUIDELINE RESOURCES

- Fraenkel, L., Bathon, J. M., England, B. R., St. Clair, E. W., Arayssi, T., Carandang, K., Deane, K. D., Genovese, M., Huston, K. K., Kerr, G., Kremer, J., Nakamura, M. C., Russell, L. A., Singh, J. A., Smith, B. J., Sparks, J. A., Venkatachalam, S., Weinblatt, M. E.,

BOX 8.3 ■ Older Adult Considerations

Rheumatoid arthritis (RA) treatment in older adults has particular challenges related to medication side effects, comorbid conditions, and the increased risk for extraarticular manifestations. Suppressing the immune system with methotrexate or disease-modifying antirheumatic drugs increases the risk of secondary infection in the already diminished immune system of the older adult. Comorbid conditions can increase the risk of complications of RA, particularly cardiovascular disease. Cardiovascular mortality is high in older adults with RA, thus making reduction of disease activity related to RA imperative to a decrease in cardiovascular events. Treatment should be tailored to negate the increased risk for complications but should also target the risk reduction of disease complication(s) (Day & Singh, 2019).

Al-Gibbawi, M., … Akl, E. A. (2021). 2021 American College of Rheumatology guideline for the treatment of rheumatoid arthritis. *Arthritis Care & Research*, *73*(7), 924–939. https://doi.org/10.1002/acr.24596

- Kolasinski, S. L., Neogi, T., Hochberg, M. C., Oatis, C., Guyatt, G., Block, J., Callahan, L., Copenhaver, C., Dodge, C., Felson, D., Gellar, K., Harvey, W. F., Hawker, G., Herzig, E., Kwoh, C. K., Nelson, A. E., Samuels, J., Scanzello, C., White, D., … Reston, J. (2020). 2019 American College of Rheumatology/Arthritis Foundation guideline for the management of osteoarthritis of the hand, hip, and knee. *Arthritis Care & Research*, *72*(2), 149–162. https://doi.org/10.1002/acr.24131

Pharmacotherapy

Osteoarthritis

Treatment choices are listed in order of strength of recommendation. Consider contraindications and maximum dosages of each medication (see Algorithm 8.1).

- Topical nonsteroidal antiinflammatory drugs (not recommended for OA of hands)
- Oral nonsteroidal antiinflammatory drugs
- Acetaminophen
- Intraarticular glucocorticoid injections

(Kolasinski et al., 2020)

Rheumatoid Arthritis

Early and aggressive treatment minimizes systemic impact. Treatment choice is based on disease severity. Rheumatology will confirm diagnosis and determine treatment (see Algorithm 8.2).

- Methotrexate
- Disease-modifying antirheumatic drugs (DMARDs) (Box 8.3)

(Fraenkel et al., 2021)

NONPHARMACOTHERAPY

Osteoarthritis

- Educate
  - Goals of therapy: Lessen pain, minimize functional loss, and preserve quality of life.
  - Adverse side effects of medication/drug interactions
  - Weight loss or weight maintenance: Prevent greater joint stress caused by increased weight.

BOX 8.4 ■ Acute Care Considerations

Up to 9% of patients presenting to the emergency department do so with symptoms related to rheumatic diseases such as rheumatoid arthritis (RA). Multiorgan system manifestations account for the need to seek acute care services. Complications associated with RA, infections caused by immunosuppressive therapy, exacerbation or new onset of a comorbid condition, and adverse drug reactions related to medication use are the most common precipitators of acute care services. Primary care providers can prevent the bulk of acute care services in persons with RA by educating them about the complications that require acute care, developing a "sick" plan in the event of infection, closely monitoring comorbid conditions in conjunction with specialty providers, and monitoring medications used for RA and other conditions (Rose, 2022; Smallheer & Reeves, 2023).

- Lifestyle
  - Exercise to improve muscle tone, ROM, and balance.
  - Modify diet to include foods high in omega-3 fatty acids, vitamin D, and vitamin K. Decrease foods that increase inflammation, such as foods with simple sugars and those that are highly processed.
- Referral
  - Physical Therapy and/or Occupational Therapy
  - Orthopedist as needed
- Follow-up
  - At 3-to-6-month intervals, or sooner if pain increases or functional ability declines

(Kolasinski et al., 2020; Smallheer & Reeves, 2023)

Rheumatoid Arthritis

- Educate
  - Goals of therapy: Pain and inflammation reduction, preservation of function and quality of life, and identification of complications (Box 8.4)
  - Medication side effects: Immunosuppression
  - Do not receive live vaccinations when taking DMARDs.
  - Vaccinations should be up to date prior to starting methotrexate or DMARDs.
  - Joint protection with use of assistive devices and/or splints as needed
  - Weight loss or weight maintenance: Prevent joint stress caused by increased weight.
- Lifestyle
  - Therapeutic exercise programs
  - Hot application (chronic phase)/cold application (acute phase)
  - Adequate rest
- Referral
  - Rheumatology
  - Occupational Therapy and/or Physical Therapy
- Follow-up
  - Routine laboratory studies done every 90 days after beginning medication (complete blood count, comprehensive metabolic panel (CMP), C-reactive protein)

(Fraenkel et al., 2021; Smallheer & Reeves, 2023)

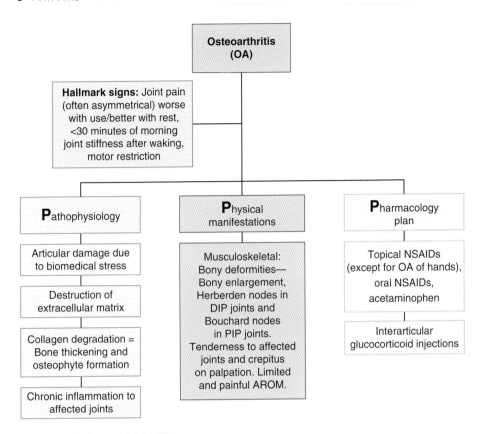

Algorithm 8.1   Osteoarthritis

Osteoarthritis (OA)

Hallmark signs: Joint pain (often asymmetrical) worse with use/better with rest, <30 minutes of morning joint stiffness after waking, motor restriction

Pathophysiology
- Articular damage due to biomedical stress
- Destruction of extracellular matrix
- Collagen degradation = Bone thickening and osteophyte formation
- Chronic inflammation to affected joints

Physical manifestations
- Musculoskeletal: Bony deformities— Bony enlargement, Herberden nodes in DIP joints and Bouchard nodes in PIP joints. Tenderness to affected joints and crepitus on palpation. Limited and painful AROM.

Pharmacology plan
- Topical NSAIDs (except for OA of hands), oral NSAIDs, acetaminophen
- Interarticular glucocorticoid injections

Distal Interphalangeal Joint = DIP
Proximal Interphalangeal Joint = PIP
Active Range of Motion = AROM
Nonsteroidal antiinflammatory = NSAID

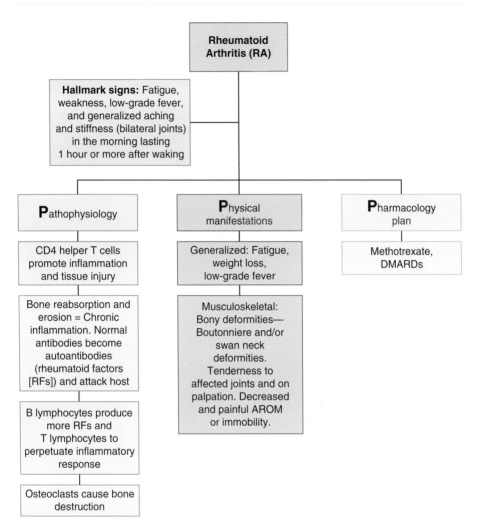

Algorithm 8.2   Rheumatoid Arthritis

References

Day, A. L., & Singh, J. A. (2019). Cardiovascular disease risk in older adults and elderly patients with rheumatoid arthritis: What role can disease-modifying antirheumatic drugs play in cardiovascular risk reduction? *Drugs & Aging, 36*(6), 493–510. https://doi.org/10.1007/s40266-019-00653-0.

Faison, W. E., Harrell, P. G., & Semel, D. (2021). Disparities across diverse populations in the health and treatment of patients with osteoarthritis. *Healthcare, 9*(11), 1421. https://doi.org/10.3390/healthcare9111421.

Fraenkel, L., Bathon, J. M., England, B. R., St. Clair, E. W., Arayssi, T., Carandang, K., Deane, K. D., Genovese, M., Huston, K. K., Kerr, G., Kremer, J., Nakamura, M. C., Russel, L. A., Singh, J. A., Smith, B. J., Sparks, J. A., Venkatachalam, S., Weinblatt, M. E., Al-Gibbawi, M., ... Aki, E. A. (2021). 2021 American College of Rheumatology guideline for the treatment of rheumatoid arthritis. *Arthritis Care & Research, 73*(7), 924–939. https://doi.org/10.1002/acr.24596.

John, R. M., & Brady, M. A. (2020). Atopic, rheumatic, and immunodeficiency disorders. In D. L. Maaks, N. Starr, M. A. Brady, N. M. Gaylord, M. Driessnack, & K. G. Duderrstadt (Eds.), *Burns' pediatric primary care* (7th ed., pp. 549–551). Elsevier.

Kolasinski, S. L., Neogi, T., Hochberg, M. C., Oatis, C., Guyatt, G., Block, J., Callahan, L., Copenhaver, C., Dodge, C., Felson, D., Gellar, K., Harvey, W. F., Hawker, G., Herzig, E., Kwoh, C. K., Nelson, A. E., Samuels, J., Scanzello, C., White, D., ... Reston, J. (2020). 2019 American College of Rheumatology/ Arthritis Foundation guideline for the management of osteoarthritis of the hand, hip, and knee. *Arthritis & Rheumatology, 72*(2), 220–233. https://doi.org/10.1002/art.41142.

Mohammed, A., Alshamarri, T., Adeyeye, T., Lazariu, V., McNutt, L. A., & Carpenter, D. O. (2020). A comparison of risk factors for osteo- and rheumatoid arthritis using NHANES data. *Preventative Medicine Reports, 20*, 101242. https://doi.org/10.1016/j.pmedr.2020.101242.

Rogers, J., & Allen, J. (2021). Understanding the most commonly billed diagnoses in primary care: Generalized musculoskeletal pain. *Nurse Practitioner, 46*(3), 38–45. http://doi.org/10.1097/01. NPR.0000733692.68427.26.

Rose, J. (2022). Autoimmune connective tissue diseases: Systemic lupus erythematosus and rheumatoid arthritis. *Emergency Medicine Clinics, 40*(1), 179–191. https://doi.org/10.1016/j.emc.2021.09.003.

Smallheer, B. A., & Reeves, G. C. (2023). Alterations of musculoskeletal function. In J. L. Rogers (Ed.), *McCance and Huether's pathophysiology: The biologic basis for disease in adults and children* (9th ed., pp. 1452–1459). Mosby-Elsevier.

Taylor, P. C. (2020). Update on the diagnosis and management of early rheumatoid arthritis. *Clinical Medicine, 20*(6), 561–564. https://doi.org/10.7861/clinmed2020-0727.

Xu, Y., & Wu, Q. (2021). Prevalence trend and disparities in rheumatoid arthritis among U.S. adults, 2005–2018. *Journal of Clinical Medicine, 10*(15), 3289. https://doi.org/10.3390/jcm10153289.

CHAPTER 9

Conditions of the Spine

Jodi Allen

Cervical and Lumbar

Conditions of the Spine

Cervical pain is typically reported to last 2 weeks or longer, common in both males and females, and a common complaint in outpatient care (Kazeminasab et al., 2022). It is estimated that 90% of all neck injuries are related to rear-end automobile accidents (Li et al., 2019). The most common cervical conditions are cervical sprain or strain (often termed whiplash) and cervical spondylosis, a general term for the chronic degeneration of the cervical vertebrae (Li et al., 2019). Occupational factors can increase the risk of cervical pain and/or sprain/strain while age is a risk factor for cervical spondylosis secondary to its degenerative nature (Li et al., 2019). Low back pain (LBP) is one of the most common reasons for persons to seek outpatient care, though 90% of persons experiencing LBP will spontaneously recover within 1 month (Institute for Health Metrics and Evaluation, 2023; Rogers & Allen, 2021). LBP is the foremost global cause of years lived with disability (Powers & Hubner, 2023). The burdens of disability are vast and impact nearly all aspects of life for persons with chronic LBP (Box 9.1). The most common causes of LBP are sprain/strain, herniated lumbar disk(s), lumbar spinal stenosis, and vertebral fracture (Powers & Hubner, 2023). Occupational factors such as those requiring repetitive lifting and exposure to vibrations by industrial machinery are risk factors for development of LBP along with obesity, osteoporosis (Box 9.2), and smoking (Powers & Hubner, 2023).

Pathophysiology

Postural control of the neck and its overall function rely on proper motor and sensory function. Structures such as muscle spindles, articular receptors, muscles, efferent motor pathways, connective tissue, and bony articulations are involved in proper sensory and motor function and work symbiotically to support the head and provide full functionality. As the supporting structures of the neck are mostly unprotected, muscles and ligaments can be easily injured (see Algorithm 9.1). Cervical musculature damage can interrupt communication between muscles and spindles of the neck and the somatosensory cortex in the brain, causing a decrease in neck muscle strength, range of motion (ROM), and overall function. Sensory impairment is manifested by scapular and upper extremity radicular symptoms, and muscle weakness is suggestive of motor branch injury (Powers & Hubner, 2023; Rogers & Allen, 2021).

The lumbosacral spine's ability to support the body is dependent on proper motor function. Upright posture is achieved through a balance between the intervertebral disks' ability to expand, the stretch placed on facet joint ligaments, and involuntary tone generated by surrounding lumbosacral and abdominal muscles. A typical amount of stress is inflicted on these structures while a person is sitting and standing, but to a greater degree when they are lifting a heavy object. When

BOX 9.1 ■ Diversity Considerations

Social determinants of health (SDOH) affect the care of low back pain (LBP). Lack of access to appropriate care providers, a person's education level, and their socioeconomic status are associated with poorer outcomes related to LBP. A lower education level has been linked to a recurrence of LBP and disability while persons considered to be in a lower socioeconomic status experience less pain control when seeking care for LBP. Public and population health initiatives can greatly impact the effects of SDOH on persons with LBP and can provide education for health care providers on the impact of SDOH on persons they care for with LBP (Karran et al., 2020).

BOX 9.2 ■ Older Adult Considerations

Osteoporosis is a common diagnosis in older adults and an underlying risk factor for cervical and lumbar pain, lumbar spinal stenosis, and vertebral fractures. Osteoporosis can occur in all persons, but those at highest risk are postmenopausal females due to a rapid decline of bone mineral density after menopause. Other risk factors for osteoporosis include low body weight, family history of the disease, estrogen deficiency, poor calcium and vitamin D intake, lack of weight bearing activities, excess alcohol use, smoking/exposure to tobacco smoke, history of corticosteroid use, and eating disorders. Screening for osteoporosis via a dual-energy X-ray (DEXA) scan for those at risk is imperative to prevent vertebral fractures and other bone fractures (such as hip fractures) that increase morbidity and mortality (Jett, 2020).

a force is placed on the spine that exceeds its stress capacity, damage to the lumbosacral spinal structures can occur (see Algorithm 9.2). Chronicity of pain and disability are highly individualized in complaints related to both cervical and lumbar spines (Powers & Hubner, 2023; Rogers & Allen, 2021).

Physical Clinical Presentation

SUBJECTIVE

Pain, which can vary from dull to sharp, will be the primary presenting symptom for both cervical and lumbar conditions, so it is imperative that a thorough history of present illness is obtained for an accurate diagnosis (Rogers & Allen, 2021). During the focused history, documentation should include the onset of symptoms; precipitating events; location, intensity, and quality of pain; progression of symptoms; alleviating and aggravating factors; previous episodes; and associated symptoms. Any musculoskeletal pain should prompt questions about functional decline and/or changes to activities of daily living caused by pain and/or injury (Rogers & Allen, 2021). Identify past medical history and family history related to the cervical and lumbar spines as well as social, occupational, and recreational activities that may contribute to or precipitate pain or injury (Rogers & Allen, 2021). Prompt identification of any musculoskeletal red flag signs and symptoms is imperative to prevent permanent disability (Tables 9.1 and 9.2). Back pain in children is always a concern (Box 9.3).

Cervical stiffness, especially reported with activity along with upper extremity paresthesias, can help to differentiate between cervical sprain/strain and cervical spondylosis. A report of unilateral radiculopathy (pain, tingling, numbness, and/or weakness) can help to differentiate between lumbar sprain/strain and a herniated lumbar disk along with reports of the inability to find a comfortable position that alleviates pain. Lumbar spinal stenosis can be differentiated with reports of pain and weakness in legs exacerbated by walking or prolonged standing as well as reporting relief when stooping over something such as a cart at the grocery store. A person will frequently

TABLE 9.1 ■ Red Flags in the Assessment of Neck Pain

- History of trauma/injury prior to onset of pain
- Associated neck stiffness with fever
- Unrelenting and/or worsening pain in persons who have tried and failed conservative treatment
- Acute, severe pain, with or without radicular symptoms, upon waking
- Pain relieved by elevating the arm above the head on the side where pain is present
- Severe pain, with or without radicular symptoms, upon flexion or extension of the neck
- Chronic neck pain with weakness of upper or lower extremities, stumbling, muscle atrophy, and/or bowel or bladder incontinence
- Pain with a personal history of malignancy

(Rogers & Allen, 2021)

TABLE 9.2 ■ Red Flags in the Assessment of Low Back Pain

- Pain associated with neurologic deficits (weakness, altered sensation, and/or bowel/bladder changes)
- Pain associated with fever and/or stiff neck
- Pain associated with unexplained weight loss with or without previous personal history of malignancy
- Pain that is worse with rest
- Pain with radiation to the abdomen or stomach area
- Pain related to a personal history of urinary tract infections, drug use, or other infections (including HIV)
- Increased pain with coughing, sneezing, or straining

(Rogers & Allen, 2021)

BOX 9.3 ■ Pediatric Considerations

Children, unlike adolescents, rarely have a complaint of low back pain that does not resolve after a brief time; therefore this complaint in a child should be evaluated swiftly. Back pain that justifies immediate attention includes a complaint of back pain in children younger than 4 years of age, persistent symptoms, presence of systemic symptoms, when a child limits their own physical activity secondary to back pain, progressive discomfort, persistent nighttime pain, neurologic symptoms, a history of cancer or tuberculosis, and back pain with unexplained weight loss. A thorough history and examination should be done to rule out pathologic conditions of the spine (Claytor, 2020).

report an injury of the spine or a fall and can specifically locate (or pinpoint) the pain in the case of a vertebral fracture (which is commonly found in the thoracic and lumbar regions of the spine) (North America Spine Society, 2010, 2020; Rogers & Allen, 2021).

OBJECTIVE*

It is imperative for the practitioner to examine the cervical and lumbar spines, without garments obscuring the exam and while still honoring the privacy of the person. During ROM testing, active

---

*Hallmark signs are bolded. Red flags are identified in Tables 9.1 and 9.2.

range of motion is preferred over passive range of motion (Rogers & Allen, 2021). Due to the motor and sensory components of both the cervical and lumbar spines, full neurologic and musculoskeletal exams should be done, looking for any weakness or neurologic deficits (Rogers & Allen, 2021).

Generalized: Fatigue

Neurological: Diminished reflexes (herniated lumbar disk/lumbar spinal stenosis); **diminished proprioception** (lumbar spinal stenosis) via assessment of position sense of lower extremities

Cardiovascular/peripheral vascular: Tachycardia (general cervical/lumbar pain)

Pulmonary: Tachypnea (general cervical/lumbar pain); bradypnea (pain due to vertebral fracture)

Musculoskeletal: <u>Inspection</u>: Lumbar scoliosis (herniated lumbar disk, lumbar spinal stenosis). <u>Palpation</u>: **Tenderness** (cervical/lumbar sprain/strain, herniated lumbar disk, vertebral fracture); **muscle spasm** (cervical or lumbar strain). <u>ROM</u>: **Decreased cervical ROM** (cervical sprain/strain); **cervical pain with resistance** (cervical sprain/strain); **weakness in shoulder abduction or general weakness in biceps or triceps** (cervical spondylosis); **decreased lumbar flexion** (lumbar sprain/strain); gait abnormality (lumbar sprain/strain, herniated lumbar disk, lumbar spinal stenosis, vertebral fracture). <u>Advanced techniques</u>: **Straight leg raise negative** (lumbar sprain/strain); **straight leg raise positive** (herniated lumbar disk) (see Algorithms 9.1 and 9.2)

Integumentary: Ecchymosis and swelling (cervical sprain/strain related to motor vehicle accident, vertebral fracture)

Psychiatric: Depression and anxiety (related to cervical/lumbar pain and fear of disability) (North American Spine Society, 2020; Rogers & Allen, 2021)

Evaluation and Differential Diagnoses

DIAGNOSTICS

Conditions of the Spine (Cervical/Lumbar)

In general, plain X-ray is the first radiographic choice (as needed), with magnetic resonance imaging (MRI) as a secondary option (as needed, unless signs of neurologic deficits are present upon examination) (American College of Radiology, 2023). Risk (radiation exposure and cost) versus benefit should be considered.

Cervical Spine

- Any evidence of neurologic deficit on examination → MRI
- Whiplash injury → Plain X-ray in all cases (anterior-posterior and lateral views)
- Laboratory testing is warranted only if systemic symptoms are present.
(American College of Radiology, 2023; North America Spine Society, 2010)

Lumbar Spine

- Any evidence of neurologic deficit on examination → MRI
- Routine imaging is not indicated in the diagnosis of persons with nonspecific LBP.
- Chronic LBP (continues for 12 weeks or more) → Plain X-ray with MRI as needed
- Vertebral fracture is suspected → Plain X-ray (anterior-posterior/lateral view) with computed tomography or MRI as needed. Consider osteoporosis as an underlying factor precipitating vertebral fracture and confirm with DEXA bone scan.
- Laboratory testing is warranted only if systemic symptoms are present.
(American College of Radiology, 2023; North American Spine Society, 2020)

DIFFERENTIAL DIAGNOSES

Differentiating between emergent and nonemergent conditions related to the cervical and lumbar spines is imperative to minimize disability (see Tables 9.1 and 9.2). Cervical spine differentials include sprain/strain, spondylosis, and other degenerative disease (e.g., spondylolisthesis, stenosis). Lumbar spine differentials include sprain/strain, degenerative joint disease (including lumbar spinal stenosis), herniated lumbar disk, and vertebral fracture.

Plan

GUIDELINE RESOURCES

- North American Spine Society. (2010). *North American Spine Society clinical guidelines: Diagnosis and treatment of cervical radiculopathy from degenerative disorders.* https://www. spine.org/Portals/0/assets/downloads/ResearchClinicalCare/Guidelines/CervicalRadiculopathy.pdf.
- North American Spine Society. (2020). *Evidence-based clinical guidelines for multidisciplinary spine care: Diagnosis and treatment of low back pain.* https://www.spine.org/Portals/0/assets/downloads/ResearchClinicalCare/Guidelines/LowBackPain.pdf.

Pharmacotherapy

- Nonsteroidal antiinflammatory drugs for no more than 10 days; can be in oral or topical form (cervical or lumbar sprain/strain, herniated lumbar disk, lumbar spinal stenosis). Consider contraindications and maximum dosages prior to prescribing (see Algorithms 9.1 and 9.2).
- Muscle relaxants if muscle spasm(s) is present upon examination (cervical or lumbar strain). Consider side effects of drowsiness and dizziness.
- Oral steroids (cervical spondylosis)
- Calcitonin nasal spray (if vertebral fracture is diagnosed within 5 days of injury and osteoporosis is underlying)
- Opioid analgesics short term (vertebral fracture, herniated lumbar disk). Consider abuse potential.
(North American Spine Society, 2010; North America Spine Society, 2020; Rogers & Allen, 2021)

NONPHARMACOTHERAPY

- Educate
  - If bowel or bladder dysfunction (saddle paresthesia) or fever arises, go to emergency department immediately (Box 9.4).
  - Importance of reporting any new or worsening symptoms immediately (specifically neurologic deficits)
  - Safe medication usage, including side effects and/or abuse potential
  - Typical success of conservative treatment on cervical and lumbar conditions
  - Reassure the person with LBP that most acute episodes are self-limited and resolve within 1 to 6 weeks
  - Activity as tolerated, avoiding full rest
  - Heat application (lumbar sprain/strain, herniated lumbar disk, lumbar spinal stenosis)
  - Avoid bending, stooping, twisting, or lifting objects over 10 pounds (4.5 kg) while recovering (vertebral fracture)
- Lifestyle
  - Physical activity such as walking or biking for 30 minutes daily improves LBP after acute phase resolves
  - Maintain healthy weight to limit additional stress to the lumbar spine
  - Stress reduction via meditation, yoga, or relaxation
  - Good posture and body mechanics at all times
  - Smoking cessation

BOX 9.4 ■ Acute Care Considerations

Cauda equina syndrome (CES) is a rare occurrence related to herniated lumbar disk(s) compressing the roots of the lower spinal canal (or cauda equina) and is a medical emergency. Persons will present with low back pain and bilateral lower extremity weakness and anesthesia or paresthesia of the perineum and buttocks (also known as saddle anesthesia/paresthesia and a hallmark sign of the syndrome). There may or may not be alteration in bowel and bladder function, but any person complaining of low back pain should be asked about their current bowel and bladder function. The person with CES may have a stumbling gait, have hip extensor weakness, and/or be unable to walk on both heels or toes, and bilateral foot drop may be observed. A full neurologic exam and musculoskeletal exam of the back and lower extremities should be performed along with assessment of sphincter tone via rectal exam. If identification of CES and subsequent decompression surgery is delayed, catastrophic consequences such as full loss of bladder, bowel, and sexual function can occur. Immediate referral to the emergency department is required for CES (Lavy et al., 2022).

■ Referral
- ■ Physical therapy, chiropractic care, and/or exercise specialists should be initiated early in the care of cervical and lumbar conditions
- ■ Orthopedist, pain management
- ■ Mental health provider for chronic cervical and lumbar conditions

■ Follow-up
- ■ As needed, unless pain does not resolve or new symptoms arise (cervical/lumbar sprain/strain)
- ■ If no symptom improvement after 6 weeks (cervical spondylosis)
- ■ 7 to 10 days after diagnosis of herniated lumbar disk, then every 2 weeks until previous functionality returns
- ■ 1 week after diagnosis of vertebral fracture

(North America Spine Society, 2010, 2020; Rogers & Allen, 2021)

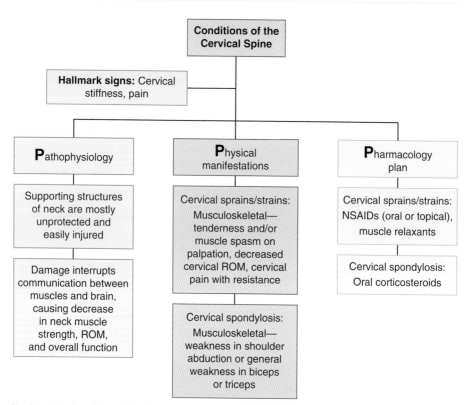

Algorithm 9.1   Conditions of the Cervical Spine. *NSAIDs*, Nonsteroidal antiinflammatory drugs; *ROM*, Range of motion.

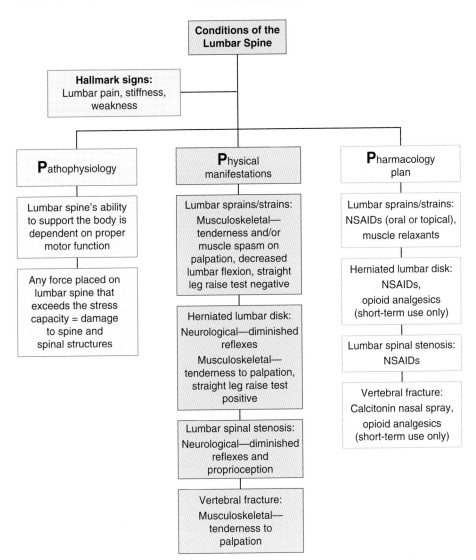

Algorithm 9.2 Conditions of the Lumbar Spine. *NSAIDs*, Nonsteroidal antiinflammatory drugs.

References

American College of Radiology. (2023). *Appropriateness criteria: Diagnostic imaging topics.* https://acsearch. acr.org/list?_

Claytor, C. M. (2020). Musculoskeletal disorders. In D. L. Maaks, N. Starr, M. A. Brady, N. M. Gaylord, M. Driessnack, & K. G. Duderrstadt (Eds.), *Burns' pediatric primary care* (7th ed., pp. 897). Elsevier.

Institute for Health Metrics and Evaluation. (2023). *The Lancet: New study shows low back pain is the leading cause of disability around the world.* https://www.healthdata.org/news-release/lancet-new-study-shows-low-back-pain-leading-cause-disability-around-world#:~:text=In%202020%20globally%2C%20 low%20back,main%20driver%20of%20YLDs%20globally.

Jett, K. (2020). Common musculoskeletal conditions. In T. A. Touhy, & K. Jett (Eds.), *Ebersole & Hess' toward healthy aging: Human needs & nursing response* (10th ed., pp. 322–323). Elsevier.

Karran, E. L., Grant, A. R., & Moseley, G. L. (2020). Low back pain and the social determinants of health: A systematic review and narrative synthesis. *Pain, 161*(11), 2476–2493. https://doi.org/10.1097/j.pain.0000000000001944.

Kazeminasab, S., Nejadghaderi, S. A., Amiri, P., Pourfathi, H., Araj-Khodaei, M., Sullman, M. J. M., Kolahi, A., & Safiri, A. (2022). Neck pain: Global epidemiology, trends and risk factors. *BMC Musculoskeletal Disorders, 23*(1), 26. https://doi.org/10.1186/s12891-021-04957-4.

Lavy, C., Marks, P., Dangas, K., & Todd, N. (2022). Cauda equina syndrome—A practical guide to definition and classification. *International Orthopaedics, 46*(2), 165–169. https://doi.org/10.1007/s00264-021-05273-1.

Li, F., Liu, N., Li, H., Zhang, B., Tian, S., Tan, M., & Sandoz, B. (2019). A review of neck injury and protection in vehicle accidents. *Transportation Safety and Environment, 1*(2), 89–105. https://doi.org/10.1093/tse/tdz012.

North American Spine Society. (2010). Evidence-based clinical guidelines for multidisciplinary spine care: Diagnosis and treatment of cervical radiculopathy from degenerative disorders. https://www.spine.org/Portals/0/assets/downloads/ResearchClinicalCare/Guidelines/CervicalRadiculopathy.pdf.

North American Spine Society. (2020). Evidence-based clinical guidelines for multidisciplinary spine care: Diagnosis and treatment of low back pain. https://www.spine.org/Portals/0/assets/downloads/Research-ClinicalCare/Guidelines/LowBackPain.pdf.

Powers, J., & Hubner, K. E. (2023). Alterations of the brain, spinal cord, and peripheral nerves. In J. L. Rogers, (Ed.), *McCance and Huether's pathophysiology: The biologic basis for disease in adults and children* (9th ed., pp. 584–588). Mosby-Elsevier.

Rogers, J., & Allen, J. (2021). Understanding the most commonly billed diagnoses in primary care: Generalized musculoskeletal pain. *Nurse Practitioner, 46*(3), 38–45. http://doi.org/10.1097/01.NPR.0000733692.68427.26.

CHAPTER 10

Soft Tissue Disorders

Jodi Allen

Sprains and Strains

Sprains/Strains

Sprains and strains of supportive musculoskeletal tissues, specifically ligaments and tendons, are two of the most common types of injuries that present with musculoskeletal pain (Rogers & Allen, 2021). Both injuries are due to inappropriate stretching, or often tearing, with a sprain occurring to muscles or tendons versus a strain occurring to ligaments (Smallheer & Reeves, 2023). Acute injuries, from either direct or indirect trauma, are frequently the cause of sprains and strains, with physical activity increasing the risk of either occurring (Box 10.1). Structures that facilitate movement are the most common sites for sprain and strain; however, the ankle is the most common site for a sprain to occur in persons living in the United States, with approximately 2 million diagnoses annually (Herzog et al., 2019; Rogers & Allen, 2021). Males and females are affected equally by sprains and strains, with the greatest risk factors being a previous sprain or strain, inappropriate footwear, limited stretching/warming up prior to activity, being overweight, and poor athletic conditioning (Box 10.2) (National Institute of Arthritis and Musculoskeletal and Skin Diseases, 2021). Sprains and strains are classified as first degree (mild), second degree (moderate), or third degree (severe) (Smallheer & Reeves, 2023). A complete separation of a tendon or ligament from where it attaches to the bone is called an avulsion (Smallheer & Reeves, 2023).

Pathophysiology

The inappropriate tearing of a muscle, tendon, or ligament is the cause of inflammation at the site of injury (Smallheer & Reeves, 2023). The gap caused by the tear becomes filled with a hematoma and inflammatory cytokines, nitric oxide, prostaglandins, and lipoxins are released, which causes necrosis of myofibrils (Rogers & Allen, 2021). Macrophages, fibroblasts, and capillary buds are present during repair of the myofibrils (see Algorithm 10.1) (Rogers & Allen, 2023). The necrotic tissue is removed via phagocytosis and remodeling of the connective tissue occurs, though scar tissue is produced during the regenerative process (Rogers & Allen, 2021). The goal is to prevent another injury during the healing process as this may cause excessive scar tissue to develop, leading to poor tendon or ligament function (Smallheer & Reeves, 2023). Ample strength is restored 8 to 12 weeks after a sprain and 4 to 5 weeks after a strain, though these time frames are dependent on the mechanism of injury, previous injury to the joint, and age and overall health of the person affected (Rogers & Allen, 2021).

Physical Clinical Presentation

SUBJECTIVE

When interviewing a person with an injury suspicious for causing a sprain or strain it is important to ask when the injury occurred, what the person was doing when it occurred, if the area of injury

---

BOX 10.1 ■ Pediatric Considerations

Musculoskeletal injuries are common in youth sports, with sprains and strains being the most common injury in active teens. Younger children have greater weakness at their growth plates versus their muscles or tendons. Therefore fractures are a concern in this age group. Utilizing Ottawa rules (Fig. 10.1 and Box 10.3) will assist the health care provider in determining the need for radiograph. Serious consideration should be given about children and radiation exposure prior to ordering an X-ray. The American College of Radiology (2023) provides recommendations based on appropriateness and relative radiation levels for children. Family should be informed of the risk versus benefit of radiation exposure at a young age (Costa E Silva et al., 2022).

BOX 10.2 ■ Diversity Considerations

It is estimated that by 2050, immigrants will make up approximately 23% of adults in the workforce. The growth of immigrants in the workforce accompanies an increased risk of occupational health disparities. Latino immigrants to the United States have a workplace fatality rate of 5.9 per 100,000 person-years, which is 50% higher than the rate for all workers. Workplace injuries (commonly sprains and strains) are even higher, though often are unreported or underreported, by Latinos in the workforce. It is crucial for health care providers to educate *all* persons cared for on ergonomics and recommended safety equipment that can decrease risk of workplace injury. Encouraging persons to advocate for themselves in the workplace as well as health care providers actively advocating within their local community/state to ensure that appropriate safety training is provided is an essential step in fighting occupational health disparities (Flynn, 2014).

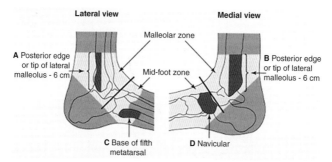

Fig. 10.1 Ottawa ankle and foot rules. From Silveira, P. C., Ip, I. K., Sumption, S., Raja, A. S., Tajmir, S., & Khorasani, R. (2016). Impact of a clinical decision support tool on adherence to the Ottawa ankle rules. *American Journal of Emergency Medicine*, 34(3), 412–418. https://doi.org/10.1016/j.ajem.2015.11.028. (Adapted from Gomes, Y. E., Chau, M., Banwell, H. A., & Causby, R. S. (2022). Diagnostic accuracy of the Ottawa ankle rule to exclude fractures in acute ankle injuries in adults: A systematic review and meta-analysis. *BMC Musculoskeletal Disorders*, 23(1), 885. https://doi.org/10.1186/s12891-022-05831-7.)

made a sound or noise (e.g., pop) when the injury occurred, and the mechanism of injury (e.g., twisting, bending, lifting, turning) (Rogers & Allen, 2021). During the focused history, documentation should include the onset of symptoms; precipitating events; location, intensity, and quality of pain (often reported as sharp); progression of symptoms; alleviating and aggravating factors; previous episodes; and associated symptoms. Any musculoskeletal pain should prompt questions about functional decline and/or changes to activities of daily living caused by the injury (Box 10.4) (Rogers & Allen, 2021). Identify medical and family histories related to the general

---

BOX 10.3 ■ Ottawa Rules

Ankle and Foot Rules

An ankle X-ray is required only if there is pain in the malleolar zone and any of these findings are present:

- Bone tenderness at A
- Bone tenderness at B
- Inability to bear weight both immediately and in the health care setting where being evaluated

A foot X-ray is required if there is pain in the midfoot zone and any of these findings are present:

- Bone tenderness at C
- Bone tenderness at D
- Inability to bear weight both immediately and in the health care setting where being evaluated

Knee Rules

A knee X-ray is only required for knee injury with any of these findings:

- Age 55 or older
- Isolated tenderness of the patella
- Tenderness at the head of the fibula
- Inability to flex to 90 degrees
- Inability to bear weight both immediately and in the health care setting where being evaluated
(Adapted from Silveira, P. C., Ip, I. K., Sumption, S., Raja, A. S., Tajmir, S., & Khorasani, R. (2016). Impact of a clinical decision support tool on adherence to the Ottawa ankle rules. *American Journal of Emergency Medicine, 34*(3), 412–418; and Stiell, I. G., Wells, G. A., Hoag, R. H., Sivilotti, M. L., Cacciotti, T. F., Verbeek, P. R., Greenway, K. T., McDowell, I., Cwinn, A. A., Greenberg, G. H., Nichol, G., & Michael, J. A. (1997). Implementation of the Ottawa knee rule for the use of radiography in acute knee injuries. *Journal of American Medical Association, 278*(23), 2075–2079.)

BOX 10.4 ■ Older Adult Considerations

Musculoskeletal pain and weakness are often considered expected age-related changes by older adults, thus leading to these complaints being unreported. Health care providers should have a systematic regimen of questions in place to identify unreported musculoskeletal symptoms that can increase risk of injury, falls, and/or loss of independence. Assessing functional ability via a Timed Up and Go test will determine lower extremity strength and transfer ability. Examination of general muscle and joint active range of motion with and without resistance provides a glimpse into the ability of the older adult to function independently with daily activities such as dressing and cooking. Expected physiologic changes in older adults lead to less flexibility of joints and a decrease in muscle mass, which increase their risk of injury. Identification of limitations and prevention of further functional loss is key in maintaining the independence and quality of life of older adults (Bishop & Harlow, 2023; Warshaw et al., 2023).

---

musculoskeletal system as well as social, occupational, and recreational activities that may contribute to or precipitate injury (Rogers & Allen, 2021). A reported inability to walk or continue activity after injury and/or swelling and discoloration within minutes after injury can indicate a severe soft-tissue injury or fracture (Smallheer & Reeves, 2023).

OBJECTIVE*

It is imperative for the practitioner to examine joints and muscles symmetrically, without garments obscuring the exam and while still honoring the privacy of the person. When assessing

---

*Hallmark signs are bolded and <u>Red flags are bolded and underlined</u>.

BOX 10.5 ■ Acute Care Considerations

Identification of an avulsion of a ligament or tendon from the bone versus a basic sprain or strain is imperative for appropriate treatment and return to preinjury functionality. Avulsion injuries occur in all age groups, but they most frequently affect athletes whose skeleton is maturing. Avulsion injuries can mimic serious conditions, including infection or neoplasm. Plain radiography is recommended to diagnose an avulsion injury, but more advanced imaging (such as ultrasound, magnetic resonance imaging, or computed tomography) is recommended to determine the extent of the damage and recommend appropriate referral for management, including surgery if needed (Choi et al., 2021).

---

the injured joint(s), the joint(s) above and below the painful joint(s) should be examined as well. During range-of-motion (ROM) testing, active range of motion is preferred over passive range of motion (Rogers & Allen, 2021).

Generalized: **Fever**

Neurological: **Hyporeflexia at area of injury**

Cardiovascular/peripheral vascular: **Decreased peripheral pulses**

Musculoskeletal: <u>Inspection</u>: **Asymmetry and/or edema of injured muscle or joint(s).** <u>Palpation</u>: **Tenderness; crepitus and/or joint effusion(s).** <u>ROM</u>: **Decreased and painful active range of motion; muscle weakness (<u>diffuse weakness</u>); joint instability; gait abnormality if lower body injury** (see Algorithm 10.1)

Integumentary: **Erythema, ecchymosis, <u>warmth</u>, and/or skin lesions to area of injury** (Rogers & Allen, 2021; Smallheer & Reeves, 2023)

Evaluation and Differential Diagnoses

DIAGNOSTICS

- Choice of diagnostic tool(s) is first based on reported mechanism of injury and physical clinical presentation (Smallheer & Reeves, 2023).
    - Use of the Ottawa rules for ankle, foot, and knee radiographic determination (see Fig. 10.1 and Box 10.3) has shown to decrease the number of unnecessary radiographs by 30% to 40% (Gomes et al., 2022).
- Plain X-ray is the first radiographic choice (if needed), with magnetic resonance imaging as a secondary option (if needed) (American College of Radiology, 2023). Risk (radiation exposure and cost) versus benefit should be considered.
    - X-rays should be ordered to provide 2 views (at minimum), specifically anterior-posterior and lateral. Certain joints may require other views.
- The need for arthroscopy or arthrography would be determined by an orthopedist (Smallheer & Reeves, 2023).
- No laboratory testing is beneficial for the diagnosis of a sprain or strain.

DIFFERENTIAL DIAGNOSES

Differentiating between sprain and strain is important as each is a differential diagnosis for the other. Other differentials include fracture, tendonitis, bursitis, and avulsion injuries of a ligament or tendon (Box 10.5).

Plan

GUIDELINE RESOURCES

No up-to-date clinical practice guidelines exist for the management of general musculoskeletal sprains and strains. Consensus for best practice in the management of sprains and strains has been provided by the American College of Sports Medicine (2011).

Pharmacotherapy

Nonpharmacologic therapy is the standard of care for sprains/strains; however, nonsteroidal anti-inflammatory drugs can be used in the short term (48 hours) for pain relief (see Algorithm 10.1). Consider contraindications and maximum dosages prior to prescribing.

NONPHARMACOTHERAPY

- Educate
  - Protection, rest, ice, compression, and elevation is the initial standard of care for the first 48 to 72 hours post injury.
  - Support the affected muscle, tendon, or ligament by use of a compression dressing or brace.
  - Restrict activity for 48 to 72 hours post injury, with gentle movement of the muscle or joint.
  - Resume activity slowly to limit risk of reinjuring muscle or joint.
- Lifestyle
  - Stretch and warm up muscles prior to activity.
  - Strengthening of muscles around affected joint can increase stability.
  - Wear properly fitting shoes when performing physical activities.
  - Wear appropriate protective gear when performing physical activities where protection is recommended (e.g., helmet, knee pads, shin guards).
- Referral
  - Physical Therapy and/or Occupational Therapy
  - Orthopedist as needed
- Follow-up
  - For persons who have persistent symptoms for more than 6 to 8 weeks, a magnetic resonance imaging scan should be done.

(American College of Sports Medicine, 2011; Smallheer & Reeves, 2023)

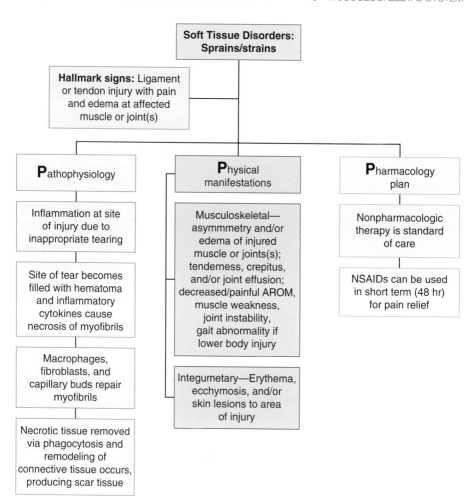

Algorithm 10.1   Soft tissue disorders: Sprains/strains. *AROM*, active range of motion; *NSAIDs*, non-steroidal anti-inflammatories; *hr*, hour.

References

American College of Radiology. (2023). *Appropriateness criteria: Diagnostic imaging topics.* https://acsearch. acr.org/list?_.

American College of Sports Medicine. (2011). *Sprains, strains, and tears.* https://www.acsm.org/docs/default-source/files-for-resource-library/sprains-strains-and-tears.pdf?sfvrsn=5b229fcf_2.

Bishop, K. I., & Harlow, E. N (2023). Geriatric assessment. In Warshaw, G. A., Potter, J. F., Flaherty, E., Heflin, M. T., McNabney, M. K., & Ham, R. J. (Eds.), *Ham's primary care geriatrics: A case-based approach* (7th ed., pp. 31). Elsevier.

Choi, C., Lee, S. J., Choo, H. J., Lee, I. S., & Kim, S. K. (2021). Avulsion injuries: An update on radiologic findings. *Yeungnam University Journal of Medicine, 38*(4), 289–307. https://doi.org/10.12701/yujm.2021.01102.

Costa E Silva, L., Teles, J., & Fragoso, I. (2022). Sports injuries patterns in children and adolescents according to their sports participation level, age, and maturation. *BMC Sports Science Medicine and Rehabilitation, 14*(1), 35. https://doi.org/10.1186/s13102-022-00431-3.

Flynn, M. A. (2014). Safety & diverse workforce: Lessons from NIOSH's work with Latino immigrants. *Professional Safety, 59*(6), 52–57.

Gomes, Y. E., Chau, M., Banwell, H. A., & Causby, R. S. (2022). Diagnostic accuracy of the Ottawa ankle rule to exclude fractures in acute ankle injuries in adults: A systematic review and meta-analysis. *BMC Musculoskeletal Disorders, 23*(1), 885. https://doi.org/10.1186/s12891-022-05831-7.

Herzog, M. M., Kerr, Z. Y., Marshall, S. W., & Wikstrom, E. A. (2019). Epidemiology of ankle sprains and chronic ankle instability. *Journal of Athletic Training, 54*(6), 603–610. https://doi.org/10.4085/1062-6050-447-17.

National Institute of Arthritis and Musculoskeletal and Skin Diseases. (2021). *Sports injuries.* National Institute of Health. https://www.niams.nih.gov/health-topics/sports-injuries.

Rogers, J., & Allen, J. (2021). Understanding the most commonly billed diagnoses in primary care: Generalized musculoskeletal pain. *Nurse Practitioner, 46*(3), 38–45. http://doi.org/10.1097/01. NPR.0000733692.68427.26.

Smallheer, B. A., & Reeves, G. C. (2023). Alterations of musculoskeletal function. In Rogers, J. L. (Ed.), *McCance and Huether's pathophysiology: The biologic basis for disease in adults and children* (9th ed., pp. 1432). Mosby-Elsevier.

Warshaw, G. A., Potter, J. F., Flaherty, E., Heflin, M. T., McNabney, M. K., Ham, R. J., & Sloane, P. D. (2023). Principles of primary care of older adults. In Warshaw, G. A., Potter, J. F., Flaherty, E., Heflin, M. T., McNabney, M. K., & Ham, R. J. (Eds.), *Ham's primary care geriatrics: A case-based approach* (7th ed., pp. 11). Elsevier.

Hematologic System

SECTION OUTLINE

11 Iron Deficiency Anemia

12 Pernicious Anemia

13 Leukocytosis

CHAPTER 11

Iron Deficiency Anemia

Jodi Allen ▓ Corrine M. Djuric

Iron Deficiency Anemia

Iron deficiency anemia (IDA), a microcytic anemia, is the most common nutritional disorder globally, affecting 10% to 20% of the world's population (McConnell & Brashers, 2023). IDA can be caused by dietary deficiency, impaired absorption, increased requirement, chronic blood loss, and/or chronic diarrhea. Toddlers (Box 11.1), adolescent females, females of childbearing age (Box 11.2), persons living in poverty, infants ingesting cow's milk, older adults with dietary restrictions, and teenagers with poor diets are most commonly afflicted (McConnell & Brashers, 2023; World Health Organization, 2023). Any person can develop IDA in response to blood loss, which is often the precipitating event that identifies disease processes such as gastric or duodenal ulcers, cirrhosis, hemorrhoids, inflammatory bowel disease, or cancer (Box 11.3). IDA in males or postmenopausal females is often the first indication of gastrointestinal (GI) disease, including *Helicobacter pylori* infection, as it impedes iron uptake (McConnell & Brashers, 2023). IDA is typically the easiest type of anemia to correct if it is not caused by a GI malignancy.

Pathophysiology

IDA is a hypochromic, microcytic anemia, meaning that the circulating red blood cells (RBCs) are smaller than the usual size of RBCs and have a decreased red color and less hemoglobin content. Insufficient dietary intake and/or excessive blood loss exhaust iron stores and reduce hemoglobin synthesis. When total body iron stores are low, erythroblasts and other tissues are deprived, causing many of the physical symptoms of IDA. The human body requires iron, balanced both in circulation (via hemoglobin) and in storage for future hemoglobin synthesis. Blood loss upsets this balance because it requires more need, pulling iron from storage without the ability to rebuild it swiftly. IDA occurs in three stages (see Algorithm 11.1). Stage I is identified by decreased bone marrow iron stores while hemoglobin and serum iron remain normal; Stage II is characterized by the loss of iron transported to bone marrow, causing iron-deficient erythropoiesis; and Stage III begins when the small (microcytic) hemoglobin cell enters circulation to replace the aged erythrocytes that are being removed from circulation. Physical manifestations of IDA occur in Stage III (McConnell & Brashers, 2023).

Physical Clinical Presentation

SUBJECTIVE

Symptoms of IDA do not typically arise until hemoglobin levels are decreased to 7 to 8 g/dL, with the first reported symptoms including fatigue, weakness, shortness of breath, and dyspnea on exertion. Persons with IDA may also complain of dizziness, poor concentration, and/or loss of appetite (McConnell & Brashers, 2023). During the focused history, documentation should include the onset of symptoms; precipitating events; location, intensity, and quality of pain (if

---

BOX 11.1 ■ Pediatric Considerations

Lead poisoning is often a comorbid condition to iron deficiency anemia (IDA) in children. If a child is determined to be at risk for IDA, they are more likely concurrently at risk for lead poisoning. Iron deficiency in children is associated with cognitive deficits that can extend into adulthood, while lead poisoning is associated with neurocognitive impairments and neurodevelopmental disorders. Many of the symptoms of IDA and lead poisoning in children can overlap, making a true diagnosis of either condition challenging without screening processes in place. The American Academy of Pediatrics Committee on Nutrition recommends universal hemoglobin screening for anemia between 9 and 12 months of age, which is also the initial recommended screening time for lead. If children are at risk for IDA or lead poisoning, repeat hemoglobin and lead testing should be performed often to negate any negative cognitive outcomes related to these two diagnoses (American Academy of Pediatrics, 2023; Giannetta, 2020).

BOX 11.2 ■ Diversity Considerations

Iron deficiency anemia (IDA) in pregnancy has a prevalence of 18% in the United States and is known to be associated with several adverse fetal and maternal health outcomes. For this reason, guidelines recommend screening for IDA during pregnancy; however, recent studies show that White females are slightly more likely to be screened than Black females. Empiric iron supplementation is often recommended without a full laboratory workup to include a ferritin level in Black females as well. Due to the preponderance of evidence that demonstrates poorer maternal and fetal outcomes for Black females in general, appropriately establishing the diagnosis of IDA and treating it effectively is paramount to aid in the improvement of these outcomes (Shevell & Sood, 2022).

BOX 11.3 ■ Older Adult Considerations

Iron deficiency anemia (IDA) is the most common anemia in older adults, most often due to gastrointestinal (GI) bleeding. A high percentage of older adults are on blood thinning antiplatelet and anticoagulant medication and many older adults take large amounts of nonsteroidal antiinflammatory drugs due to musculoskeletal pain. These two types of medication can directly affect the GI tract, increase the incidence of it bleeding, and are often the underlying cause of IDA in older adults. Any older adult who presents with IDA should be evaluated for underlying pathology in addition to GI malignancies. Medication review and alteration may be required to prevent further GI bleeding, but education is equally important to ensure that older persons with IDA understand side effects of seemingly benign medication, such as over-the-counter nonsteroidal antiinflammatory drugs (Prochaska & Artz, 2022).

---

any); progression of symptoms; alleviating and aggravating factors; previous episodes; and associated symptoms. Personal and family history should be reviewed to identify potential GI disease processes as the cause of IDA, such as Crohn's disease or ulcerative colitis, as these tend to be familial. Family history of cancer should be noted as well. Surgical history should be evaluated for gastric bypass. Social history, including diet recall, can identify consumption habits or recent diet changes that can incite gastric ulcers as a precipitating factor for IDA. Medication review, including prescription, over-the-counter (e.g., nonsteroidal antiinflammatory drugs), herbal, and illicit drug use, is imperative to ensure that one or more medications are not a cause of a disease process that precipitates IDA. Review of systems should highlight the GI system, asking if there has been any noticeable blood in the stool or abdominal (epigastric) pain, and the reproductive system for females, asking about menstrual blood flow.

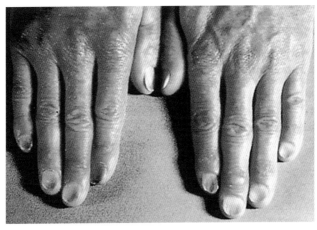

Fig. 11.1 Koilonychia, or spoon-shaped fingernails, is a common objective finding in iron deficiency anemia. Notice how the nails are concave, ridged, and brittle. (From Rogers, J. L. (2022). *McCance and Huether's pathophysiology: The biologic basis for disease in adults and children* (9th ed.). Mosby-Elsevier.)

OBJECTIVE*

Generalized: **Malaise**; weight loss

Neurological: Diminished ability to concentrate

HEENT: **Pale conjunctiva**; **pale mucus membranes**; <u>**stomatitis**</u>; ulcerations of the mouth; smooth/beefy tongue

Cardiovascular/peripheral vascular: **Tachycardia**; **palpitations**; <u>**hemic murmur**</u>

Pulmonary: **Tachypnea**; decreased capillary refill

Gastrointestinal: Epigastric pain/abdominal pain with palpation

Integumentary: **Pallor**; **koilonychia** (spoon-shaped fingernails [Fig. 11.1]); brittle/thin nails; hair loss (see Algorithm 11.1)

(Ko et al., 2020; McConnell & Brashers, 2023)

Evaluation and Differential Diagnoses

DIAGNOSTICS (TABLE 11.1)

- Complete blood count
- Reticulocyte count
- Ferritin
- Iron level, total iron binding capacity, transferrin
  - Anemia is defined as hemoglobin <13 g/dL in males and <12 g/dL in nonpregnant females. Serum ferritin <45 ng/mL is diagnostic for IDA (Ko et al., 2020).
  - The white blood cell count may be low and the platelet count may be high or low, but neither one is diagnostic specifically for IDA (American Society of Hematology, 2023).
  - Mean corpuscle volume reflects the size of an RBC, mean corpuscle hemoglobin is the measure of the average amount of hemoglobin in an RBC, mean cell hemoglobin concentration is the measure of the average concentration of hemoglobin in an RBC, and red cell distribution width is an indication of the variation in RBC size (Pagana et al., 2021).

---

*Hallmark signs are bolded and <u>Red flags are bolded and underlined</u>.

TABLE 11.1 ▪ Iron Deficiency Anemia Workup Laboratory Expected Values and Findings in Adults

Complete blood count	Male	Female	Iron deficiency anemia
Hemoglobin (g/dL)	14–18	12–16	↓
Hematocrit (%)	42–52	37–47	↓
Red blood cell count (x10⁶/µL)	4.7–6.1	4.2–5.4	↓
Red blood cell indices			
Mean corpuscle hemoglobin	27–31		↓
Mean corpuscle volume (fL)	80–95		↓
Mean cell hemoglobin concentration (g/dL)	32–36		↓
Red cell distribution width (%)	11–14.5		↑
White blood cell count (mm³)	5000–10,000		Normal or ↓
Platelet count (mm³)	150,000–400,000		↑ or ↓
Reticulocyte count (%)	0.5–2		↓
Ferritin (ng/mL)	12–300	10–150	↓
Iron (mcg/dL)	80–180	60–160	↓
Total iron binding capacity (mcg/dL)	250–460		↑
Transferrin (mg/dL)	215–365	250–380	↑

(American Society of Hematology, 2023; Pagana et al., 2021)

- If IDA is diagnosed, the next step is to determine the cause, most commonly via the following:
  - Fecal occult blood test
  - Endoscopy and/or colonoscopy
  - *H. pylori* testing
  - Urinalysis
  - Pelvic ultrasound in females with menorrhagia

(Ko et al., 2020)

DIFFERENTIAL DIAGNOSES

- There are other forms of microcytic anemias, and they should all be differential diagnoses for IDA, including anemia of chronic disease, sideroblastic anemia, and thalassemia.

Plan

GUIDELINE RESOURCES

Ko, C. W., Siddique, S. M., Patel, A., Harris, A., Sultan, S., Altayar, O., & Falck-Ytter, Y. (2020). AGA clinical practice guidelines on the gastrointestinal evaluation of iron deficiency anemia. *Gastroenterology*, *159*(3), 1085–1094. https://doi.org/10.1053/j.gastro.2020.06.046

Pharmacotherapy

The first step in treatment of IDA is to identify and eliminate the source(s) of blood loss if there is the underlying cause.

BOX 11.4 ■ Acute Care Considerations

Persons with iron deficiency anemia who are severely symptomatic often present to the emergency department (ED). For those who are hemodynamically unstable due to acute hemorrhage, the gold standard is a blood transfusion. For those who are well compensated, the recommendations have changed to prioritize intravenous iron as first-line therapy for persons with severe iron deficiency anemia. Studies identify intravenous iron therapy in the ED to be a cost-effective, time-saving (2-hour reduction in patient ED stay) therapeutic approach (Beverina et al., 2022).

- Oral iron (ferrous sulfate) 150 to 200 mg every 12 hours, though a lower dosage or every-other-day dosing may improve tolerability of the medication (see Algorithm 11.1).
- Parenteral iron replacement is only recommended in severe IDA, uncontrolled or chronic blood loss, intolerance to oral iron replacement, intestinal malabsorption, or poor adherence to oral therapy (Box 11.4).

(Ko et al., 2020; McConnell & Brashers, 2023)

NONPHARMACOTHERAPY

- Educate
  - Person and their family on the diagnosis of IDA, treatments (including length of treatment), possible side effects of treatment, importance of adherence to both pharmacologic and nonpharmacologic therapy, and underlying cause
  - Take ferrous sulfate on an empty stomach or at most with a small snack.
  - Taking a vitamin C supplement with ferrous sulfate can improve absorption.
  - Importance of eating iron-rich foods, including animal proteins, legumes, and dark, leafy, green vegetables; importance of eating foods rich in vitamin C and B-complex vitamins to promote RBC development
  - Avoid or limit foods that interfere with iron absorption, including coffee, tea, soda, and dairy.
  - Avoid antacids 2 hours before or 4 hours after taking oral iron as this can also interfere with its absorption.
  - Constipation is a common side effect of oral iron use. Therefore increase water and activity as able to promote consistent bowel habits.
- Lifestyle
  - Smoking cessation
  - Dietary recommendations as above
  - Regular physical activity (150 minutes/week)
- Referral
  - Persons with a family history of colon cancer should be referred to a gastroenterologist for a diagnostic colonoscopy, regardless of age; persons aged 50 and older should be referred to gastroenterologist for a diagnostic colonoscopy, regardless of family history; Gastroenterology will determine if an upper endoscopy is needed.
  - Gynecology if a female's IDA is related to a diagnosis requiring procedural intervention
- Follow-up
  - Laboratory testing (complete blood count and ferritin) at 1, 2, 4, and 6 months to ensure full recovery. Serum ferritin is a precise measurement of IDA improvement.
  - Keep in mind that typical improvement in treated IDA can take 1 to 3 months, and an additional 4 to 5 months to fully replenish iron stores in the body.

(Ko et al., 2020; McConnell & Brashers, 2023)

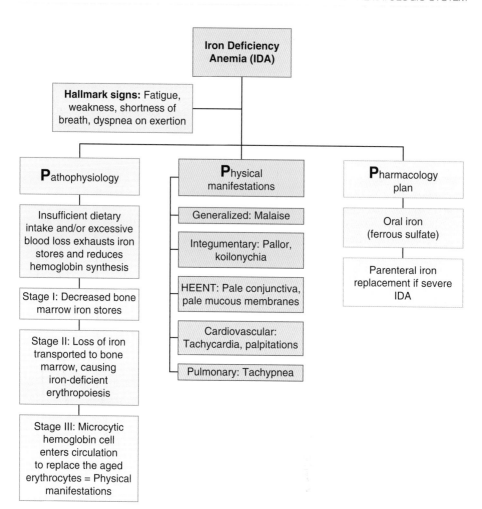

Algorithm 11.1   Iron Deficiency Anemia

References

American Academy of Pediatrics. (2023). Recommendations for preventive pediatric health care. https://downloads.aap.org/AAP/PDF/periodicity_schedule.pdf.

American Society of Hematology. (2023). Iron deficiency anemia. https://www.hematology.org/education/patients/anemia/iron-deficiency.

Beverina, O., Razionale, G., Ranzini, M., Aloni, A., Finazzi, S., & Brando, B. (2022). Early intravenous iron administration in the emergency department reduces red blood cell unit transfusion, hospitalization, re-transfusion, length of stay and costs. *Blood Transfusion, 18*(2), 106–116. https://doi.org/10.2450/2019.0248-19.

Giannetta, T. (2020). Hematologic disorders. In D. L. Maaks, N. Starr, M. A. Brady, N. M. Gaylord, M. Driessnack, & K. G. Duderrstadt (Eds.), *Burns' pediatric primary care* (7th ed., pp. 748–750). Elsevier.

Ko, C. W., Siddique, S. M., Patel, A., Harris, A., Sultan, S., Altayar, O., & Falck-Ytter, Y. (2020). AGA clinical practice guidelines on the gastrointestinal evaluation of iron deficiency anemia. *Clinical Practice Guidelines, 159*(3), P1085–P1094. https://doi.org/10.1053/j.gastro.2020.06.046.

McConnell, S., & Brashers, V. L. (2023). Alterations of hematologic function. In J. L. Rogers (Ed.), *McCance and Huether's pathophysiology: The biologic basis for disease in adults and children* (9th ed., pp. 925–942). Mosby-Elsevier.

Pagana, K. D., Pagana, T. J., & Pagana, T. N. (2021). *Mosby's diagnostic & laboratory test reference* (15th ed.). Elsevier.

Prochaska, M. T., & Artz, A (2022). Anemia in older adults. In G. A. Warshaw, J. F. Potter, E. Flaherty, M. T. Heflin, M. K. McNabney, & R. J. Ham (Eds.), *Ham's primary care geriatrics* (7th ed., pp. 449–451). Elsevier.

Shevell, L., & Sood, S. L. (2022). Racial disparities in screening and management of anemia among pregnancy women. *Blood, 140*(Supplement 1), 7979–7980. https://doi.org/10.1182/blood-2022-169188.

World Health Organization. (2023). Anaemia. https://www.who.int/health-topics/anaemia#tab=tab_1.

CHAPTER 12

Pernicious Anemia

Jodi Allen

Pernicious Anemia

Pernicious anemia (PA), a severe form of vitamin B12 deficiency, is a macrocytic (megaloblastic) anemia. The cause of vitamin B12 (or cobalamin) malabsorption is the absence of intrinsic factor (IF). PA affects females more than males at a rate of five to one, and onset occurs most often after the age of 40 (McConnell & Brashers, 2023). It can take 10 to 12 years to clinically develop symptomatic PA, so there is concern that subclinical PA is more common than previously understood (Esposito et al., 2022). PA is more prominent in females of northern European ethnicity; however, recent studies reflect a similar prevalence of PA in females of African descent (Box 12.1), with an earlier onset of the condition (Esposito et al., 2022). Disorders that decrease absorption of vitamin B12 and folate in the gut (e.g., Chron's disease) and conditions that require an increased need of these vitamins, such as in pregnancy, hyperthyroidism, chronic infection, and cancer, increase the risk of developing vitamin B12 deficiency and PA (McConnell & Brashers, 2023). PA related to the absence of IF can be congenital, with approximately 20% of persons with PA noting a family member with PA. Since there is an autoimmune component to PA, other autoimmune disorders can increase the risk of developing PA. Chronic infection with *Helicobacter pylori*, surgical removal of the stomach, resection of the ileum, tapeworm infection, excessive alcohol intake, and smoking are all additional causes of PA (Esposito et al., 2022; McConnell & Brashers, 2023).

Pathophysiology

Persons with autoimmune PA have two types of antibodies: one to parietal cells and the other to IF or its binding site in the small intestine. In the absence of IF, autoantibodies destroy parietal and zymogenic cells, leading to gastric atrophy. Early in the disease, the gastric submucosa becomes inundated with inflammatory cells including autoreactive T cells, which instigates gastric mucosal injury. This injury results in a deficiency in the stomach secretions, specifically hydrochloric acid, pepsin, and IF. Without adequate IF, vitamin B12 malabsorption occurs (see Algorithm 12.1). Nuclear maturation and DNA synthesis in red blood cells (RBCs) require the presence of vitamin B12. PA is characterized by abnormal RBC precursor cells in the bone marrow (megaloblasts) and enlarged mature RBCs in circulation (McConnell & Brashers, 2023).

Physical Clinical Presentation

SUBJECTIVE

PA develops slowly. Therefore persons seeking care often report severe symptoms. Early symptoms are frequently ignored because they are vague, often thought to be related to age (McConnell & Brashers, 2023). These vague symptoms include decreased appetite and fatigue. When the hemoglobin level has decreased to 7 to 8 g/dL, the person will experience general anemia symptoms such as weakness, fatigue, and shortness of breath. Classic PA symptoms include paresthesia of the

BOX 12.1 ■ Diversity Considerations

Pernicious anemia (PA) is well-known for its high prevalence in persons of northern European descent, but many studies also demonstrate high prevalence in persons of African descent. Despite this knowledge, few studies have been conducted and little knowledge has been gained since the 1970s about the risk of PA in those of African descent. Ensuring proper diagnosis of PA is imperative due to both its inability to be cured and the consequences of it being untreated. Further research needs to be done surrounding the prevalence of PA in those of African descent, including identification and treatment in this population (Htut et al., 2021).

BOX 12.2 ■ Older Adult Considerations

Pernicious anemia in older adults appears to be increasing in prevalence, with the suspected cause being the use of acid-reducing agents (e.g., proton pump inhibitors [PPIs]) and *H. pylori* infections. Studies are identifying that a reduction in vitamin B12 occurs in older adults using long-term PPIs, but not in those using long-term histamine H2–receptor antagonists (H2 blockers). It is important to note that vitamin B12 supplementation does not appear to prevent a reduction in circulating vitamin B12. Screening older adults on long-term PPI therapy can identify pernicious anemia so that appropriate treatment can occur (Mumtaz et al., 2022).

feet and fingers, difficulty walking, loss of balance, abdominal pain, weight loss, and a sore tongue (McConnell & Brashers, 2023). During the focused history, documentation should include the onset of symptoms; precipitating events; location, intensity, and quality of pain (if any); progression of symptoms; alleviating and aggravating factors; previous episodes; and associated symptoms. Personal and family histories of anemias along with gastric disease and autoimmune disease should be ascertained. Identify whether the person with suspected PA has had a previous gastric surgery. Social history should be evaluated for excessive alcohol use and smoking, as these increase the risk of PA. Diet recall may be beneficial to determine if dietary intake (or lack thereof) is the cause of vitamin B12 deficiency. Medication review is imperative, as certain medications can impede vitamin B12 absorption, such as allopurinol, metformin, proton pump inhibitors, histamine H2–receptor antagonists (H2 blockers), and many chemotherapeutics (Box 12.2). Review of systems should include the neurologic system, as cognitive impairment is common in PA, including memory impairment, attention deficit, and slow mentation (Esposito, 2022).

OBJECTIVE*

Generalized: **Malaise**; weight loss

Neurological: Diminished ability to concentrate; diminished immediate and recent memory recall; **decreased vibratory and position sense**; **positive Romberg sign**; **variable Babinski sign**; **ataxia** (see Algorithm 12.1)

HEENT: **Pale conjunctiva**; **pale mucus membranes**; **stomatitis**; ulcerations of the mouth; **smooth/beefy tongue (glossitis)** (Fig. 12.1)

Cardiovascular/peripheral vascular: **Tachycardia**; **palpitations**; **hemic murmur**

Pulmonary: **Tachypnea**

Gastrointestinal: Epigastric pain/abdominal pain with palpation

Integumentary: **Pallor**

(Esposito et al., 2022; McConnell & Brashers, 2023)

---

*Hallmark signs are bolded** and **Red flags are bolded and underlined**.

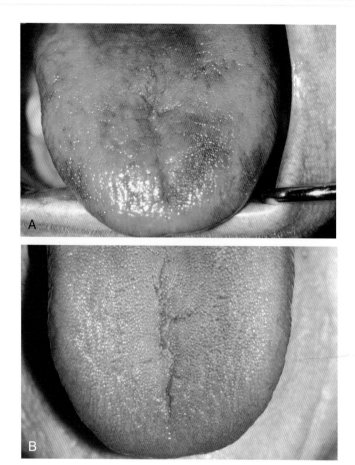

Fig. 12.1   (A) Glossitis (erythema, smooth/beefy tongue) related to pernicious anemia. (B) After therapy with vitamin B12, the mucosal alteration is resolved. (From Neville, B. W., Damm, D. D., Allen, C. M., & Chi, A. C. (2024). *Oral and maxillofacial pathology* (5th ed.). Elsevier.)

Evaluation and Differential Diagnoses

DIAGNOSTICS

Diagnosis is based on clinical manifestations as well as the following:

- Complete blood count demonstrating anemia with ↑ mean corpuscle volume and normal mean cell hemoglobin concentration (Table 11.1). Often persons with PA will develop iron deficiency anemia.
- Vitamin B12 level ↓ (normal value is 160–950 pg/mL)
- Folic acid level ↑ in PA (normal value is 5–25 ng/mL)
- IF antibody is positive (normal value is negative), though a negative result cannot rule out the possibility of PA

(Ammouri et al., 2020; Pagana et al., 2021)

Of note, vitamin B12 deficiency is an independent risk factor for atherosclerosis and venous thromboembolism. Therefore a lipid panel should be obtained in those with PA (Ammouri et al., 2020).

DIFFERENTIAL DIAGNOSES

- There are other forms of macrocytic anemias, and they should all be differential diagnoses for PA, including folic acid deficiency and megaloblastic anemia caused by medication.
  - With PA, folic acid deficiency will present with a decreased folic acid level versus an elevated level.

Plan

GUIDELINE RESOURCES

- Ammouri, W., Harmouche, H., Khibri, H., Benkirane, S., Masrar, A., Tazi, Z., Maamar, M., & Adnaoui, M. (2020). Pernicious anaemia: Mechanisms, diagnosis, and management. *European Medical Journal Hematology*, *1*(1), 71–80. https://doi.org/10.33590/emjhematolus/19-00187.

Pharmacotherapy

- Vitamin B12 1000 mcg intramuscular injection daily or every other day for the first week, then weekly for 1 month, then monthly thereafter is the gold standard (see Algorithm 12.1).
- Vitamin B12 nasal spray 500 mcg; 1 spray in only 1 nostril weekly is an option.
- High-dose oral vitamin B12 is an option, but consider the ineffectiveness of absorption via the oral route.
  - Vitamin B12 1000 to 2000 mcg orally daily

(Ammouri et al., 2020)

NONPHARMACOTHERAPY

- Educate
  - Person and their family about the diagnosis of PA, treatments (noting need for lifetime treatment), possible side effects of treatment, and importance of adherence to therapy (Box 12.3)
  - Importance of eating foods high in vitamin B12 including fish/shellfish; red meat (in moderation); dairy products such as milk, yogurt, and cheese; poultry; eggs; and fortified cereals (Box 12.4)
  - Risk of developing iron deficiency anemia and gastric cancer
- Lifestyle
  - Smoking cessation
  - Dietary recommendations as above
  - Regular physical activity (150 minutes/week)
- Referral
  - Hematology if person is not responding to typical PA treatment
  - Gastroenterologist due to increased risk of gastric cancer
- Follow-up
  - Laboratory testing (complete blood count and vitamin B12 level) every 2 weeks if receiving vitamin B12 parenterally; every month if receiving vitamin B12 orally

(Ammouri et al., 2020)

BOX 12.3 ■ Acute Care Considerations

Pernicious anemia (PA) was once a deadly disease. In fact, the word *pernicious* means having harmful effects, especially in a gradual way. In the 1920s it was discovered that feeding persons raw or very lightly cooked liver could keep those with PA alive. Even today, without treatment PA can lead to problems of the heart, nerves, and other body systems, which can be permanent and increase morbidity and mortality. Through the use of vitamin B12 supplementation mortality has been limited, though the risk for long-term complications remains and lifetime supplementation is required (Pernicious Anaemia Society, 2023).

BOX 12.4 ■ Pediatric Considerations

While juvenile pernicious anemia (PA) is rare, it is not impossible. Most commonly, a vitamin B12 deficiency exists secondary to infant consumption of powdered cow's milk and/or alternative milk sources such as goat's milk, or in the older child who has a strict vegetarian or vegan diet. However, if a child lacks gastric intrinsic factor, they in fact have PA. Management of juvenile PA is best accomplished in conjunction with a pediatric hematologist. Treatment is centered on dietary supplementation and correction of an underlying disorder (such as infection), if possible (Giannetta, 2020).

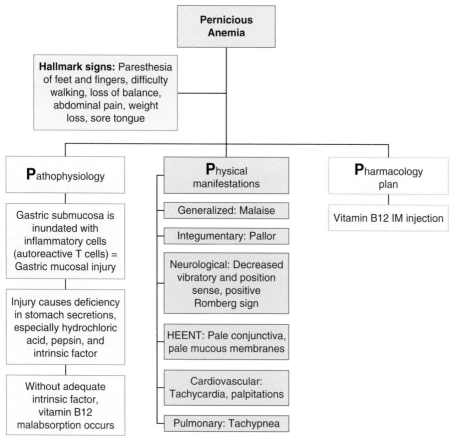

Algorithm 12.1   Pernicious Anemia

References

Ammouri, W., Harmouche, H., Khibri, H., Benkirane, S., Aziarab, M., Tazi, Z. M., Maamar, M., & Adnaoui, M. (2020). Pernicious anemia: Mechanisms, diagnosis, and management. *European Medical Journal Hematology, 1*(1), 71–80. https://www.emjreviews.com/hematology/article/pernicious-anaemia-mechanisms-diagnosis-and-management.

Esposito, G., Dottor, L., Pivetta, G., Ligato, I., Dilaghi, E., & Lahner, E. (2022). Pernicious anemia: The hematological presentation of a multifaceted disorder caused by cobalamin deficiency. *Nutrients, 14*(8), 1672. https://doi.org/10.3390/nu14081672.

Giannetta, T. (2020). Hematologic disorders. In Maaks, D. L., Starr, N., Brady, M. A., Gaylord, N. M., Driessnack, M., & Duderrstadt, K. G. (Eds.), *Burns' pediatric primary care* (7th ed., pp. 752). Elsevier.

Htut, T. W., Thein, K. Z., & Oo, T. H. (2021). Pernicious anemia: Pathophysiology and diagnostic difficulties. *Journal of Evidence-Based Medicine, 14*(2), 161–169. https://doi.org/10.1111/jebm.12435.

McConnell, S., & Brashers, V. L. (2023). Alterations of hematologic function. In Rogers, J. L. (Ed.), *McCance and Huether's pathophysiology: The biologic basis for disease in adults and children* (9th ed., pp. 929–932). Mosby-Elsevier.

Mumtaz, H., Ghafoor, B., Saghir, H., Tariq, M., Dahar, K., Ali, S. H., Waheed, S. T., & Syed, A. A. (2022). Association of vitamin B12 deficiency with long-term PPI use: A cohort study. *Annals of Medicine and Surgery, 82*, 104762. https://doi.org/10.1016/j.amsu.2022.104762.

Pagana, K. D., Pagana, T. J., & Pagana, T. N. (2021). *Mosby's diagnostic & laboratory test reference* (15th ed.). Elsevier.

Pernicious Anaemia Society. (2023). What is pernicious anaemia? https://pernicious-anaemia-society.org/pernicious-anaemia.

CHAPTER 13

Leukocytosis

Jodi Allen ■ Corrine M. Djuric

Leukocytosis

Leukocytosis is a broad term for an increased leukocyte count, typically above 11,000 mm³ (Pagana et al., 2021). Leukocyte function, which is to fight infections, is affected if too many white blood cells (WBCs) are present in the blood or if the cells that are present are structurally or functionally defective (McConnell & Brashers, 2023). Many benign conditions can cause leukocytosis, such as strenuous exercise, emotional changes, temperature changes, anesthesia, surgery, and pregnancy; however, pathologic conditions such as malignancies and hematologic disorders can also be the cause. Some drugs, hormones, and toxins can contribute to leukocytosis as well (McConnell & Brashers, 2023). Essentially any entity that can cause severe stress on the body can be the cause of leukocytosis, which makes determining prevalence challenging. The most common infections to cause leukocytosis are pneumonia, urinary tract infection, pyelonephritis, and abscesses, making identification of these diagnoses paramount to preventing complications (Viner et al., 2023). Any person at any age and of any ethnicity can develop leukocytosis; however, it is important to know that the total WBC count is higher in children under the age of 2 and newborns (Box 13.1) (Pagana et al., 2021).

Pathophysiology

In a person's bone marrow, stem cells differentiate into megakaryoblasts (which become platelet-producing megakaryocytes), erythroblasts (which become erythrocytes and red blood cells), myeloblasts (which become eosinophils, basophils, and neutrophils), monoblasts (which become monocytes), and lymphoid progenitor cells (which become B or T lymphocytes) (Mank et al., 2023; Trzebanski & Jung, 2020). Leukocytosis can be classified based on the cell line that is elevated. Neutrophilia is the most common form of leukocytosis, but lymphocytosis, monocytosis, eosinophilia, and basophilia are possible depending on the underlying cause (Mank et al., 2023; Pagana et al., 2021). Leukocytosis can occur acutely, transiently, or chronically, depending on the underlying cause (see Algorithm 13.1).

Physical Clinical Presentation

SUBJECTIVE

Persons presenting with leukocytosis may have no complaints and the discovery may be an incidental finding, especially in the case of stress and physical exercise as the cause. Persons can present with fever, chills, night sweats, unintended weight loss, fatigue, and/or easy bruising, which should prompt questions related to underlying malignancy as the cause (Box 13.2) (Mank et al., 2023). During the focused history, documentation should include the onset of symptoms; precipitating events; location, intensity, and quality of pain (if any); progression of symptoms; alleviating and aggravating factors; previous episodes; and associated symptoms. Past medical and family

---

BOX 13.1 ■ Pediatric Considerations

Expected white blood cell counts are vastly different in younger children and newborns. White blood cell counts in children under 2 years of age can range from 6200 to 17,000 mm^3 and in newborns from 9000 to 30,000 mm^3. These high expected ranges should impress upon the health care provider the type of infection or malignancy that could cause leukocytosis and the importance of prompt identification. Evaluation of leukocytosis in the pediatric population follows the same pathway as with adults, though with children, referral to a pediatric hematologist and/or oncologist should be expedited (Giannetta, 2020).

BOX 13.2 ■ Diversity Considerations

The American Cancer Society suspected that approximately 185,840 persons would be diagnosed with hematologic malignancies in the United States in 2020; however, disparities were identified in cancer outcomes. Medically underserved populations, including racial and ethnic minorities, those without insurance, and those with lower socioeconomic status and lower health literacy, experienced the greatest disparity in cancer outcomes. This disparity is multifactorial and complicated, but increasing access to health care is a key factor in increasing hematologic cancer identification and referral to appropriate treatment. Health care providers caring for medically underserved populations should be assisting with systemwide changes that allow for cost-effective methods enabling swift identification of hematologic malignancies (Smith-Graziani & Flowers, 2021).

BOX 13.3 ■ Older Adult Considerations

Age is not associated with changes in white blood cell counts; therefore leukocytosis should be evaluated in all older adults. After ruling out conditions that increase morbidity and mortality, consider medication. Medications are common causes of leukocytosis, due to both polypharmacy and independent medication side effects. Identifying older adults who take allopurinol, aspirin, heparin, or steroids (singularly or in combination) and have leukocytosis should prompt medication change or dose adjustment to improve symptoms (Jett, 2020).

---

histories should be reviewed, particularly for previous malignancies, as so many malignancies have a genetic predisposition. Note whether the person has had a splenectomy, as this can cause persistent, mild elevation of WBCs (Pagana et al., 2021). Social history should be assessed, as smoking and occupational exposure to chemicals including benzene, pesticides, and other industrial chemicals have been linked to a higher risk of bone marrow malignancy (Mank et al., 2023). Medication review should take place, as medications such as allopurinol, aspirin, heparin, and steroids can cause leukocytosis (Box 13.3) (Pagana et al., 2021). A review of systems should be undertaken based on symptomatology.

OBJECTIVE*

Generalized: Malaise; **fever**; <u>**unintended weight loss**</u>
　　HEENT: Lymphadenopathy (secondary to infection as cause)
　　Cardiovascular/peripheral vascular: Tachycardia
　　Pulmonary: Increased tactile fremitus; dullness to percussion; decreased breath sounds (secondary to pneumonia as cause)

***Hallmark signs are bolded** and <u>**Red flags are bolded and underlined**</u>.

Gastrointestinal: Splenomegaly; abdominal pain with palpation; costovertebral angle (CVA) tenderness

Integumentary: Pallor; petechiae; ecchymosis

(Mank et al., 2023)

Evaluation and Differential Diagnoses

DIAGNOSTICS (TABLE 13.1)

- Complete blood count (CBC), specifically looking at the total number of WBCs, differential, and peripheral blood smear (see Algorithm 13.1)
- Prior CBCs should be reviewed, identifying trends.
- Presence of immature or lymphoma cells on peripheral blood smear is indicative of malignancy.
- Presence of immature neutrophils, known as bands, on peripheral blood smear demonstrates a *left shift* in WBC production and is commonly found in acute bacterial infections (Fig. 13.1).
- Further laboratory testing and imaging will be based on the cell line that is elevated and on the patient's history and physical examination findings.

(Mank et al., 2023; Pagana et al., 2021)

DIFFERENTIAL DIAGNOSES

- There are numerous etiologies for leukocytosis, and they are all differentials for each other. It is important to first determine if leukocytosis is acute versus chronic and the degree of leukocytosis (Box 13.4). The more elevated the WBC count, the greater the risk of significant infection or malignancy.

(Mank et al., 2023)

Plan

GUIDELINE RESOURCES

- NHS. (2020). *Adult Haematology GP Pathway Guides*. https://mft.nhs.uk/app/uploads/2020/08/Haematology-GP-Pathway-Guide.pdf

Underlying causes of leukocytosis should be treated based on the clinical guideline for each disease, many of which are found in this textbook.

TABLE 13.1 ■ **Leukocytosis Workup Laboratory Expected Values and Abnormal Findings**

	Expected		Abnormal
Total white blood cell count in adult/child >2 years of age	4000–11,000 mm³	Leukocytosis	>11,000 mm³
Neutrophils	2500–7500 mm³	Neutrophilia	>7500 mm³
Lymphocytes	1000–4000 mm³	Lymphocytosis	>4000 mm³
Monocytes	100–700 mm³	Monocytosis	>700 mm³
Eosinophils	50–500 mm³	Eosinophilia	>500 mm³
Basophils	25–100 mm³	Basophilia	>100 mm³

(Pagana et al., 2021)

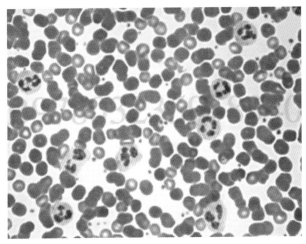

Fig. 13.1 Microscopic neutrophilic leukocytosis without a left shift. Neutrophils are the cells that have two to five lobes joined together and are scant here. You can see the large number of generalized white blood cells, but a smaller than expected proportion are neutrophils, hence neutrophilic leukocytosis. From Hudnall, S. D. (2024). *Hematology: A pathophysiologic approach* (2nd ed.). Elsevier.

BOX 13.4 ▪ Acute Care Considerations

Acute or chronic significant leukocytosis, known as hyperleukocytosis, is a total white blood cell count exceeding 100,000 mm³. This condition is potentially fatal due to the extreme elevation in white blood cell count, causing a hyperviscosity syndrome often seen in leukemia, lymphoma, and myeloproliferative disorders. Persons will present with bleeding, stroke or neurological changes, vision changes, infarction, ischemia, and/or multiorgan failure. Quick recognition and prompt treatment can prevent death and reduce long-term complications (Mank et al., 2023).

Pharmacotherapy

Pharmacologic management of leukocytosis is dependent upon the underlying cause (see Algorithm 13.1).

NONPHARMACOTHERAPY

- Educate
  - Person and family about leukocytosis as a common laboratory finding, how it can resolve with little to no treatment, and how further workup may be needed to identify an underlying cause
- Lifestyle
  - Smoking cessation
  - Proper occupational risk reduction if industrial chemical exposure is possible
  - Handwashing and age-appropriate vaccinations to decrease risk of communicable disease and infection
  - Allergen avoidance as necessary and based on known allergic triggers
  - Stress reduction practices
- Referral
  - Infectious disease if underlying infection as cause of acute leukocytosis
  - Hematology if persistent leukocytosis with an unknown underlying cause

- Oncology if presence of immature or lymphoma cells on peripheral blood smear
- Follow-up
- Based upon the underlying cause of leukocytosis and if no specific cause is identified, recheck CBC with differential and blood smear in 4 to 6 weeks.

(Mank et al., 2023; National Health Service, 2020)

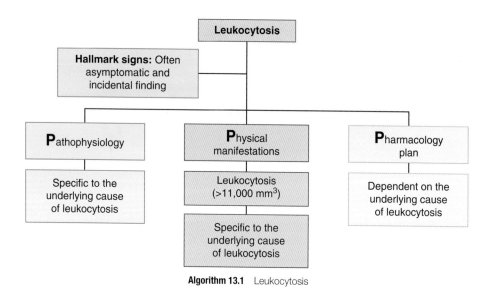

Algorithm 13.1 Leukocytosis

References

Giannetta, T. (2020). Hematologic disorders. In D. L. Maaks, N. Starr, M. A. Brady, N. M. Gaylord, M. Driessnack, & K. G. Duderrstadt (Eds.), *Burns' pediatric primary care* (7th ed., pp. 740–742). Elsevier.

Jett, K. (2020). Laboratory diagnostics and geriatrics. In T. A. Touhy, & K. Jett (Eds.), *Ebersole & Hess' toward healthy aging* (10th ed., p. 93). Elsevier.

Mank, V., Azhar, Q., & Brown, K. (2023). Leukocytosis. In *StatPearls*. National Library of Medicine. https://www.ncbi.nlm.nih.gov/books/NBK560882.

McConnell, S., & Brashers, V. L. (2023). Alterations of hematologic function. In J. L. Rogers (Ed.), *McCance and Huether's pathophysiology: The biologic basis for disease in adults and children* (9th ed., p. 943). Mosby-Elsevier.

National Health Service (NHS). (2020). Adult haematology GP pathway guides. https://mft.nhs.uk/app/uploads/2020/08/Haematology-GP-Pathway-Guide.pdf.

Pagana, K. D., Pagana, T. J., & Pagana, T. N. (2021). *Mosby's diagnostic & laboratory test reference* (15th ed.). Elsevier.

Smith-Graziani, D., & Flowers, C. F. (2021). Understanding and addressing disparities in patients with hematologic malignancies: Approaches for clinicians. *American Society of Clinical Oncology Educational Book, 41*, 351–357. https://doi.org/10.1200/EDBK_320079.

Trzebanski, S., & Jung, S. (2020). Plasticity of monocyte development and monocyte fates. *Immunology Letters, 227*, 66–78. https://doi.org/10.1016/j.imlet.2020.07.007.

Viner, E., Berger, J., & Bengualid, V. (2023). Etiologies of extreme leukocytosis. *Cureus, 15*(4), e38062. http://doi.org/10.7759/cureus.38062.

Endocrine System

SECTION OUTLINE

14 Diabetes Mellitus Type 2

15 Hypothyroidism

CHAPTER 14

Diabetes Mellitus Type 2

Jodi Allen

Diabetes Mellitus Type 2

Diabetes mellitus type 2 (DMT2) is a metabolic disease characterized by hyperglycemia caused by insulin resistance and impaired insulin secretion by the beta islet cells of the pancreas (Allen, 2023). A worldwide health concern affecting over 400 million people, DMT2 prevalence is highest in adults but is rising in children (Khan et al., 2020). A disproportionate number of Black, Latinx, and Native American persons have DMT2, which highlights the environmental and socioeconomic factors related to this diagnosis (Box 14.1) (Elsayed et al., 2022). Environmental factors combine with genetic factors to incite the pathophysiologic mechanisms of DMT2. Persons who have a first-degree relative diagnosed with DMT2 have a significantly increased risk of developing the disease in their lifetime; however, age, obesity, hypertension, and history of gestational diabetes can be independent risk factors of development (Box 14.2) (Elsayed et al., 2022). Diets high in simple carbohydrates, saturated fats, and red meat as well as physical inactivity are factors that can contribute to the risk for DMT2 (Allen, 2023). The comorbidities associated with DMT2, including micro- and macrovascular complications (see Chapters 19 and 20), negatively impact the health outcomes and prognosis for persons diagnosed with DMT2. Prevention of DMT2 with lifestyle modifications is essential.

Pathophysiology

Insulin resistance is the inappropriate response of insulin-sensitive tissues, particularly adipose tissue, liver, and muscle, to insulin (Rogers & Allen, 2020). As insulin resistance escalates, glucose levels remain normal while insulin levels rise, causing a state of hyperinsulinemia (Rogers & Allen, 2020). Beta cell function further diminishes, leading to deficient insulin secretion and prolonged hyperglycemia (Allen, 2023). Prolonged hyperglycemia leads to further destruction of pancreatic beta cells and thus the cascade of negative effects and comorbid conditions related to hyperglycemia (see Algorithm 14.1) (Rogers & Allen, 2020).

Insulin resistance is amplified by elevated levels of proinflammatory cytokines and free fatty acids, which are linked to aging and obesity (Rogers & Allen, 2020). Proinflammatory cytokines are also associated with DMT2 comorbid conditions such as dyslipidemia, atherosclerosis, and nonalcoholic fatty liver disease (see Chapter 19) (Rogers & Allen, 2020). Gastrointestinal incretins such as glucagon-like peptides and gastric inhibitory polypeptides are reduced in DMT2, which significantly reduces the satiating effect of insulin, causing appetite dysregulation and weight gain (Rogers & Allen, 2020). Kidney function is altered in the presence of hyperglycemia, so the increased reabsorption of glucose increases the risk for microvascular renal complications (Rogers & Allen, 2020). Understanding the pathophysiology of DMT2 provides valuable insight into the consequences of chronic hyperglycemia and how various medication classes work to effectively treat DMT2.

BOX 14.1 ■ Diversity Considerations

Racial and ethnic minority and low-income adult populations in the United States are dispropor-tionately affected by diabetes. Nonclinical influences, known as social determinants of health, directly impact the prevention and early diagnosis of diabetes mellitus type 2. Addressing social determinants of health is a priority to understand how each person's food environment (food access), health care (access, affordability, quality), physical environment (housing, environmental exposures), social environment (social support), and socioeconomic status (education, income, occupation) can contribute to diabetes mellitus type 2 and its negative health effects. Identifying these social influences and mitigating their impact promotes health equity and should be a focus of total care of persons with diabetes (Centers for Disease Control and Prevention [CDC], 2022a; Hills-Briggs et al., 2021).

BOX 14.2 ■ Pediatric Considerations

The incidence of youths in the United States under the age of 20 diagnosed with diabetes mellitus type 2 (DMT2) has increased at a rate of 4.8% per year between 2015 and 2022. It is estimated that this number will nearly quadruple by 2050. Risk of micro- and macrovascular complications related to diabetes increases over time; therefore a significant number of young adults are experiencing poor glycemic control and early complications related to youth-onset DMT2. Early identification is key, but be mindful that symptoms of DMT2 in youths are likely absent or subtle. Any child at risk should be screened. Metformin is currently the only oral antihyperglycemic agent approved by the US Food and Drug Administration for pediatric use. Lifestyle modification remains the mainstay for glycemic improvement, with a focus on behaviors that can impact weight, nutrition, and activity throughout the lifespan (Centers for Disease Control and Prevention [CDC], 2022b; TODAY Study Group, 2021).

Physical Clinical Presentation

SUBJECTIVE

A thorough health history is imperative to identify risk factors for DMT2. It is most common for persons to be asymptomatic (Rogers & Allen, 2020). During the focused history, documenta-tion should include the onset of symptoms; precipitating events; location, intensity, and qual-ity of pain; progression of symptoms; alleviating and aggravating factors; previous episodes; and associated symptoms. Document allergies and medical, social, and family histories including any form of diabetes, pancreatic disease, or other endocrine dysfunction. The medication list should be reviewed for the presence of drugs that worsen insulin resistance. DMT2 should be suspected in persons who report fatigue, recurrent infections, slow wound healing, blurred vision, polydipsia, polyphagia, polyuria, and/or paresthesia/weakness (Allen, 2023). Cardiovascular, neurologic, and renal symptoms should be evaluated, as complications of DMT2 often manifest prior to diagnosis (see Chapters 19 and 20) (Rogers & Allen, 2020).

OBJECTIVE*

Abnormal findings may be absent in patients with undiagnosed or newly diagnosed DMT2.
    Generalized: **Fatigue**; obesity
    Neurological: **Decreased sensation to upper and/or lower extremities** via monofilament and/or vibratory sensation assessment; <u>**confusion**</u>

---

*Hallmark signs are bolded and <u>**Red flags are bolded and underlined**</u>.

BOX 14.3 ■ Acute Care Considerations

Diabetic hyperglycemic hyperosmolar state (HHS) occurs more commonly in patients with diabetes mellitus type 2 (DMT2) versus diabetic ketoacidosis, which occurs more commonly in patients with diabetes mellitus type 1. The patient experience is similar, though, with glucose levels often greater than 1000 mg/dL due to the beta cells of persons with DMT2 having enough insulin to produce energy. Extreme diuresis and dehydration occur, with an average fluid deficit of 8 to 12 L. Infection is the most common cause of HHS, particularly pneumonia and urinary tract infection. Myocardial infarction and stroke may precipitate HHS, and glucocorticoid use may be an underlying cause of development as well. Patients present with severe dehydration and will be hypotensive and tachycardic with focal neurologic deficits and potentially seizures. Patients with HHS will not present with Kussmaul respirations due to the lack of metabolic acidosis so often seen with diabetic ketoacidosis. Patients with suspected HHS need immediate determination of cause and aggressive fluid replacement (Brown et al., 2018; Hassan et al., 2022).

HEENT: **Soft and hard exudates** on dilated ophthalmologic examination related to diabetic retinopathy; dry mucus membranes; **fruity-smelling breath**; enlarged thyroid

Cardiovascular/peripheral vascular: Elevated blood pressure; abnormal Ankle-Brachial Index; **tachycardia**; **hypotension** (Box 14.3)

Gastrointestinal: Hypoactive bowel sounds

Genitourinary: Urinary tract infection (recurring)

Reproductive: Vaginitis (recurring)

Musculoskeletal: Decreased muscle mass

Integumentary: **Slow-healing wounds**; **acanthosis nigricans** (Fig. 14.1); poor skin turgor (see Algorithm 14.1)

Psychiatric: Disordered eating

(Allen, 2023; Rogers & Allen, 2020)

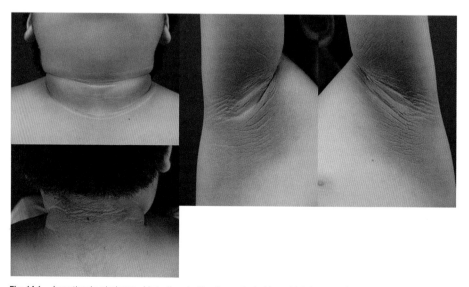

Fig. 14.1 Acanthosis nigricans. Note the darkly pigmented skin, which has a velvety appearance and texture. This is a common finding in patients with obesity, insulin resistance, hyperinsulinemia, and diabetes mellitus type 2. (From Karadağ, A. S., You, Y., Danarti, R., Al-Khuzaei, S., & Chen, W. (2018). Acanthosis nigricans and the metabolic syndrome. *Clinics in Dermatology, 36*(1), 48–53. https://doi.org/10.1016/j.clindermatol.2017.09.008.)

Evaluation and Differential Diagnoses

DIAGNOSTICS

Differentiating between prediabetes, DMT1, and DMT2 is imperative to appropriate treatment and subsequent health outcomes.

Diagnostic Criteria for DMT2

- *Fasting plasma glucose ≥126 mg/dL
OR
- 2-hour plasma glucose ≥200 mg/dL during oral glucose tolerance test
OR
- Glycosylated Hgb ≥6.5%
OR
- Random plasma glucose ≥200 mg/dL in patients with classic symptoms of hyperglycemia or hyperglycemic crisis
*Fasting is defined as no caloric intake for at least 8 hours.

Categories of Increased Risk for Diabetes or Prediabetes

- *Fasting plasma glucose 100 to 125 mg/dL
- 2-hour plasma glucose 140 to 199 mg/dL during oral glucose tolerance test
- Glycosylated Hgb 5.7% to 6.4%

DIFFERENTIAL DIAGNOSES

- Prediabetes or impaired glucose tolerance
  - Increased risk for diabetes mellitus and cardiovascular disease based on family history and lifestyle
  - Diagnosed based on diagnostic criteria noted earlier
- Diabetes mellitus type 1 (DMT1)
  - Acute symptoms of diabetes present with markedly elevated blood glucose levels.
  - To differentiate between DMT1 and DMT2, a C-peptide test should be ordered. In the presence of DMT2 the C-peptide level will be normal or elevated whereas in the presence of DMT1 the C-peptide level will be decreased.

Plan

GUIDELINE RESOURCES

- ElSayed, N. A., Aleppo, G., Aroda, V. R., Bannuru, R. R., Brown, F. M., Bruemmer, D., Collins, B. S., Cusi, K., Das, S. R., Gibbons, C. H., Giurini, J. M., Hilliard, M. E., Isaacs, D., Johnson, E. L., Kahan, S., Khunti, K., Kosiborod, M., Leon, J., Lyons, S. K., ... on behalf of the American Diabetes Association. (2022). Introduction and methodology: *Standards of Care in Diabetes—2023. Diabetes Care, 46*(Supplement_1), S1–S4. https://doi.org/10.2337/dc23-sint
- Samson, S. L., Vellanki, P., Blonde, L., Christofides, E. A., Galindo, R. J., Hirsch, I. B., Isaacs, S. D., Izuora, K. E., Low Wang, C. C., Twining, C. L., Umpierrez, G. E., & Valencia, W. M. (2023). American Association of Clinical Endocrinology consensus statement: Comprehensive type 2 diabetes management algorithm—2023 update. *Endocrine Practice, 29*(5), 305–340.

Following are three keys for a successful management plan for persons with DMT2:

1. Lifestyle modification underlies *all* therapy.
2. Evaluate for diabetes mellitus complications, including micro-/macrovascular complications and target organ damage. Prevent and/or manage these expediently with comprehensive care.
3. Engage the person with diabetes in the development of their management plan, including shared decision making and goal setting.

Pharmacotherapy

Choice of pharmacologic management for DMT2 should be based on a complication-centric or glucose-centric model depending on the presence of atherosclerotic cardiovascular disease (ASCVD, see Chapter 19) (see Algorithm 14.1) (Samson et al., 2023).

- ASCVD is the leading cause of mortality in persons with DMT2, so with high risk or an established presence, including heart failure, stroke/transient ischemic attack, or chronic kidney disease, the complication-centric algorithm will guide medication choices (Samson et al., 2023).
- Without established or high risk of ASCVD, metformin should be started (if no contraindication), and the glucose-centric algorithm will guide further medication choices (Samson et al., 2023).
- Glycosylated Hgb ≤6.5% should be the goal for most persons, but if there is high risk for adverse effects from hypoglycemia and/or limited life expectancy, the goal should be 7% to 8% (Box 14.4) (Samson et al., 2023).
- Prescribers must be aware of the risks, benefits, contraindications, and cost of each type of pharmacologic intervention. Ease of use and access to medication must also be considered (Rogers & Allen, 2020).
- DMT2 is a progressive disease and often requires more than one antihyperglycemic agent for optimal treatment (Elsayed et al., 2022).

Nonpharmacotherapy

- Educate
  - Risks and need for assessment of diabetes complications:
    - ASCVD and heart failure (see Chapters 18 and 19)
    - Chronic kidney disease
    - Retinopathy
    - Neuropathy
  - Importance of vaccinations for disease/complication prevention:
    - Hepatitis B
    - Human papilloma virus
    - Influenza
    - Pneumonia
    - Tetanus, diphtheria, pertussis
    - Zoster
    - COVID-19
  - Hypoglycemia signs/symptoms and how to prevent/manage
  - Home monitoring of blood glucose
- Lifestyle
  - Reduce carbohydrate intake, increase fiber intake, and limit processed foods. Mediterranean eating pattern may improve glucose metabolism and lower cardiovascular disease risk.
  - Engage in 150 minutes or more of moderate-to-vigorous aerobic activity per week and two or three sessions of resistance exercise per week.

BOX 14.4 ■ Older Adult Considerations

Management of diabetes mellitus type 2 in older adults requires a focus on overall health status, cognitive and functional status, social factors, and personal preference. Ensuring the safety of older adults requires careful attention to blood glucose levels and blood pressure and minimization of medication side effects. The American Diabetic Association recommends selecting treatment goals based on the older adult's health, functional status, and life expectancy. A suggested glycosylated Hgb of <7.5% is recommended for those older adults who are healthy with few chronic illnesses and intact cognitive and functional status. The glycosylated Hgb recommendations rise in older adults with complex health issues, multiple chronic illnesses, activities of daily living impairments, or cognitive and functional impairments. As older adults experience a decline in health, deprescribing of antihyperglycemic medication may be required (Elsayed et al., 2022).

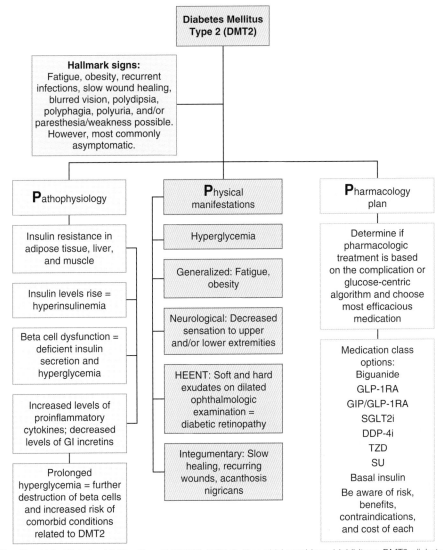

Algorithm 14.1   Diabetes Mellitus Type 2 (DMT2). *DDP-4i*, Dipeptidyl peptidase 4 inhibitors; *DMT2*, diabetes mellitus type 2; *GI*, gastrointestinal; *GIP/GLP-1RA*, glucose-dependent insulinotropic polypeptide/glucagon-like peptide-1 receptor agonists; *GLP-1RA*, glucagon-like peptide-1 receptor agonists; *SGLT2i*, sodium-glucose cotransporter 2 inhibitors; *SU*, sulfonylureas; *TZD*, thiazolidinediones.

- Smoking cessation
- Sleep 6 to 8 hours per night.
- Referral
  - Diabetes self-management education
  - Registered dietician for medical nutrition therapy
  - Ophthalmologist for annual dilated eye exam
  - Dentist for comprehensive dental and periodontal exam
  - Family Planning for persons of childbearing potential
  - Social worker/community resources, as needed
  - Mental health professional, as needed
- Follow-up
  - HgbA1C every 3 months until target is reached, then every 6 months

(Elsayed et al., 2022)

References

Allen, J. A. (2023). Alterations of hormonal regulation. In J. L. Rogers (Ed.), *McCance and Huether's pathophysiology: The biologic basis for disease in adults and children* (9th ed., pp. 702–715). Mosby-Elsevier.

Samson, S. L., Vellanki, P., Blonde, L., Christofides, E. A., Galindo, R. J., Hirsch, I. B., Isaacs, S. D., Izuora, K. E., Low Wang, C. C., Twining, C. L., Umpierrez, G. E., & Valencia, W. M. (2023). American Association of Clinical Endocrinology consensus statement: Comprehensive type 2 diabetes management algorithm—2023 update. *Endocrine Practice, 29*(5), 305–340. https://doi.org/10.1016/j.eprac.2023.02.001.

ElSayed, N. A., Aleppo, G., Aroda, V. R., Bannuru, R. R., Brown, F. M., Bruemmer, D., Collins, B. S., Cusi, K., Das, D. R., Gibbons, C. H., Giurini, J. M., Hilliard, M. E., Isaacs, D., Johnson, E. L., Kahan, S., Khunti, K., Kosiborod, M., Leon, J., & Lyons, S. K., ... on behalf of the American Diabetes Association. (2022). Standards of care in diabetes—2023. *Diabetes Care, 46*(Supplement_1), S1–S4.

Brown, A., Clouse, A. L., Slovis, C. M., & Dingle, H. E. (2018). Assessment and treatment of five diabetic emergencies. *Journal of Emergency Medical Services.* https://www.jems.com/patient-care/assessment-treatment-of-five-diabetic-emergencies.

Centers for Disease Control and Prevention. (2022a). Why is addressing social determinants of health important for CDC and public health? https://www.cdc.gov/about/sdoh/addressing-sdoh.html.

Centers for Disease Control and Prevention (2022b). Rates of new diagnosed cases of type 1 and type 2 diabetes continue to rise among children, teens. https://www.cdc.gov/diabetes/research/reports/children-diabetes-rates-rise.html.

Hassan, E. M., Mushtag, H., Mahmoud, E. E., Chhibber, S., Saleem, S., Issa, A., Nitesh, J., Jama, A. B., Khedr, A., Boike, S., Mir, M., Attallah, N., Surani, S., & Khan, S. A. (2022). Overlap of diabetic ketoacidosis and hyperosmolar hyperglycemic state. *World Journal of Clinical Cases, 10*(32), 11702–11711. https://doi.org/10.12998/wjcc.v10.i32.11702.

Hills-Briggs, F., Adler, N. E., Berkowitz, S. A., Chin, M. H., Gary-Webb, T. L., Nacas-Acien, A., Thornton, P. L., & Haire-Joshu, D. (2021). Social determinants of health and diabetes: A scientific review. *Diabetes Care, 44*(1), 258–279. https://doi.org/10.2337/dci20-0053.

Khan, M. A. B., Hashim, M. J., King, J. K., Govender, R. D., Mustafa, H., & Al Kaabi, J. (2020). Epidemiology of type 2 diabetes—Global burden of disease and forecasted trends. *Journal of Epidemiology and Global Health, 10*(1), 107–111. https://doi.org/10.2991/jegh.k.191028.001.

Rogers, J., & Allen, J. (2020). Understanding the most commonly billed diagnoses in primary care: Diabetes mellitus. *Nurse Practitioner, 45*(9), 48–54. http://doi.org/10.1097/01.NPR.0000694716.14005.93.

TODAY Study Group. (2021). Long-term complications in youth-onset type 2 diabetes. *New England Journal of Medicine, 385*(5), 416–426. http://doi.org/10.1056/NEJMoa2100165.

CHAPTER 15

Hypothyroidism

Jodi Allen

Hypothyroidism

Hypothyroidism is a common disorder of thyroid hypofunction due to thyroid hormone deficiency. Thyroid hypofunction can be due to the thyroid itself or the result of pituitary or hypothalamic alterations (Allen, 2023). Globally iodine deficiency is the most common cause of hypothyroidism, including approximately 5% of the US population (Hatch-McChesney & Lieberman, 2022). Iodine is required for thyroid hormone production but is not produced by the body naturally; therefore dietary intake plays a key socioeconomic factor in prevention (Box 15.1). The prevalence of hypothyroidism in the United States has risen to 11.7% as of 2019 and the incidence is significantly higher in females than males and in older adults (Wyne et al., 2022). Primary hypothyroidism accounts for the majority of all cases while central (secondary) hypothyroidism is less common (Allen, 2023). Chronic autoimmune thyroiditis, known as Hashimoto's thyroiditis, is the most common cause of primary hypothyroidism in the United States (Rogers, 2020). Persons with a family history of thyroid disease; personal history of radiation treatment(s) to head, neck, or chest; autoimmune diseases; presence of antithyroid antibodies; advanced age; and/or the use of lithium, amiodarone, or iodine are at increased risk for hypothyroidism (Rogers, 2020). As an endocrine disorder, hypothyroidism is associated with other metabolic disorders including hyperglycemia, dyslipidemia, and obesity, increasing cardiovascular risk. (see Chapters 14 and 19)

Pathophysiology

General hypofunction of the thyroid is directly related to a deficiency of hormones produced by the thyroid gland, specifically thyroxine (T4) and triiodothyronine (T3). The regulatory negative feedback system of the thyroid begins in the hypothalamus, where thyrotropin-releasing hormone (TRH) is released into the hypothalamic-hypophyseal portal system and transported to the anterior pituitary gland. TRH stimulates the pituitary gland to release thyroid-stimulating hormone (TSH), which then moves to the thyroid gland, binds to receptors, and triggers the release of T3 and T4. As T3 and T4 levels increase in systemic circulation, the hypothalamus and pituitary stop releasing TRH and TSH (see Algorithm 15.1). Inversely, when systemic levels of T3 and T4 decrease, the hypothalamus and pituitary secrete TRH and TSH (Rogers, 2020).

Primary Hypothyroidism

Hashimoto's thyroiditis is an immune-mediated inflammatory process that destroys thyroid tissue in persons who are genetically inclined (Rogers, 2020). As thyroid function declines, less T3 and T4 are produced, which leads to an increase in TRH and TSH secretion (Allen, 2023). Antithyroid antibodies are present, including antithyroglobulin antibodies (TgAb), antimicrosomal/antithyroid peroxidase antibodies (TPOAb), and TSH receptor antibodies (TSHRAb) (Rogers, 2020). Due to the autoimmune nature of Hashimoto's thyroiditis, there is an increased incidence of other autoimmune disorders seen in tandem (Rogers, 2020).

BOX 15.1 ■ Diversity Considerations

The undertreatment of hypothyroidism is associated with adverse clinical outcomes, with disparities in treatment leading to a higher risk of adverse outcomes. The greatest proportion of disparities are related to gender (males with untreated subclinical hypothyroidism), age (those aged 22 to 44 years with untreated subclinical hypothyroidism), and access to care (those unable to access routine care for any form of hypothyroidism). There are inconsistencies in screening recommendations and this could be a precipitating factor for the lack of treatment of subclinical hypothyroidism in males and in those aged 20 to 35 years. The American Thyroid Association recommends all adults over the age of 35 years be screened every 5 years for hypothyroidism, while the American Association of Clinical Endocrinologists recommends routine screening in older adults, especially females. Ensuring that practitioners are recognizing common signs and symptoms of hypothyroidism in all persons, regardless of gender and age, and identifying persons who lack access to care are paramount to equitable care in hypothyroidism (Ettleson et al., 2021; Rogers, 2020).

Subclinical hypothyroidism is considered a mild failure of the thyroid gland characterized by an elevated TSH with normal serum-free T3 and serum-free T4. Overt hypothyroidism reflecting near total failure of the thyroid gland is characterized by an elevated TSH with low serum-free T4 (Rogers, 2020). Progression from subclinical to overt hypothyroidism is common over time (Allen, 2023).

Central (Secondary) Hypothyroidism

The direct cause of central hypothyroidism is either the pituitary gland's failure to synthesize proper amounts of TSH or a general lack of TRH in the pituitary. The hypothalamic dysfunction causing central hypothyroidism will be characterized by low levels of T3, T4, TSH, and TRH (Allen, 2023).

Physical Clinical Presentation
SUBJECTIVE

The clinical manifestations of hypothyroidism occur insidiously and can affect all body systems (Rogers, 2020). During the focused history, documentation should include the onset of symptoms; precipitating events; location, intensity, and quality of pain; progression of symptoms; alleviating and aggravating factors; previous episodes; and associated symptoms. The person's medical history should identify autoimmune disorders, metabolic disorders, hyperlipidemia, radiation exposure (including occupational), and any family history of autoimmune or thyroid disorders (Rogers, 2020). Increased fatigue, lethargy, weight gain, constipation, oligomenorrhea, and cold intolerance are common early symptoms of hypothyroidism (Rogers, 2020). Alopecia, hoarseness, dysphagia, headache, arthralgia, hypersomnia, and depression are symptoms commonly reported later in the disease process (Allen, 2023). Older adults may not report symptoms of hypothyroidism as they can mimic expected age-related changes (Box 15.2). The pediatric population, depending on age, can present quite differently than the adult population (Box 15.3).

OBJECTIVE*

Generalized: **Weight gain; decreased body temperature**; flat affect
    Neurological: <u>**Decreased level of consciousness**</u>; hyporeflexia; bradykinesia
    HEENT: **Course, thinning hair; periorbital edema; enlarged thyroid**

---

*Hallmark signs are bolded and <u>**Red flags are bolded and underlined**</u>.

Cardiovascular/peripheral vascular: **Bradycardia**; elevated diastolic blood pressure; peripheral edema; **hypotension** (see Algorithm 15.1)

Pulmonary: **Hypoventilation**

Gastrointestinal: Hypoactive bowel sounds

Integumentary: **Cool, pale, dry, and rough skin with brittle nails; dry, course, thick hair**

Psychiatric: Memory impairment, depression

(Allen, 2023; Rogers, 2020)

Evaluation and Differential Diagnoses

DIAGNOSTICS

- Primary hypothyroidism → elevated serum TSH and low serum-free T4 (Fig. 15.1).
- Hashimoto's thyroiditis (chronic autoimmune thyroiditis) will present as primary hypothyroidism with elevation of antithyroid antibodies (TgAb, TPOAb, and TSHRAb).
- Subclinical hypothyroidism → serum TSH above the upper reference limit with a normal serum-free T4. Measure antithyroid antibodies (TgAb, TPOAb, and TSHRAb).
- Overt hypothyroidism → TSH >10 mU/L with decreased serum-free T4
- Central hypothyroidism → TSH may be normal or low with a low serum-free T4.
  (Garber et al., 2012)

For any person who presents with a firm goiter or palpable mass, or when nodular thyroid disease is suspicious for chronic autoimmune thyroid disease, TPOAb should be measured and thyroid ultrasound performed. Fine needle aspiration may be needed to confirm diagnosis (Garber et al., 2012).

Euthyroid	Hyperthyroid	Hypothyroid
↑ Free T4	↑ Free T4	↓ Free T4
↑ TSH (typically <10 mU/L and transient)	↓ TSH (undetectable)	↑ TSH (typically >10 mU/L)
↓ Total T3	↑ Total T3	↓ Total T3
	+/− Antithyroid antibodies	+ Antithyroid antibodies

Fig. 15.1 Thyroid laboratory testing results in euthyroid and thyroid disease. *TSH*, Thyroid-stimulating hormone. (From Robertson, R. P. (2023). DeGroot's endocrinology: Basic science and clinical practice (8th ed.). Elsevier.)

Laboratory testing is recommended for identification of common comorbid conditions related to hypothyroidism including lipid panel (dyslipidemia, see Chapter 19), comprehensive metabolic panel (altered renal function), complete blood count (anemia, see Chapter 11), and urinalysis (renal impairment). An electrocardiogram is advised for patients with known cardiovascular disease and those with prolonged hypothyroidism (Garber et al., 2012).

DIFFERENTIAL DIAGNOSES

- Subacute thyroiditis: Nonbacterial inflammation of the thyroid gland frequently preceded by a viral infection
- Postpartum thyroiditis: Can occur up to 6 months after birthing a child and can progress to hypothyroidism
- Iatrogenic thyroiditis: Consequence of thyroid ablation during treatment for hyperthyroidism (Allen, 2023)

Plan

GUIDELINE RESOURCES

- Garber, J. R., Cobin, R. H., Gharib, H., Hennessey, J. V., Klein, I., Mechanick, J. I., Pessah-Pollack, R., Singer, P., & Woeber, K. A. (2012). Clinical practice guidelines for hypothyroidism in adults: Cosponsored by the American Association of Clinical Endocrinologists and the American Thyroid Association. *Endocrine Practice, 18*(6), 988–1028. https://doi.org/10.4158/ep12280.gl.

Pharmacotherapy

The goal of thyroid hormone replacement in primary hypothyroidism is to decrease the serum TSH and increase serum-free T4 levels to normal values while the goal in central hypothyroidism is to increase serum-free T4 levels (Garber et al., 2012; Rogers, 2020).

- Levothyroxine (synthetic T4) as monotherapy (see Algorithm 15.1)
  - Dose is dependent on person's age, lean body mass, duration and severity of disease, and presence of comorbid conditions, especially cardiovascular disease.
  - Young, healthy persons can be started on a full dose (1.6 mcg/kg daily).
  - Subclinical hypothyroidism requires lower doses (0.5–1.0 mcg/kg daily).
  - Start with a lower initial dose and titrate upward for older adults.
  (Garber et al., 2012)

- Levothyroxine dose adjustments are guided by serum TSH levels 4 to 8 weeks following initiation of medication, after dosage adjustments, or after a change in the levothyroxine preparation (Garber et al., 2012).
- Once the TSH normalizes, a repeat level can be done at 6 months, and if the TSH level remains within normal limits, levels can be repeated annually. Any significant change in weight or return of symptoms should prompt a serum TSH level to be done (Rogers, 2020).

NONPHARMACOTHERAPY

- Educate
  - Appropriate medication administration. Levothyroxine should be taken on an empty stomach with water, either 30 minutes to 1 hour before breakfast or at bedtime 4 hours after the last meal. Wait at least 1 hour before consuming other medications or foods (Garber et al., 2012).
  - Medications that interfere with levothyroxine's metabolism should be taken 4 hours before or after levothyroxine (Rogers, 2020).
  - Importance of *not* taking levothyroxine the morning of blood draws (Garber et al., 2012)
  - Thyrotoxicity signs/symptoms (Box 15.4)
  - Dose adjustments often needed during severe illness, prior to major surgery, and during pregnancy
- Lifestyle
  - Healthy diet, emphasizing low-fat, high-fiber foods, particularly raw fruits and vegetables, to combat constipation and decrease cardiovascular risk
  - Increase water intake to 6 to 8 glasses daily to combat constipation.
  - Increase physical activity.
- Referral
  - Endocrinology if:
    - Cardiac disease, symptoms of myxedema, adrenal or pituitary disorders, or central hypothyroidism are present
    - Difficulty titrating the correct dose of levothyroxine to normalize serum TSH levels or maintaining a euthyroid state
    - Under the age of 18
    - Presence of goiter, nodule, or other structural changes in the thyroid gland
    - Female and pregnant, postpartum, or planning contraception
    - Taking lithium or amiodarone
- Follow-up
  - 4 to 8 weeks after levothyroxine initiation, dosage adjustment, or change in levothyroxine preparation where serum TSH measurement is obtained
  - 6 months after normalization of serum TSH level

(Garber et al., 2012; Rogers, 2020)

BOX 15.4 ■ Acute Care Considerations

Myxedema coma is a medical emergency associated with severe hypothyroidism that can lead to death. Signs include diminished level of consciousness, hypothermia without shivering, hypotension, hypoventilation, hypoglycemia, lactic acidosis, and coma. Infection or acute illness in persons with hypothyroidism, cessation of thyroid medications, overuse of narcotics or sedatives, or undiagnosed hypothyroidism can provoke myxedema coma. Older adults with comorbid conditions are at greater risk for developing myxedema coma (Allen, 2023; Rogers, 2020).

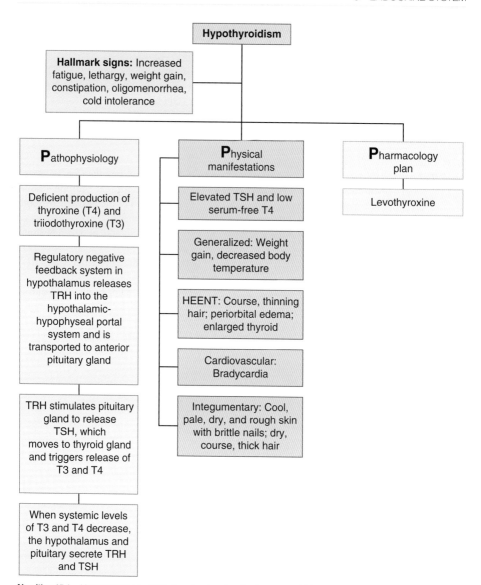

Algorithm 15.1 Hypothyroidism. *TRH*, thyrotropin-releasing hormone; *TSH*, thyroid-stimulating hormone.

References

Allen, J. A. (2023). Alterations of hormonal regulation. In J. L. Rogers (Ed.), *McCance and Huether's patho-physiology: The biologic basis for disease in adults and children* (9th ed., pp. 694–700). Mosby-Elsevier.

Ettleson, M. D., Bianco, A. C., Zhu, M., & Laiteerapong, N. (2021). Sociodemographic disparities in the treatment of hypothyroidism: NHANES 2007–2012. *Journal of the Endocrine Society, 5*(7), bvab041. https://doi.org/10.1210/jendso/bvab041.

Garber, J. R., Cobin, R. H., Gharib, H., Hennessey, J. V., Klein, I., Mechanick, J. I., Pessah-Pollack, R., Singer, P., & Woeber, K. A. (2012). Clinical practice guidelines for hypothyroidism in adults: Cosponsored by the American Association of Clinical Endocrinologists and the American thyroid association. *Endocrine Practice, 18*(6), 988–1028. https://doi.org/10.4158/EP12280.GL.

Hatch-McChesney, A., & Lieberman, H. R. (2022). Iodine and iodine deficiency: A comprehensive review of a re-emerging issue. *Nutrients, 14*(17), 3474. https://doi.org/10.3390/nu14173474.

Lage, M. J., Espaillat, R., Vora, J., & Hepp, Z. (2020). Hypothyroidism treatment among older adults: Evidence from a claims database. *Advances in Therapy, 37,* 2275–2287. https://doi.org/10.1007/s12325-020-01296-z.

Rogers, J. (2020). Understanding the most commonly billed diagnoses in primary care: Hypothyroidism. *Nurse Practitioner, 45*(12), 36–42. http://doi.org/10.1097/01.NPR.0000722320.87129.51.

Rose, S. R., Wassner, A. J., Wintergerst, K. A., Yayah-Jones, N. H., Hopkin, R. J., Chuang, J., Smith, J. R., Abell, K., & LaFranchi, S. H. (2023). Congenital hypothyroidism: Screening and management. *Pediatrics, 151*(1), e2022060419. http://doi.org/10.1542/peds.2022-060419.

Wyne, K. L., Nair, L., Schneiderman, C. P., Pinsky, B., Antunez Flores, O., Guo, D., Barger, B., & Tessnow, A. H (2022). Hypothyroidism prevalence in the United States: A retrospective study combining national health and nutrition examination survey and claims data, 2009–2019. *Journal of the Endocrine Society, 7*(1), bvac172. https://doi.org/10.1210/jendso/bvac172.

Cardiovascular System

SECTION OUTLINE

16 Angina

17 Dysrhythmias

18 Heart Failure

19 Hyperlipidemia

20 Hypertension

CHAPTER 16

Angina

Julia L. Rogers

Stable, Unstable, and Vasospastic

Angina

Angina, commonly called chest pain, is a symptom of myocardial ischemia. Angina can present as three distinct types: stable angina, unstable angina, or vasospastic angina. Stable angina is the most common and is defined as the occurrence of symptoms with exertion only, whereas unstable angina occurs at rest. Chronic stable angina affects approximately 112 million people worldwide and 9 million people in the United States (Kureshi et al., 2017). Recognition of symptoms and prompt evaluation and management in an acute care setting are imperative in improving patient outcomes (Box 16.1). Modifiable risk factors for angina include hyperlipidemia, hypertension, tobacco use, diabetes mellitus, obesity, and metabolic syndrome. Increasing body mass index is an independent risk factor for coronary artery disease (CAD). Nonmodifiable risk factors include increasing age, male gender, family history of CAD, and ethnic origin (Box 16.2).

Pathophysiology

Angina is the result of an imbalance between myocardial oxygen demand and myocardial oxygen supply. Four main factors contribute to oxygen demand: heart rate, systolic blood pressure, myocardial wall tension, and myocardial contractility (see Algorithm 16.1) (Brashers, 2023; Gulati et al., 2021). These factors can be associated with periods of illness, stress, and exercise. The four main factors that contribute to myocardial oxygen supply include coronary artery diameter and tone, collateral blood flow, perfusion pressure, and heart rate (Brashers, 2023; Gulati et al., 2021).

During times of increased myocardial oxygen demand, atherosclerotic plaques, injury or impairment of the endothelial lining, and stenosis can prevent adequate oxygenation to the myocardium (see Algorithm 16.1) (Brashers, 2023; Gulati et al., 2021). Narrowing of the coronary arteries is the primary cause of reduced oxygen supply to the heart. Atherosclerotic plaques can partially obstruct coronary vessels, limiting the ability to dilate. This restriction prevents adequate oxygen supply to the heart muscle during periods of increased myocardial demand from physical exertion or stress (Brashers, 2023; Gulati et al., 2021). Multiple mechanisms can result in injury or impairment of the endothelial lining, including stress, hypertension, hypercholesterolemia, viruses, bacteria, and immune complexes. Other conditions that can prevent adequate oxygen delivery to the myocardium include coronary artery vasospasm, embolism, dissection, and microvascular disease (Brashers, 2023; Gulati et al., 2021). When the myocardial oxygen demand exceeds the myocardial oxygen supply, this will often manifest with symptoms such as chest pain or angina, which is often one of the first manifestations or warning signs of underlying coronary disease (see Chapter 19).

The classic finding with angina is ischemia due to an inadequate amount of oxygen reaching the myocardium, endocardium, or endothelium. This ischemia is thought to trigger release of adenosine, bradykinin, and other molecules that stimulate nerve fibers in the myocardium and result

---

BOX 16.1 ■ Acute Care Considerations

The initial emergency department assessment of patients presenting with acute chest pain is focused on the rapid identification of life-threatening conditions such as acute coronary syndrome (ACS), myocardial infarction (MI), acute coronary syndromes, pulmonary emboli, aortic dissection, or esophageal rupture. ST-segment elevation myocardial infarction (STEMI) can be easily recognized on the electrocardiogram, however, it can be a challenge to distinguish between a non–STEMI and noncardiac chest pain. The clinical clue associated with aortic dissection is the sudden onset of severe chest pain or back pain associated with limb pulse differential. Manifestations associated with pulmonary emboli are tachycardia, dyspnea, and accentuated P2. Pericarditis is another life-threatening condition requiring emergent care. Individuals have chest pain that increases in the supine position and a friction rub may be present. Chest pain accompanied by a painful tympanic abdomen may indicate a potentially life-threatening gastrointestinal etiology such as esophageal rupture. All life-threatening etiologies require emergent care and hospital admission (Gulati et al., 2021).

BOX 16.2 ■ Diversity Considerations

There are racial, ethnic, and socioeconomic disparities that exist in healthcare among patients who present for the evaluation of chest pain. Black and Hispanic patients presenting with angina pectoris relative to other races are less likely to be treated urgently. Individuals without health care insurance or with Medicaid are less likely to have a comprehensive diagnostic workup with an electrocardiogram, labs for cardiac biomarkers drawn, cardiac monitoring, or pulse oximetry measured. These disparities are linked to increased incidence of acute myocardial infarction, higher rates of fatal coronary events, and overall worse clinical outcomes. Health care professionals in the outpatient and inpatient evaluation of symptomatic patients must consider race, ethnicity, and sociocultural differences in the evaluation and management of patients with suspected acute coronary syndrome. Cultural competency training of providers is crucial to improve diagnosis, treatment, and outcomes for diverse patient populations. Providers should address any language barriers and provide access to translation services, which is vital to obtain an accurate and complete patient history. The first step is to be aware of the disparities and then take proactive steps to ensure equitable care for all patients (Gulati et al., 2021).

---

in the sensation of chest pain. Myocardial ischemia stimulates chemosensitive and mechanoreceptive receptors within the cardiac muscle fibers and surrounding the coronary vessels (Brashers, 2023; Gulati et al., 2021). The activation of these receptors triggers impulses through the sympathetic afferent pathways from the heart to the cervical and thoracic spines (Brashers, 2023). Each spinal level has a corresponding dermatome; the discomfort described by the patient will often follow the specific dermatomal pattern (Brashers, 2023; Gulati et al., 2021).

STABLE ANGINA

Stable angina is the most common type of chest pain. It occurs when one or more arteries have 70% or greater stenosis from plaque buildup (Brashers, 2023; Gulati et al., 2021). The heart is able to meet metabolic demands at rest; however, if the body demands more blood and oxygen during exertional activities or stressful situations, the heart compensates by pumping harder and faster. It is during these times of stress that chest pains occur because blood flow is not meeting the metabolic demands of the heart muscle or myocardium. If the pain and symptoms last less than 20 minutes and subside after the exertion or stress is taken away, it is considered stable angina (Brashers, 2023; Gulati et al., 2021). Another potential condition that can cause stable angina is a thickened muscle cell wall from hypertrophic cardiomyopathy or aortic stenosis. The increase in muscle size can be due to a genetic cause or the heart having to pump against higher pressure, as is the case in aortic stenosis or hypertension (Brashers, 2023; Gulati et al., 2021). These larger, thicker heart muscles require more oxygen and if the body cannot meet the demands, chest pain occurs.

UNSTABLE ANGINA

Unstable angina is grouped under the classification of non–ST-segment elevation ACS because it does cause myocardial injury (Gulati et al., 2021). Unstable angina signals the rupture of an atherosclerotic plaque and possible impending infarction. The damaged area within the vessel that has an eroded plaque can become occluded or vasoconstricted, causing transient episodes of pain lasting no more than 10 to 20 minutes (Brashers, 2023; Gulati et al., 2021). A key feature of unstable angina is pain occurring at rest.

VASOSPASTIC ANGINA

Vasospastic angina is chest pain attributable to transient ischemia of the myocardium that occurs unpredictably and often at rest (Gulati et al., 2021). Pain is caused by vasospasm of one or more major coronary arteries and can occur in those with or without CAD. The spasm may involve the large epicardial coronary arteries or may occur in the microvasculature. Vasospasm may result from coronary smooth muscle hypercontractility, decreased vagal activity, endothelial dysfunction, magnesium deficiency, inflammation, oxidative stress, or hyperactivity of the sympathetic nervous system (Brashers, 2023; Gulati et al., 2021). It can be triggered by hyperventilation, mental stress, smoking, alcohol, use of stimulants, or rapid eye movement (REM) sleep (Brashers, 2023; Gulati et al., 2021).

Physical Clinical Presentation

SUBJECTIVE

Chest pain can be due to cardiac or noncardiac causes. That is why a thorough history and physical is critical in differentiating the cause and identifying any person experiencing ACS (see Chapter 19). It is important to remeber that while ACS is often seen in older persons, it can also be observed in the pediatric population (Boxes 16.3 and 16.4).

A comprehensive history should capture all the characteristics of chest pain including onset of symptoms; duration of symptoms; precipitating events; intensity and quality of pain; location and radiation of pain; progression of symptoms; alleviating and aggravating factors; previous episodes; and associated symptoms. Pain, pressure, tightness, or discomfort in the chest, shoulders,

---

BOX 16.3 ■ Pediatric Considerations

Chest pain due to cardiac disease in pediatric patients is rare; however, it does present a diagnostic challenge due to its diverse etiologies. While often benign, it necessitates a thorough evaluation to rule out potentially serious underlying conditions. The most common etiology is musculoskeletal pain followed by pulmonary conditions such as asthma or pneumonia. Two cardiac causes of chest pain in children are (1) coronary artery–type chest pain or angina pectoris and (2) pericarditis, an inflammation around the heart. Pediatric patients may have congenital coronary artery abnormalities that may cause an imbalance between the delivery of oxygenated blood and the needs of the heart. Other children may have a diagnosis of cardiomyopathy. Narrowing or blockage of the coronary artery similar to that in adults is rare but can occur after certain diseases involving the coronary arteries such as Kawasaki disease or due to familial hypercholesterolemia, a genetic elevation of cholesterol levels (Ann & Robert H. Lurie Children's Hospital of Chicago, 2024).

BOX 16.4 ■ Older Adult Considerations

Advanced age is a significant risk factor for acute coronary syndrome (ACS). Older persons also have an increased likelihood of being diagnosed with comorbid conditions which may be the cause of chest pain. As a result, a more extensive history, physical examination and diagnostic workup is required in this patient population. Although patients older than age 75 years represent approximately one-third of ACS cases, it is imperative to seek alternative diagnoses because non-cardiac causes of chest pain are still more prevalent in this age group upon initial presentation. A substudy of the PROMISE trial suggests that patients older than age 75 years with stable symptoms indicative of coronary artery disease are more likely to show higher amounts of coronary artery calcification as compared to younger individuals. Positive results on noninvasive tests (i.e., computed tomography [CT]) and reveal. For older patients (over age 75 years), a positive stress test was associated with increased risk of mortality or myocardial infarction, when compared to positive anatomical imaging (i.e., cardiac CT) detecting obstructive coronary artery disease. Older patients may present with vague symptoms or unexplained manifestations such as dyspnea, syncope, change in cognition, abdominal pain or report an unexplained fall (Gulati et al., 2021).

---

arms, neck, back, upper abdomen, or jaw as well as shortness of breath and fatigue should all be considered anginal equivalents (Gulati et al., 2021). Document allergies and recent ill contacts. A detailed assessment of cardiovascular risk factors, review of systems, and past medical, family, and social histories should complement the assessment of presenting symptoms (Ball et al., 2023; Gulati et al., 2021). Stable angina or angina pectoris is typically described as transient retrosternal chest discomfort that builds gradually in intensity (over several minutes), ranging from chest heaviness or pressure to moderately severe pain (Gulati et al., 2021). The pain is usually precipitated by physical or emotional stress or occurs at rest with characteristic radiation to the left arm, neck, or jaw. Individuals often have associated symptoms such as dyspnea, nausea or vomiting, lightheadedness, confusion, presyncope, or syncope (Gulati et al., 2021). Vague abdominal pain may be reported and is more frequent among patients with diabetes, females, and the elderly (Gulati et al., 2021). The discomfort may be mistaken for indigestion. Individuals may also report diaphoresis, pallor, and dyspnea when the pain is present (Brashers, 2023; Gulati et al., 2021). When actively treated or spontaneously resolving, the pain usually dissipates over a few minutes.

Unstable angina presents as substernal intense pain or pressure radiating to the neck, jaws, and arms, particularly the left. Unstable angina is not relieved by rest and is often accompanied by shortness of breath, fatigue, diaphoresis, faintness, and syncope (Ball et al., 2023). Chest pain may be described as pressure or squeezing and can radiate to the left arm, shoulders, jaw, and back. Individuals with unstable angina may report increased anxiety as the angina worsens (Gulati et al., 2021). Vasospastic angina presents as transient pain that occurs unpredictably and often at rest. The sensation produced by myocardial ischemia is characteristically deep, difficult to localize, and usually diffuse. Point tenderness renders ischemia less likely (Gulati et al., 2021). The terms *cardiac*, *possible cardiac*, and *noncardiac* should be used to describe the suspected cause of chest pain (Gulati et al., 2021).

OBJECTIVE*

Many individuals with reversible myocardial ischemia will have a normal physical examination between events. No definitive examination findings suggest angina myocardial ischemia (see Algorithm 16.1).

Generalized: Weakness; fatigue

Neurological: Alert and oriented to person, place, and time

---

*Hallmark signs are bolded and <u>Red flags are bolded and underlined</u>.

HEENT: Xanthelasmas (suggest severe dyslipidemia and possible atherosclerosis)
Neck: Bruits (presence of peripheral or carotid artery bruits suggests atherosclerotic disease); jugular venous distention
Cardiovascular: Chest pain; tachycardia; hypertension; reduction in the S1 intensity or an S4; abnormal pulsations on palpation over precordium; arrhythmia; murmurs
Pulmonary: *Inspection:* Tachypnea, labored respirations; use of accessory muscles
Auscultation: **Rales** from pulmonary congestion/edema **indicating impaired left ventricular function**; wheezing
Integumentary: Diaphoresis; pallor
Extremities: Edema
Psychiatric: Anxious
(Ball et al., 2023; Brashers, 2023; Dains et al., 2024)

Evaluation and Differential Diagnoses

DIAGNOSTICS

- Electrocardiogram (transient ST-segment depression and T wave inversion are characteristic signs of stable angina involving the endocardium; ST elevation is indicative of ischemia involving the full myocardial wall)
- High-sensitivity troponin I
- Chest radiography
- Stress radionucleotide imaging with single-photon emission computerized tomography is effective at identifying ischemia and estimating coronary risk.
- Stress echocardiography
- Coronary computed tomography angiography

DIFFERENTIAL DIAGNOSIS

- Pericarditis (acute onset angina)
- Myocardial infarction (angina)
- Pneumonia (fine crackles auscultated; localized pleuritic chest pain accompanied by a friction rub)
- Gastroesophageal reflux disease (angina)
- Aortic dissection (sudden onset of severe chest pain or back pain associated with limb pulse differential suggests aortic dissection)
- Pulmonary embolism (tachycardia, dyspnea, and accentuated P2)

Fig. 16.1 shows the risks, manifestations, diagnostics, and differential diagnoses for the evaluation of chest pain.

Plan

GUIDELINE RESOURCES

- Gulati, M., Levy, P. D., Mukherjee, D., Amsterdam, E., Bhatt, D. L., Birtcher, K. K., Blankstein, R., Boyd, J., Bullock-Palmer, R. P., Conejo, T., Diercks, D. B., Gentile, F., Greenwood, J. P., Hess, E. P., Hollenberg, S. M., Jaber, W. A., Jneid, H., Joglar, J. A., Morrow, D. A., … Shaw, L. J. (2021). 2021 AHA/ACC/ASE/CHEST/SAEM/SCCT/SCMR guideline for the evaluation and diagnosis of chest pain: A report of the American College of Cardiology/American Heart Association Joint Committee on Clinical Practice Guidelines. *Circulation, 144*(22), e368–e454. https://doi.org/10.1161/cir.0000000000001029.

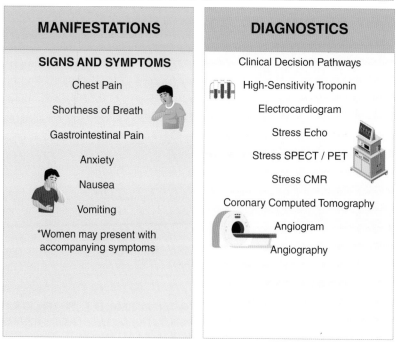

RISKS

Structured Risk Assessment

HEART score   TIMI score
GRACE score   ADAPT score
EDACS score

Modifiable   **Nonmodifiable**

Smoking   Age

Depression   Gender

Hypertension

Dyslipidemia

Diabetes Mellitus

Obesity

Chronic Kidney Disease

DIFFERENTIAL DIAGNOSIS

Angina

Acute Coronary Syndrome

Myocardial Infarction

Arrythmia

Pericarditis

Pulmonary Embolism

Costochondritis

Aortic Stenosis

Esophageal Etiology

MANIFESTATIONS

SIGNS AND SYMPTOMS

Chest Pain

Shortness of Breath

Gastrointestinal Pain

Anxiety

Nausea

Vomiting

*Women may present with accompanying symptoms

DIAGNOSTICS

Clinical Decision Pathways

High-Sensitivity Troponin

Electrocardiogram

Stress Echo

Stress SPECT / PET

Stress CMR

Coronary Computed Tomography

Angiogram

Angiography

Fig. 16.1   Evaluation and diagnosis of chest pain. From Gulati, M., et al., 2021.

- Goal-directed medical therapy: Treatment approach that focuses on achieving specific, measurable objectives to improve patient outcomes.
- The goals for patients presenting to the office or emergency care centers with acute chest pain are:
  - Identify life-threatening causes
  - Determine clinical stability
  - Assess need for hospitalization versus safety of outpatient evaluation and management

Pharmacotherapy

- Goal-directed medical therapy
- Medications
  - Dependent on cause of chest pain and risk (ST-segment elevation myocardial infarction, non–ST-segment elevation ACS, angina)
  - Review the 2021 AHA/ACC/ASE/CHEST/SAEM/SCCT/SCMR Guideline for the Evaluation and Diagnosis of Chest Pain (See guideline resources above).
- Management of unstable angina requires immediate hospitalization with administration of nitrates and antithrombotic.
- Anticoagulants (low molecular weight heparin, bivalirudin or fondaparinux)
- Beta-blockers, calcium channel blockers, and angiotensin-converting enzyme inhibitors: Choices based on symptoms, underlying conditions, and planned interventions
- Lipid-lowering medications (statins)
- Rapid intervention with percutaneous coronary intervention (PCI) if the individual's condition is refractory to medical treatment
- Smoking cessation aids should be offered to any person currently smoking tobacco.
- Vaccines: Influenza annually, pneumococcal, COVID-19, and zoster according to Centers for Disease Control and Prevention guidelines and recommendations

NONPHARMACOTHERAPY

- Educate
  - Identification and elimination of stressors
  - Self-management
  - Disease progression and red flags
  - Importance of vaccines
- Lifestyle and behavioral modifications
  - Smoking cessation
  - Exercise
  - Heart-healthy diet
- Complementary treatment
  - Co-Q 10
  - Fish oil
  - Complementary and alternative therapies with natural medicines and supplements may interact with prescription medications. Obtain a complete medication history.
- Referral (identify and refer for treatment of comorbid conditions*)
  - Cardiologist
  - Pulmonologist* (chronic obstructive pulmonary disease, pulmonary hypertension)
  - Gastroenterologist* (gastroesophageal reflux disease)
- Follow-up
  - 1 to 2 weeks after hospital discharge
  - 1 month after new medications initiated
  - Office visit every 3 to 6 months

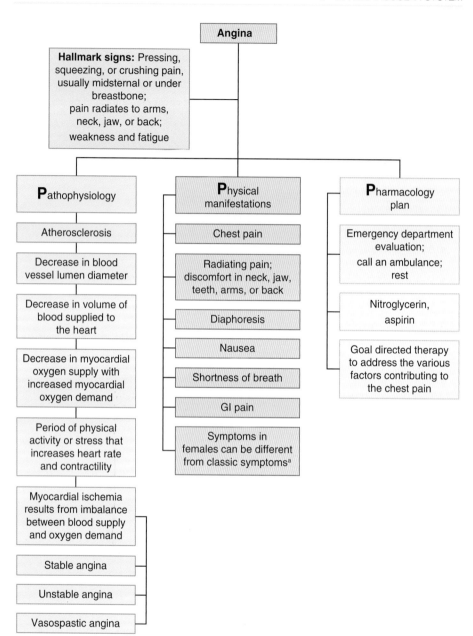

Algorithm 16.1   Angina
aFemales may present with indigestion, back pain, or possibly absence of obvious chest pain. Classic symptoms are considered to be chest pressure or chest pain that radiates to the jaw, neck, or arm.
GI, Gastrointestinal.

References

Ann & Robert H. Lurie Children's Hospital of Chicago. (2024). Chest pain in children & teenagers. https://www.luriechildrens.org/en/specialties-conditions/chest-pain/.

Ball, J. W., Dains, J. E., Flynn, J. A., Solomon, B. S., & Stewart, R. W. (2023). *Seidel's guide to physical examination* (10th ed.). Elsevier.

Brashers, V. (2023). Alterations of cardiac function. In J. L. Rogers (Ed.), *McCance & Huether's pathophysiology: The biologic basis for disease in adults and children* (9th ed., pp. 1059–1108). Elsevier.

Dains, J. E., Baumann, L. C., & Scheibel, P. (2024). *Advanced health assessment & clinical diagnosis in primary care* (7th ed.). Elsevier.

Gulati, M., Levy, P. D., Mukherjee, D., Amsterdam, E., Bhatt, D. L., Birtcher, K. K., Blankstein, R., Boyd, J., Bullock-Palmer, R. P., Conejo, T., Diercks, D. B., Gentile, F., Greenwood, J. P., Hess, E. P., Hollenberg, S. M., Jaber, W. A., Jneid, H., Joglar, J. A., Morrow, D. A., … Shaw, L. J. (2021). 2021 AHA/ACC/ASE/CHEST/SAEM/SCCT/SCMR guideline for the evaluation and diagnosis of chest pain: A report of the American College of Cardiology/American Heart Association Joint Committee on Clinical Practice Guidelines. *Journal of the American College of Cardiology, 78*(22), e187–e285.

Kureshi, F., Shafiq, A., Arnold, S. V., Gosch, K., Breeding, T., Kumar, A. S., Jones, P. G., & Spertus, J. A. (2017). The prevalence and management of angina among patients with chronic coronary artery disease across US outpatient cardiology practices: Insights from the Angina Prevalence and Provider Evaluation of Angina Relief (APPEAR) study. *Clinical Cardiology, 40*(1), 6–10.

CHAPTER 17

Dysrhythmias

Julia L. Rogers

Atrial, Ventricular, and Sinus

Dysrhythmia

Cardiac dysrhythmia is a common problem seen in health care with a wide range of outcomes. A dysrhythmia is an irregularity of the heartbeat and disturbances of rate and conduction. The term is often used interchangeably with *arrhythmia*. Normal heart rhythms are generated by the sinoatrial (SA) node and travel through the heart's conduction system, causing the atrial and ventricular myocardium to contract and relax at a regular rate that is appropriate to maintain circulation at various levels of physical activity (Brashers, 2023). A dysrhythmia results from abnormal impulse initiation or disordered electrical activity along the conduction system or myocardium. There are multiple etiologies for disorders affecting heart conduction including congenital abnormalities, ischemia (myocardial infarction [MI]), infection, comorbidities (coronary artery disease [CAD], heart failure [HF], valvular disorders, obstructive sleep apnea), medications, iatrogenic injury from surgery or percutaneous interventions, and advancing age (Brashers, 2023). Dysrhythmias are categorized as arterial dysrhythmias, ventricular dysrhythmias, and sinus node conduction dysfunction. Individuals may seek evaluation by a health care provider if symptoms are present, or a dysrhythmia may incidentally be found on annual screening or physical exam through a pulse rate check, an electrocardiogram (ECG), or a stress test. Common diagnosed dysrhythmias include premature atrial contractions, atrial fibrillation (AF), atrial flutter, premature ventricular contractions (PVC), bradycardia, ventricular tachycardia, supraventricular tachycardia, and atrioventricular (AV) block (Lévy et al., 2022). Some arrhythmias require urgent evaluation in an acute care setting (Box 17.1) and others will need further workup to determine underlying cardiovascular pathology.

ATRIAL FIBRILLATION

AF is a common dysrhythmia affecting 3 million to 5 million people in the United States (Centers for Disease Control and Prevention [CDC], 2022) (Boxes 17.2 and 17.3). The highest risk factor is hypertension, with other risks being increased body mass index, smoking, cardiac disease, and diabetes (Tsao et al., 2022; Tsao et al., 2023). Other risk factors include thyroid disease, chronic kidney disease, moderate to heavy alcohol consumption, obstructive sleep apnea, and psychosocial factors (posttraumatic stress disorder, depression) (Algorithm 17.1). AF and HF share many risk factors, and 40% of individuals with either AF or HF will develop the other condition (see Chapter 18) (CDC, 2022; Tsao et al., 2022; Tsao et al., 2023).

Pathophysiology

The conduction pathway is initiated in the SA node, travels through the atria to the AV node, then to the bundle of His, the right and left bundle branches, and the Purkinje fibers, and ends at the

---

BOX 17.1 ■ Acute Care Considerations

The following presentation of an individual requires an immediate evaluation in the emergency department: sudden collapse, blackout, or syncope; chest pain; family history of sudden cardiac death; palpitations associated with dizziness or lightheadedness; symptomatic bradycardia; atrial fibrillation with rapid ventricular response; and sustained ventricular tachycardia. Early diagnosis and treatment may prevent stroke. Left atrial appendage occlusion devices such as the Watchman device can be placed in acute care for patients with increased risk of stroke or bleeding and to avoid complications associated with anticoagulation. This is an option for an older patient with a history of falls who may have severe bleeding while on anticoagulation if a fall is sustained (Gharacholou & Bungo, 2022; Tsao et al., 2022).

BOX 17.2 ■ Older Adult Considerations

Age is an independent risk factor for atrial fibrillation (AF) due to atrial fibrosis and myocardium structural remodeling. This may be the reason AF is the most common cardiac dysrhythmia encountered in outpatient clinical practice. The incidence of atrial fibrillation increases with age, with 30% of individuals being diagnosed with AF by age 90 years. Older adults have significant cognitive decline, physical disabilities, and increased falls due to AF (Gharacholou & Bungo, 2022; Tsao et al., 2022).

BOX 17.3 ■ Diversity Considerations

Individuals with European ancestry are at an increased risk of developing atrial fibrillation. While arrhythmias in athletes are rarely fatal, they require careful evaluation to screen for risk of ventricular tachycardia and sudden cardiac death (Virani et al., 2021). School sports physicals play a crucial role in identifying potential arrhythmias in diverse racial and ethnic populations that could lead to sudden cardiac death in young athletes. These routine examinations provide a valuable opportunity for healthcare professionals to detect subtle signs of heart abnormalities, such as irregular heartbeats or murmurs, which might otherwise go unnoticed. By thoroughly evaluating an athlete's cardiovascular health during these physicals, healthcare providers can potentially prevent tragic incidents on the field and save young lives through early intervention and appropriate management of any discovered cardiac conditions.

---

ventricular muscle (Brashers, 2023). A normal sinus rhythm is when that electrical impulse travels through this pathway at a rate of 60 to 100 bpm (Dains et al., 2024). A cardiac dysrhythmia is an alteration of the electrical flow of this coordinated electrical system (Algorithm 17.2). Conduction defects can occur within the heart; this is a primary cause or result from external problems and is related to secondary causes. It is important to differentiate between primary and secondary causes because treating the secondary cause will eliminate the dysrhythmia. Secondary causes include anxiety, exercise, hyperthyroidism, and anemia (Goolsby & Grubbs, 2019).

Dysrhythmias are classified by the location of the conduction defect in the heart (atrial, ventricle, or AV node), the rate (bradycardia or tachycardia), and the regularity (regular or irregular) (Table 17.1 and Fig. 17.1).

Physical Clinical Presentation

SUBJECTIVE

The primary clinical manifestations for dysrhythmias are the result of changes in the delivery of blood to vital tissues due to changes in pulse rate, cardiac output, and blood pressure. These changes can range from asymptomatic to life threatening. Initial evaluation is aimed at identifying

TABLE 17.1 ■ Dysrhythmia Differential Diagnoses

Dysrhythmia	Pathophysiology	Physical Manifestations	Pharmacology Plan	Etiology
Sinus dysrhythmia (Fig. 17.1A)				
Bradycardia (Fig. 17.1B)	Slow, regular conduction reducing heart rate	Heart rate <60 bpm, with every P wave followed by a QRS complex	No treatment if asymptomatic	Physical fitness, beta-blocker toxicity, or sinus disease
Tachycardia Figure 17.1C	Rapid, regular conduction increasing heart rate	Heart rate >100 bpm, with every P wave followed by a QRS complex	No treatment if asymptomatic; beta-blockers or calcium channel blockers to control heart rate	Metabolic: Fever, medications, hyperthyroidism, anemia, HF, hypovolemia, shock, anxiety, pulmonary embolus
Atrial dysrhythmia				
Atrial tachycardia (Fig. 17.1D)	Electrical impulses originating within the atria Multifocal P waves appear different based on the origination site in the atrium and become irregular, with rates >100 bpm. Focal P waves appear regular, with rates around 100–250 bpm. Enhanced automaticity, triggered, or reentry	Palpitations, sensations of rapid heart rate, lightheadedness, chest pain or pressure, or shortness of breath	Address underlying cause (acute illness, stimulants, stress, digoxin toxicity, or chronic disease). Ventricular rate is controllable with beta-blockers or calcium channel blockers, antiarrhythmic medications, or ablation of the ectopic focus.	Structural heart disease, heart failure, or ischemic CAD Multifocal: Elderly, COPD, hypoxia, metabolic and electrolyte disorders Focal: Stimulants (cocaine, caffeine, chocolate, ephedra, alcohol), mitral valve or rheumatic heart disease, acute MI, pulmonary disease, hypokalemia, and digitalis toxicity
Premature atrial contraction (Fig. 17.1E)	Premature contraction initiated in the atrial conduction pathways but occurs before the next expected SA node impulse	Heart "skipping" beats, anxiety, or shortness of breath	Address underlying cause.	Stress, alcohol, tobacco, or caffeine; MI, digitalis toxicity, low serum potassium or magnesium levels, hypoxia

TABLE 17.1 ▪ Dysrhythmia Differential Diagnoses—cont'd

Dysrhythmia	Pathophysiology	Physical Manifestations	Pharmacology Plan	Etiology
Atrial fibrillation (Fig. 17.1F)	Rapid disorganized atrial activation with random conduction through the AV node and uncoordinated contraction by the atria Characterized as paroxysmal (self-terminates, lasts <7 days) Persistent or permanent	Disorganized pattern of atrial electrical activity producing irregular rate and rhythm with absent P waves QRS complexes appear in an irregular pattern. May be controlled ventricular response Asymptomatic, lightheadedness, palpitations, or dyspnea	Cardioversion, anticoagulants, antiarrhythmics, ablation	CAD, MV disease, ischemic heart disease, HTN, MI, pericarditis, CHF, digitalis toxicity, hyperthyroidism
Atrial flutter (Fig. 17.1G)	Reentry circuit within the right atrium Ectopic beat that depolarizes one segment of the pathway of the circuits that become refractory and starts the tachycardia from a no-refractory segment, resulting in an atrial rate of 200–400 bpm Not all the atrial impulses conduct to the ventricles, resulting in a rate less than the atrial rate May be regular or irregular	Atrial rate often >250 bpm with variable ventricular response (2:1 or 3:1) Asymptomatic, lightheadedness, palpitations, or dyspnea	Medications to control rhythm, rate, and anticoagulation for embolization risk Calcium channel blockers, beta-blockers, or digoxin	Presence of a reentry mechanism: Areas with fast and slow velocities of conduction; different refractory periods; a functional core where the circuit exists Most common prototypic macro reentrant atrial tachycardia is atrial flutter

Continued

TABLE 17.1 ■ Dysrhythmia Differential Diagnoses—cont'd

Dysrhythmia	Pathophysiology	Physical Manifestations	Pharmacology Plan	Etiology
Ventricular dysrhythmia				
Supraventricular tachycardia (Fig. 17.1H)	Arises from above the level of the bundle of His and encompasses regular atrial, irregular atrial, and regular atrioventricular tachycardias	HR 140–240 bpm Occurs suddenly and lasts from a few seconds to several hours Dizziness, syncope, nausea, dyspnea, intermittent palpitations, pain or discomfort in the neck, pain or discomfort in the chest, anxiety, fatigue, diaphoresis, and polyuria	Ablation	Digitalis toxicity; reentry, initiated by PAC or PVC
Premature ventricular contraction (Fig. 17.1I)	Contraction originates prematurely in the ventricles; as a result, they are not preceded by a premature P wave, and the QRS is broad. A pause normally follows them. Ectopic nodal automaticity, reentrant signaling, or triggered beats occur due to after-depolarizations.	Skipped or extra heartbeat sensation, dizziness, near-fainting, anxiety, or pounding sensation in the neck	Frequent and/or symptomatic PVCs include antiarrhythmics, beta-blockers, and calcium channel blockers.	Occurs in healthy individuals and more common with heart disease Excess caffeine or alcohol consumption, tobacco or illicit drug use, high levels of anxiety, and electrolyte abnormalities
Ventricular fibrillation/ flutter (Fig. 17.1J)	Areas of ventricular myocardium depolarize erratically in an uncoordinated manner. VF results from abnormal impulse formation from increased automaticity, or a triggered activity and impulse conduction where functional and anatomical reentry circuits help sustain ventricular arrhythmia.	Chest pain, shortness of breath, nausea, and vomiting before sudden collapse from cardiac arrest; unconscious, unresponsive, and no palpable pulse	ACLS protocol Initial assessment while receiving quality CPR Shock immediately with 120–200 joules on a biphasic defibrillator or 360 joules using a monophasic defibrillator.	Underlying structural heart disease MI may lead to VF during the acute phase Electrolyte abnormalities, hypoxia, cardiomyopathies, family history of sudden cardiac death, congenital abnormalities, Brugada syndrome, and alcohol abuse are risk factors.

TABLE 17.1 ■ Dysrhythmia Differential Diagnoses—cont'd

Dysrhythmia	Pathophysiology	Physical Manifestations	Pharmacology Plan	Etiology
Ventricular tachycardia (Fig. 17.1K)	A potentially life-threatening dysrhythmia arising in the ventricles Reentry is the most common mechanism followed by triggered activity and enhanced automaticity.	Palpitations, shortness of breath, chest pain, and syncope May occur during exercise or emotional stress Broad and bizarre QRS complexes that are not preceded by P waves A fast rhythm, usually 120–250 bpm	Amiodarone, beta-blocker, implantable cardiac defibrillator, ablation	Occurs most commonly in people with significant structural heart disease Other causes include ischemic or nonischemic dilated cardiomyopathy, adult and congenital structural heart disease, inherited cardiac channelopathies, infiltrative cardiomyopathy, electrolyte imbalances, illicit drug use, or digitalis toxicity.
Heart block				
AV block, 1st degree (Fig. 17.1L)	A conduction delay located at the atrioventricular node, right atrium, or His-Purkinje system	A prolonged PR interval >0.30 seconds Generally asymptomatic, dyspnea, malaise, lightheadedness, chest pain, syncope	Usually requires no treatment, just monitoring Pacemaker if symptomatic and PR >.30 seconds	May indicate beta-blocker toxicity
AV block, 2nd degree, Mobitz I (Fig. 17.1M)	A reversible suppression of AV conduction or block at the level of the AV node	The PR interval lengthens in successive beats until a QRS complex is dropped. This sequence then typically repeats.	Close monitoring if asymptomatic If associated with symptoms, atropine may be used and rarely may be an indication for pacemaker implantation.	Benign finding generally, may be due to increased vagal tone Reversible ischemia, myocarditis, status postcardiac surgery, or medications that slow AV nodal conduction (e.g., beta-blockers, nondihydropyridine calcium channel blockers, adenosine, digitalis, and amiodarone)

Continued

TABLE 17.1 ■ Dysrhythmia Differential Diagnoses—cont'd

Dysrhythmia	Pathophysiology	Physical Manifestations	Pharmacology Plan	Etiology
AV block, 2nd degree, Mobitz II (Fig. 17.1N)	Block below the AV node occurring at the level of the bundle of His, both bundles branches, or the three fascicles (i.e., left anterior fascicle, left posterior fascicle, and right bundle branch)	Regular PR interval with absent QRS on regular interval Respiratory distress and hypoperfusion such as diaphoresis, tachypnea, altered mental status, cool skin, and decreased capillary refill	Implantation of a permanent pacemaker Risk of progressing to complete AV block, 3rd degree	Associated with progressive disease of the heart's conduction system seen from MI, fibrosis, or necrosis
Complete AV block, 3rd degree (Fig. 17.1O)	No atrial impulses conduct to the ventricles. A complete absence of AV conduction in complete heart block, with none of the supraventricular impulses conducted to the ventricles. The three hallmarks of complete heart block on the ECG are the atrial rate is faster than the ventricular rate; the pace of the ventricles is slow and consistent; and there is no relationship between the atrial impulse and the ventricular impulse.	Dissociation between atrial and ventricular rhythms No conduction from SA or AV through the ventricles Syncope (if self-terminating) or sudden cardiac death (if prolonged)	Transcutaneous pacing; permanent pacemaker	Idiopathic fibrosis, underlying chronic cardiac diseases, medication toxicity, nodal ablation, electrolyte abnormalities, and postoperative heart block; Lyme disease; collagen vascular disorders; amyloidosis, sarcoidosis, and systemic lupus erythematosus

(Alkhaqani, 2022; Brashers, 2023; Dains et al., 2024; Goolsby & Grubbs, 2019)

ACLS, Advanced cardiovascular life support; *AV*, atrioventricular; *bpm*, beats per minute; *CAD*, coronary artery disease; *CHF*, congestive heart failure; *COPD*, chronic obstructive pulmonary disease; *CPR*, cardiopulmonary resuscitation; *ECG*, electrocardiogram; *HF*, heart failure; *HR*, heart rate; *HTN*, hypertension; *MI*, myocardial infarction; *MV*, mitral valve; *PAC*, premature atrial contraction; *PVC*, premature ventricular contraction; *VF*, ventricular fibrillation.

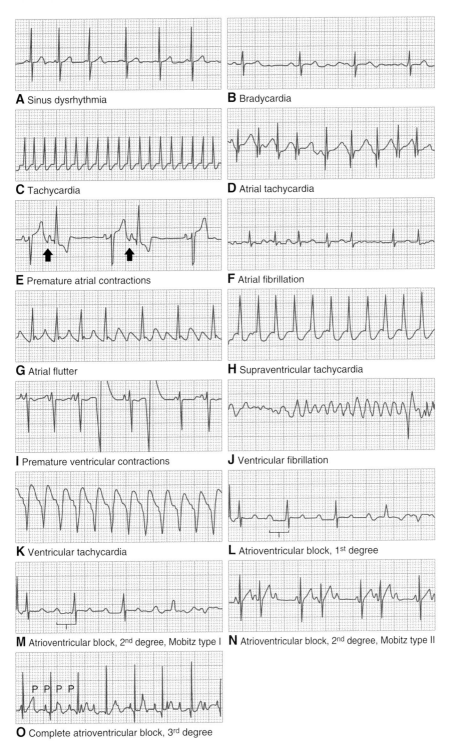

Fig. 17.1 Various cardiac dysrhythmias as they would appear in an electrocardiogram strip recording.

the symptoms, timing of the dysrhythmia, and potential underlying diseases (Algorithm 17.2). The type and severity of clinical manifestations help identify the need for urgent treatment. However, the seriousness of symptoms does not always correlate to cardiac pathology or a potential for lethal dysrhythmia. The most frequent presenting symptoms include palpitations (rapid, fluttering, or pounding), lightheadedness or dizziness, extreme fatigue, shortness of breath, chest pain, and irregular heartbeat. However, many dysrhythmias can also be asymptomatic. Symptoms often correlate with underlying etiology, heart rate abnormality, or other comorbidities.

During the focused history, documentation should include the onset of symptoms; precipitating events; location, intensity, and quality of pain; progression of symptoms; alleviating and aggravating factors; previous episodes; and associated symptoms. Document allergies, ill contacts, congenital aberrations, and medical, social, and family histories. Palpitations may be precipitated by stress, alcohol, medications (including over-the-counter and drugs of abuse), frequency of associated symptoms (i.e., lightheadedness, dizziness, shortness of breath), and relieving factors such as bearing down/vagal tone. The quality may be described as fluttering in the chest or overt chest pain that may radiate from midsternal to neck or back. Ask the individual about the frequency of palpitations or irregular heart rate. Past medical history may include hypertension, CAD, rheumatic fever, and a stressful home or work environment. Surgical history might include implanted cardiac devices (i.e., pacemaker or defibrillator), cardiac stents, valvular surgery, and coronary artery bypass graft. Document any family history of dysrhythmia, premature, sudden, or unexpected cardiac death, thyroid disease, congenital abnormalities, or autoimmune diseases. Social history should include any use of nicotine, tobacco products, vaping, caffeine, or illegal drugs; unexplained blackout or syncopal episodes; heart palpitations with chest pain; or palpitations precipitated by exercise.

OBJECTIVE*

Generalized: Weakness; **fatigue**; **obese**
  Neurological: <u>Syncope</u>, dizziness, vertigo, **<u>confusion</u>**; **<u>paresthesia</u>**
  Neck: Assess thyroid size and nodules; jugular venous distention, bruits
  Cardiovascular: Irregular heart rate and/or rhythm; **irregular apical pulse**; **irregular radial pulse to palpation**, murmur; rub; gallop
  Pulmonary: *Inspection:* **<u>Labored respirations</u>**; **tachypnea**; **<u>use of accessory muscles</u>**
  Auscultation: Wheezing; coarse rhonchi; rales; diminished
  Genitourinary: Hematuria; hesitancy
  Integumentary: **<u>Diaphoretic</u>**
  Extremities: Edema; clubbing; **<u>cyanosis</u>**
  Psychiatric: Anxious
  (See Box 17.4 for differences in pediatric physical manifestations.)
(Ball et al., 2023; Brashers, 2023; Dains et al., 2024; Goolsby & Grubbs, 2019)

Evaluation and Differential Diagnoses
DIAGNOSTICS

- ECG: Diagnosis begins with documenting characteristic changes in the ECG (Brashers, 2023; Lévy et al., 2022).

---

*Hallmark signs are bolded and <u>Red flags are bolded and underlined</u>.

> **BOX 17.4 ■ Pediatric Considerations**
>
> Dysrhythmias have a multitude of etiologies ranging from benign to lethal. A dysrhythmia in the pediatric population requires a thorough history, physical exam, and electrocardiogram. It is imperative to ask the parents of the child about any family history of sudden cardiac death or congenital abnormalities. History should focus on the clinical manifestations of cardiac disease to differentiate the etiology, which may include palpitations, syncope, or chest pain. The physical exam is the same as for an adult and includes inspection, palpitation, and auscultation of the heart and lungs. In primary care, most asymptomatic arrhythmias are benign and include sinus arrhythmia, premature ventricular contraction, and premature atrial contraction. Premature ventricular contractions become concerning when they increase in frequency, are related to bradycardia, or coincide with depressed left ventricular function. Symptomatic arrhythmias may present with intermittent palpitations or with worse symptoms such as syncope and chest pain, up to sudden cardiac death. Symptomatic atrial arrhythmias include atrial tachycardia, atrial flutter, atrial fibrillation, and supraventricular tachycardia (Wolf–Parkinson–White syndrome). A referral to Pediatric Cardiology is necessary if the initial evaluation does not result in a diagnosis, the patient is symptomatic, or there is a clinically significant abnormality seen on the electrocardiogram (Blaufox, 2023).

- Arrhythmias are often paroxysmal and if not present on office ECG, further testing using an ambulatory monitor is necessary (Lévy et al., 2022).
  - Holter monitor (24 to 48 hours)
  - Event recorder (30 days)
  - Implantable cardiac monitor (loop recorder)
- Echocardiogram
- Labs: Ordered to evaluate for secondary causes of arrhythmia
  - Complete blood count
  - Comprehensive metabolic panel
  - B natriuretic peptide
  - Troponin
  - Thyroid panel (thyroid-stimulating hormone, T_3, T_4)
- Other tests may be ordered if dysrhythmia is not found on the above tests or coincides with physical or emotional stress
  - Stress test
  - Tilt table
- Chest X-ray

DIFFERENTIAL DIAGNOSIS

- See Table 17.1.
- Medications such as cold and allergy medications; alcohol or caffeine; drugs of abuse

Plan

GUIDELINE RESOURCES

- Al-Khatib, S. M., Stevenson, W. G., Ackerman, M. J., Bryant, W. J., Callans, D. J., Curtis, A. B., Deal, B. J., Dickfeld, T., Field, M. E., Fonarow, G. C., Gillis, A. M., Granger, C. B., Hammill, S. C., Hlatky, M. A., Joglar, J. A., Kay, G. N., Matlock, D. D., Myerburg, R. J., & Page, R. L. (2018). 2017 AHA/ACC/HRS guideline for management of patients with ventricular arrhythmias and the prevention of sudden cardiac death. *Circulation*, *138*(13), e272–e391. https://doi.org/10.1161/cir.0000000000000549.

■ January, C. T., Samuel Wann, L., Calkins, H., Chen, L. Y., Cigarroa, J. E., Cleveland, J. C. Jr, Ellinor, P. T., Ezekowitz, M. D., Field, M. E., Furie, K. L., Heidenreich, P. A., Murray, K. T., Shea, J. B., Tracy, C M., & Yancy, C. W. (2019). 2019 AHA/ACC/HRS focused update of the 2014 AHA/ACC/HRS guideline for the management of patients with atrial fibrillation: A report of the American College of Cardiology/American Heart Association Task Force on Clinical Practice Guidelines and the Heart Rhythm Society in collaboration with the Society of Thoracic Surgeons. *Circulation*, *140*(2), e125–e151. https://doi.org/10.1161/cir.0000000000000665.

■ Hindricks, G., Potpara, T., Dagres, N., Arbelo, E., Bax, J. J., Blomström-Lundqvist, C., Boriani, G., Castella, M., Dan, G.-A., Dilaveris, P. E., Fauchier, L., Filippatos, G., Kalman, J. M., La Meir, M., Lane, D. A., Lebeau, J.-P., Lettino, M., Lip, G. Y. H., Pinto, F. J., … ESC Scientific Document Group. (2020). 2020 ESC guidelines for the diagnosis and management of atrial fibrillation developed in collaboration with the European Association for Cardio-Thoracic Surgery (EACTS). *European Heart Journal*, *42*(5), 373–498. https://doi.org/10.1093/eurheartj/ehaa612.

The goal in dysrhythmia treatment includes alleviating symptoms, optimizing cardiac output and hemodynamics, assessing the future risk of developing lethal arrhythmias, reducing the risk of consequences of the arrhythmia (reduce stroke in AF), and preventing death (life-threatening arrhythmias) (Lévy et al., 2022).

Pharmacotherapy

■ Medications
  ▪ Anticoagulation for AF
  ▪ Remove offending medication if known. For example, discontinue beta-blocker if the patient has symptomatic bradycardia.
■ Smoking cessation aids should be offered to any person currently smoking tobacco.
■ Vaccines: Influenza annually, pneumococcal, COVID-19, and zoster according to Centers for Disease Control and Prevention guidelines and recommendations

NONPHARMACOTHERAPY

■ Educate
  ▪ Importance of compliance with medications
  ▪ Keep a log of symptoms and when the symptoms occur
  ▪ Ways to decrease a stressful work or home environment
  ▪ Eliminate environmental and occupational irritants
  ▪ Importance of vaccines
  ▪ Self-management
  ▪ Disease progression
■ Lifestyle and behavioral modifications
  ▪ Heart-healthy Dietary Approaches to Stop Hypertension (DASH) diet
  ▪ Limit or avoid alcohol and caffeine
  ▪ Smoking cessation
  ▪ Stress reduction (environmental and occupational)
  ▪ Maintain healthy body mass index
  ▪ Exercise at a moderate intensity for at least 150 minutes weekly and perform muscle strengthening at least 2 days weekly

- Complementary treatment
  - Psychosocial rehabilitation
  - Complementary and alternative therapies with natural medicines and supplements may interact with prescription medications. Obtain a complete medication history.
- Referral (identify and refer for treatment of comorbid conditions*)
  - Cardiologist if pharmacology therapy is needed or patient remains in an uncontrolled dysrhythmia
  - Cardiology interventionalist/electrophysiologist:
    - Electrical stimulation (cardioversion, pacemaker insertion, cardiac resynchronization techniques) while attempting to reverse the underlying etiology (Brashers, 2023; Lévy et al., 2022)
  - Heart transplant center
  - Pulmonologist* for comorbid pulmonary disease (chronic obstructive pulmonary disease, asthma, pulmonary hypertension)
- Follow-up
  - Office visit every 1 to 2 weeks after hospital discharge
  - Follow-up every 3 to 6 months
  - Long-term arrhythmia management is collaborative after the diagnosis is confirmed and management is stable.

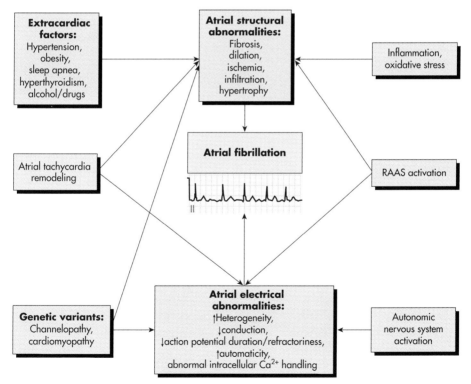

Algorithm 17.1   Mechanisms of Atrial Fibrillation. *RAAS*, Renin-angiotensin-aldosterone system. (From Parrillo, J. E., & Dellinger, R. P. (2019). *Critical care medicine, principles of diagnosis and management in the adult* (5th ed.). Philadelphia, Elsevier.)

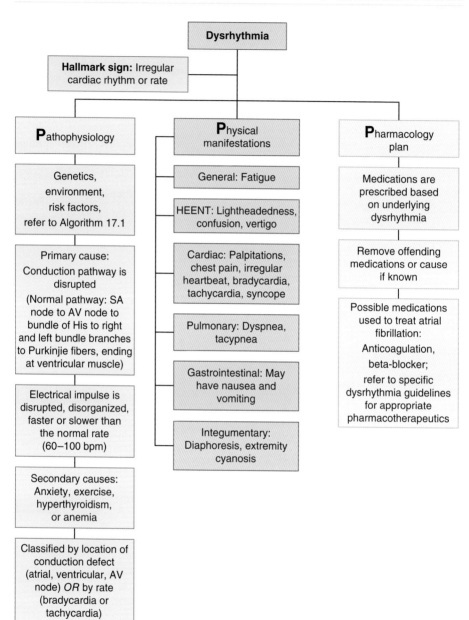

Algorithm 17.2   Dysrhythmia. *AV,* Atrioventricular; *bpm,* beats per minute; *SA,* sinoatrial.

References

Alkhaqani, A. L. (2022). Recognizing and management of arrhythmia: Overview of nurses' role. *International Journal of Nursing and Health Science, 4*(1), 33–40.

Ball, J. W., Dains, J. E., Flynn, J. A., Solomon, B. S., & Stewart, R. W. (2023). *Seidel's guide to physical examination* (10th ed.). Elsevier.

Blaufox, A. D. (2023). *Irregular heart rhythm (arrhythmias) in children.* UpToDate. Retrieved August 28, 2023, from. https://www.uptodate.com/contents/irregular-heart-rhythm-arrhythmias-in-children.

Brashers, V. L. (2023). Alterations of cardiovascular function. In J. L. Rogers (Ed.), *McCance and Huether's pathophysiology: The biologic basis for disease in adults and children* (9th ed., pp. 1059–1103). Elsevier.

Centers for Disease Control and Prevention. (2022). Atrial fibrillation: What is atrial fibrillation? Accessed September 6, 2023, from https://www.cdc.gov/heartdisease/atrial_fibrillation.htm#:~:text=Facts%20About%20AFib,will%20have%20AFib%20in%202030.&text=In%202019%2C%20AFib%20was%20mentioned,in%2026%2C535%20of%20those%20deaths.&text=People%20of%20European%20descent%20are,have%20AFib%20than%20African%20Americans.

Dains, J. E., Baumann, L. C., & Scheibel, P. (2024). *Advanced health assessment & clinical diagnosis in primary care* (7th ed.). Elsevier.

Gharacholou, M., & Bungo, C (2022). Coronary artery disease and atrial fibrillation. In G. A. Warshaw, J. F. Potter, E. Flaherty, M. T. Heflin, M. K. McNabney, & R. J. Ham (Eds.), *Ham's primary care geriatrics* (7th ed., pp. 361–378). Elsevier.

Goolsby, M. J., & Grubbs, G. L. (2019). *Advanced assessment: Interpreting findings and formulating differential diagnoses* (4th ed.). F. A. Davis Company.

Lévy, S., Steinbeck, G., Santini, L., Nabauer, M., Maceda, D. P., Kantharia, B. K., Saksena, S., & Cappato, R. (2022). Management of atrial fibrillation: Two decades of progress—A scientific statement from the European Cardiac Arrhythmia Society. *Journal of Interventional Cardiac Electrophysiology, 65*(1), 287–326.

Tsao, C. W., Aday, A. W., Almarzooq, Z. I., Alonso, A., Beaton, A. Z., Bittencourt, M. S., Boehme, A. K., Buxton, A. E., Carson, A. P., Commodore-Mensah, Y., Elkind, M. S. V., Evenson, K. R., Eze-Nliam, C., Ferguson, J. F., Generoso, G., Ho, J. E., Kalani, R., Khan, S. S., & Kissela, B. M., … American Heart Association Council on Epidemiology and Prevention Statistics Committee and Stroke Statistics Subcommittee. (2022). Heart disease and stroke statistics—2022 update: A report from the American Heart Association. *Circulation, 145*(8), e153–e639.

Tsao, C. W., Aday, A. W., Almarzooq, Z. I., Anderson, C. A., Arora, P., Avery, C. L., Baker-Smith, C. M., Beaton, A. Z., Boehme, A. K., Buxton, A. E., Commodore-Mensah, Y., Elkind, M. S. V., Evenson, K. R., Eze-Nliam, C., Fugar, S., Generoso, G., Heard, D. G., Hiremath, S., & Ho, J. E., … American Heart Association Council on Epidemiology and Prevention Statistics Committee and Stroke Statistics Subcommittee. (2023). Heart disease and stroke statistics—2023 update: A report from the American Heart Association. *Circulation,, 147*(8), e93–e621.

Virani, S. S., Alonso, A., Aparicio, H. J., Benjamin, E. J., Bittencourt, M. S., Callaway, C. W., Carson, A. P., Chamberlain, A. M., Cheng, S., Delling, F. N., Elkind, M. S. V., Evenson, K. R., Ferguson, J. F., Gupta, D. K., Khan, S. S., Kissela, B. M., Knutson, K. L., Lee, C. D., Lewis, T. T., … Tsao, C. W. (2021). Heart disease and stroke statistics—2021 update: A report from the American Heart Association. *Circulation, 143*(8), CIR0000000000000950. https://www.ahajournals.org/doi/10.1161/CIR.0000000000000950.

Heart Failure

Julia L. Rogers

Heart Failure

Heart failure (HF) is the result of different pathophysiologic processes that cause abnormalities in systolic function, diastolic function, or both due to structural and/or functional irregularities resulting in inadequate ventricular filling and reduced cardiac output (Harrington et al., 2023; Heidenreich et al., 2022; McDonagh et al., 2022). HF affects approximately 6.7 million Americans and causes 1 in 9 deaths in the United States (American Heart Association [AHA], 2024a; Brashers, 2023a; Tsao et al., 2023) (Box 18.1).

HF is classified as acute (Fig. 18.1 and Box 18.2) or chronic, left sided or right sided, and HF with preserved ejection fraction (HFpEF), HF with reduced ejection fraction (HFrEF), or HF with mildly reduced ejection fraction (HFmEF) (Table 18.1). Acute HF develops very suddenly whereas chronic HF is a long-term condition that gradually worsens over time. Chronic HF may suddenly worsen or exacerbate, in which case the individual may have acute on chronic HF. HFrEF is defined as having a left ventricular ejection failure (LVEF) of 40% or lower and HFpEF is defined as having an LVEF of 50% or higher (Heidenreich et al., 2022). HF and an LVEF between the HFrEF and HFpEF range are termed as HF with midrange EF or HF with mildly reduced EF (HFmrEF) (Heidenreich et al., 2022). The classification of HF is also differentiated by whether the right side or left side of the circulatory system is affected. Left-sided HF is associated with underlying risk factors such as coronary artery disease (CAD), hypertension (HTN), myocarditis, and valvular disease whereas right-sided HF is associated with chronic obstructive pulmonary disease (COPD), pulmonary hypertension, pulmonary valve stenosis, pulmonary embolism (PE), and pericardial effusion.

Other disease processes or conditions can be worsened by the decreased blood flow and oxygenation that result from HF or can contribute to the development of HF by placing added strain on the heart muscle. There are several risk factors for HF, including HTN (see Chapter 20), CAD (see Chapter 16), atherosclerotic cardiovascular disease (ASCVD) (see Chapter 19), diabetes (see Chapter 14), and obesity. Every 3.36 pounds per feet (5 kg/m) increase in body mass index (BMI) is associated with a 41% increased risk for HF (Tsao et al., 2023). Other contributing factors include underlying systemic illnesses or connective tissue disease such as sarcoidosis, lupus, rheumatoid arthritis (see Chapter 8), scleroderma, and hypothyroidism (see Chapter 15) (Harrington et al., 2023). Medications and/or substances such as cardiotoxic chemotherapy, cocaine, alcohol, and methamphetamines can also increase the risk for HF (Harrington et al., 2023).

Pathophysiology

HF is due to myocardial dysfunction resulting in a failure to pump (systolic) or elevated filling pressures (diastolic). Contributing factors include structural abnormalities of the valves, pericardium, and endocardium and functional irregularities of heart rhythm and conduction (see Chapter 17) (Harrington et al., 2023; McDonagh et al., 2022). The heart attempts to compensate by contracting more quickly to increase output. Over time, the heart develops more muscle mass as the

BOX 18.1 ■ Diversity Considerations

There are important differences in heart failure (HF) incidence, risk factors, clinical care needs, and outcomes among specific patient populations. It is important for health care providers to be aware of the biological factors, social determinants of health, and implicit biases that impact the burden of disease, clinical decision making, and effective delivery of medical care directed by guidelines. HF may look different in females than in males because of differing heart and artery size and the effect of estrogen on females. It has been shown that an estimated 59% of females with hypertension are diagnosed with HF and that females with HF are more likely to have diabetes than males. Also concerning are the racial and ethnic disparities in mortality rates from HF, with non-Hispanic Black patients having the highest death rate per capita. Survival rates for females with HF are more favorable despite presenting with HF later in life, having more comorbidities, and having a lower patient-reported health status than males. The highest incidence of HF is observed in self-identified Black patients with higher hospitalization and mortality rates than for White patients. Important strategies to remove biases among health care professionals and systems impacting minority and socioeconomically disadvantaged patient populations include implicit bias training, recruiting a diverse workforce, and promoting broad access to HF care (Nayak et al., 2020).

BOX 18.2 ■ Acute Care Considerations

Acute decompensated heart failure is a life-threatening medical condition that requires acute care treatment with a multidisciplinary approach. Patients should understand the importance of going to the hospital for care when an acute exacerbation occurs. Patients should be assessed for dyspnea severity, hemodynamic status, heart rhythm, and fluid status. Providers should carefully assess for clinical manifestations associated with hypoperfusion, cardiac and pulmonary congestion, peripheral edema, and jugular venous dilatation (JVD). Diagnostic testing should include electrocardiogram, thoracic ultrasound, chest X-ray, echocardiogram, and computed tomography (CT) scan. Monitoring labs of brain natriuretic peptide (BNP), troponin, renal function tests, liver function tests, and complete blood count (CBC) are important to determine severity. Immediate therapy should be provided if the patient has hypoxemia by ordering noninvasive oxygen therapy. Loop diuretics are key in treatment to reduce the amount of congestion and fluid. If there is an underlying cause such as an infection, it should be treated as soon as it is known. The criteria to move a patient from a telemetry floor to the intensive care unit are (1) if the patient requires intubation, (2) has evidence of hypoperfusion with hypoxemia, (3) has increased respirations with accessary muscle use, (4) has symptomatic bradycardia or tachycardia, and/or (5) has systolic blood pressure less than 90 mm Hg (Njoroge & Teerlink, 2021).

contracting cells become larger, and the heart stretches to contract more forcefully to keep up with the demand to pump more blood (AHA, 2024a). This eventually is followed by the inability of the left ventricle to contract properly, resulting in HF. The body will attempt to maintain homeostasis by activating the renin-angiotensin-aldosterone system (RAAS), a compensatory mechanism for maintaining adequate cardiac output. RAAS leads to vasoconstriction and fluid and sodium retention, which aids in oxygen perfusion by maintaining blood pressure and flow. However, over the long term this mechanism causes more cardiac dysfunction and negative remodeling. Another mechanism, activation of the sympathetic nervous system, improves stroke volume by increasing heart rate and myocardial contractility. However, this also eventually leads to negative remodeling and left ventricular dysfunction from the increased afterload (Harrington et al., 2023).

HFrEF AND HFpEF

HFrEF and HFpEF represent two distinct disease entities, each with a different pathophysiology. HFrEF is initiated by an insult to the heart muscle, leading to reduced cardiac output triggering a cascade of maladaptive processes (Simmonds et al., 2020). An increased cardiac workload results

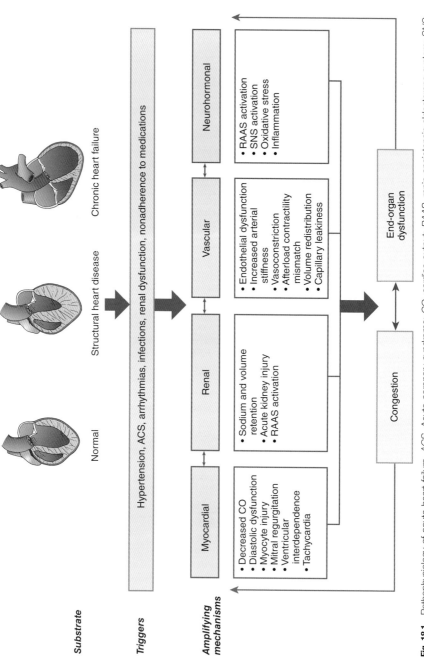

Fig. 18.1 Pathophysiology of acute heart failure. *ACS*, Acute coronary syndrome; *CO*, cardiac output; *RAAS*, renin-angiotensin-aldosterone system; *SNS*, sympathetic nervous system. (From Zipes, D. P. (2019). *Braunwald's heart disease, a textbook of cardiovascular medicine* (11th ed.). Philadelphia, Elsevier.)

TABLE 18.1 ■ Classification and Treatment of Heart Failure

Stage A: At risk for HF	Stage B: Pre-HF	Stage C: Symptomatic HF (current or previous manifestations) Stage D: Advanced HF (manifestations that interfere with ADLs and/or recurrent hospitalizations)			
		HFrEF	HFmrEF: Evidence of spontaneous or provokable LV filling pressures	HFimpEF: Previous diagnosis of HFrEF and evidence of spontaneous or provokable LV filling pressures	HFpEF: Evidence of spontaneous or provokable LV filling pressures
No structural or functional heart disease; no biomarker abnormalities	No current or previous clinical manifestations of HF, but has one of the following: Structural heart disease, evidence of increased filling pressures, risk factors, and increased BNP OR				
No current or previous clinical manifestations of HF, but with risk factors: Hypertension, CVD, DM, obesity, toxic exposure, genetic variant or family history of cardiomyopathy	Persistently elevated troponin in the absence of comorbid diagnosis				
LVEF ≥50%	LVEF ≥50%	LVEF ≤40%	LVEF 41%–49%	LVEF >40%	LVEF ≥50%
Treatment					
SGL2i with DM	SGL2i with DM	ARNi in NYHA II and III	Diuretics PRN		Diuretics PRN
Blood pressure control	ACEi	ACEi or ARB in NYHA II–IV	SGL2i		SGL2i
CVD management	ARB if ACEi intolerant	Beta-blocker			
	Beta-blocker	MRA	ACEi, ARB, ARNi		ARNi
	Blood pressure control	SGL2i	MRA		MRA
	CVD management	Diuretics PRN			ARB
		Hydral nitrates in NYHA III and IV in Black patients	Beta-blockers for HFrEF		
		Ivabradine			
		Vericiguat			
		Digoxin			
		PUFA			
		Potassium binders			

Continued

TABLE 18.1 ■ Classification and Treatment of Heart Failure—cont'd

| | | Stage C: Symptomatic HF (current or previous manifestations) Stage D: Advanced HF (manifestations that interfere with ADLs and/or recurrent hospitalizations) | | | |
Stage A: At risk for HF	Stage B: Pre-HF				
Steps					
Step 1	Step 2	Step 3	Step 4	Step 5	Step 6
Establish diagnosis (HFrEF).	Titrate medication as tolerated to target dose.	Consider patient scenarios.	Implement additional GDMT and device therapy as indicated.	Reassess symptoms, labs, health status, and LVEF.	Refer to HF specialist.
Evaluate and treat fluid overload/congestion.	Obtain initial labs, evaluate current health status, and determine LVEF.	Discuss palliative care, end-of-life care, and treatment targets.	Discuss treatment targets.	Discuss palliative care, end-of-life care, and treatment targets.	Discuss palliative care, end-of-life care, and treatment targets.
Initiate GDMT.	Discuss treatment targets.	Establish health goals, adherence, and optimizing therapy.	Establish health goals, adherence, and optimizing therapy.	Establish health goals, adherence, and optimizing therapy.	Establish health goals, adherence, and optimizing therapy.
Discuss treatment targets.	Establish health goals, adherence, and optimizing therapy.				
Establish health goals, adherence, and optimizing therapy.					

ACEi, Angiotensin-converting enzyme inhibitor; *ADLs*, activities of daily living; *ARB*, angiotensin receptor blocker; *ARNi*, angiotensin receptor-neprilysin inhibitor; *BNP*, brain natriuretic peptide; *CVD*, cardiovascular disease; *DM*, diabetes mellitus; *EF*, ejection fraction; *GDMT*, guideline-directed medical therapy; *HFimpEF*, heart failure with improved ejection fraction; *HFmrEF*, heart failure with mildly reduced ejection fraction; *HFpEF*, heart failure with preserved ejection; *HFrEF*, heart failure with reduced ejection fraction; *LV*, left ventricular; *LVEF*, left ventricular ejection failure; *MRA*, mineralocorticoid receptor antagonists; *NYHA*, New York Heart Association; *PRN*, as needed; *SGL2i*, sodium/glucose cotransporter-2 inhibitor.

(Harrington et al., 2023; Heidenreich et al., 2022)

from dysregulation of cardiac muscle contractions, which reduces the ability of the heart to pump enough blood to meet the body's need for blood and oxygen.

The pathophysiology of HFpEF is not fully understood, partially due to the heterogeneity of the underlying chronic comorbidity causes, such as left ventricular hypertrophy, arterial hypertension, diastolic dysfunction, type 2 diabetes mellitus, obesity, renal insufficiency, fibrosis, pulmonary disease (see Chapters 22 and 23), liver disease, sleep apnea, gout, and cancer. HFpEF is characterized by structural and cellular alterations (e.g., cardiomyocyte hypertrophy and intercellular fibrosis) that lead to inflammation, altered cardiomyocyte relaxation, and an inability of the left ventricle to relax properly. The inflammatory process in HFpEF is a common link to the comorbidities, which also activate inflammation (Brashers, 2023a).

HF is also classified according to whether the right side or left side of the circulatory system is affected. Left-sided dysfunction is related to volume overload and increases pulmonary pressure. This causes the clinical manifestations associated with pulmonary congestion such as dyspnea, tachypnea, and rales (Harrington et al., 2023). Peripheral edema of the lower extremities is associated with right sided HF and results from increased capillary pressures in the peripheral circulation caused by overfilling of the vascular system due to impaired cardiac output (Ellinas, 2019)

The pathophysiologic processes are directly related to the physical clinical manifestations assessed in HF. Low cardiac output combined with impaired pulmonary gas exchange result in a multitude of clinical manifestations. In response to hypoxic cell metabolism, sinus tachycardia ensues as a compensatory mechanism to adapt to the physiologic and hemodynamic deficits. An S4 gallop may result from atrial contraction with rapid ejection of blood into the rigid and noncompliant ventricle in late diastole (Brashers, 2023a). Fluid accumulates in the alveoli and airways from shifting capillary fluid, resulting in pulmonary edema (increased afterload) and causing a cough with white or pink frothy sputum. The movement of air through the alveolar fluid produces pulmonary crackles or rales during auscultation of breath sounds. Diminished breath sounds can be an indication of a pleural effusion from the excess fluid (Ellinas, 2019). Pulmonary edema causes lung stiffness and poor lung expansion and impairs gas exchange. Since the lungs have a decreased ability to oxygenate the blood, hemoglobin leaves the pulmonary circulation without being fully oxygenated, resulting in shortness of breath and peripheral cyanosis from poorly oxygenated peripheral tissues (Ellinas, 2019). Hepatomegaly, abdominal tenderness, or ascites may occur with venous distention, congestion, and/or pressure of the hepatic veins (Ellinas, 2019). This usually reflects right ventricular failure and chronic elevation of systemic venous pressure in HF.

Medications are directly linked to inhibiting the pathophysiologic processes involved in HF. For example, the angiotensin receptor-neprilysin inhibitor (angiotensin II receptor blocker [ARB] + neprilysin inhibitor) blocks angiotensin II–mediated activity while the neprilysin inhibitor prevents degradation of atrial natriuretic peptide (ANP), brain natriuretic peptide (BNP), and bradykinin, allowing low blood pressure and lower contractility while improving vasodilation and permeability (Heidenreich et al., 2022). Angiotensin-converting enzyme (ACE) inhibitors reduce preload and afterload by stopping the RAAS cycle from converting angiotensin I to angiotensin II, which allows improved cardiac output by controlling the compensatory action (vasoconstriction) of the RAAS. Finally, ARBs work by inhibiting angiotensin II from binding to its target cell receptors, disrupting its effects. Diuretics are able to reduce preload by eliminating excess fluid through micturition and are considered a mainstay of therapy. Sodium restriction and aldosterone blockers can also be incorporated into treatment plans (Brashers, 2023a).

Physical Clinical Presentation

SUBJECTIVE

The history and physical examination provide useful information to the health care provider about the cause of an underlying cardiomyopathy, including the possibility of an inherited or congenital link. A thorough history can provide clues as to the reason why a stable chronic patient developed an acute

BOX 18.3 ■ Pediatric Considerations

There are risk factors associated with congenital heart disease that the health care provider should include in the family, maternal, fetal, neonatal, and infant medical histories when performing a physical examination in school-age children. The risk factors to assess in the medical history are (1) deviation from normal growth and development, (2) activity less than peers, (3) frequent infections, and (4) illnesses lasting longer than usual in the age group. Physical examination findings may include the presence of a murmur, hypertension, chest pain with exertion, shortness of breath with minimal activity, dizziness or syncope, and fluttering in the chest (tachycardia, bradycardia, bounding pulse, or irregular rhythm).

BOX 18.4 ■ Older Adult Considerations

The incidence of heart failure (HF) increases with age. Approximately 10% of all persons aged 65 years and older have a diagnosis of HF. The geriatric population continues to have a high mortality rate despite promising medications and treatments over the past decade. The 5-year survival rate is only 50%. HF leads to more than 1 million hospital admissions annually, contributing to chronic disability in this population. The geriatric patient may present with atypical symptoms such as abdominal pain and bloating, anorexia, chest pain, delirium, irritability, insomnia, and depression. There are concerns about the diagnostic utility of the brain natriuretic peptide (BNP) and probrain natriuretic peptide (pBNP) because these values can be altered due to age, gender, and renal function. Furthermore, when initiating or changing treatment, it is best to start low and slow due to a decreased ability for elderly patients to metabolize the medications. It is important to discuss both pharmacotherapy and nonpharmacotherapy options. One important educational topic is diet. Patients should be informed about the appropriate amount of dietary salt intake as well as monitoring fluid intake. Older patients with HF are especially vulnerable to polypharmacy, multimorbidity, cognitive decline, and frailty, all of which the health care provider should address (Dixon & Rich, 2022).

exacerbation leading to decompensated HF. A critical component is to assess for clinical manifestations resulting from elevated cardiac filling pressures and congestion (Heidenreich et al., 2022).

The cardinal subjective symptoms that individuals report with HF are dyspnea, lower extremity peripheral edema bilaterally, and fatigue. Other common complaints include chest pain, pressure, or heaviness; palpitations; and cough (Goolsby & Grubbs, 2019). During the focused cardiovascular history, documentation should include the onset of symptoms, precipitating events, and location, intensity, quality, and progression of pain and symptoms. Specifically, ask about orthopnea and how many pillows are used in bed or if the patient sleeps in a recliner.

Investigate alleviating and aggravating factors, documenting whether chest pain resolves with rest and/or worsens with increased exertional activity or with routine activities of daily living. Ask if the individual experienced previous episodes and list all associated symptoms. Document allergies and past medical, social, and family histories. This is important when caring for pediatric and older adult patients (Boxes 18.3 and 18.4).

Past medical history is important to obtain, evaluating the presence of common causes of HF such as CAD, angina (see Chapter 16), acute coronary syndrome, ischemic heart disease, myocardial infarction (MI), HTN, arrythmias (see Chapter 17), or valvular heart disease. Other important information to collect includes history of autoimmune diseases such as amyloidosis or sarcoidosis; previous cardiotoxicity from chemotherapy or other treatments; history of iron overload including hemochromatosis (see Chapter 11); previous tachycardia, right ventricular pacing, or stress-induced cardiomyopathies; peripartum cardiomyopathy; or myocarditis. Also ask about endocrine (thyroid or diabetes mellitus) (see Chapters 14 and 15), metabolic, or nutritional causes related to HF (Heidenreich et al., 2022). List any cardiovascular-related procedures or surgeries (e.g., angiography, angioplasty, stent placement, or coronary artery bypass graft) (Centers for Disease Control and Prevention [CDC], 2024).

Social history plays an integral role in the development of HF. Therefore, document any current or previous tobacco use (cigarettes, cigars, vaping) and substance abuse with alcohol, cocaine, methamphetamines, or illegal substances. Home and work environments should also be evaluated for a causal relationship to HF including sedentary lifestyle, social environment, change in seasons, sunlight exposure, circadian rhythms, green space, air pollution, noise pollution, and social determinants of health (Bhatnagar, 2017; Czepluch et al., 2018).

An essential step in preventing heart disease and associated complications is documenting the family history. If a genetic or inherited cardiomyopathy is suspected, document at least three generations, listing any first- and second-degree relatives with CVD or congenital heart disease. Health care providers should ask about any family history of CAD, MI, HTN, angina, arrhythmias, cardiomyopathy, HF, cerebral vascular accidents, and sudden cardiac death, making sure to provide the age at diagnosis (Goolsby & Grubbs, 2019; Heidenreich et al., 2022).

OBJECTIVE*

Generalized: Fatigue; generalized weakness; activity intolerance

   Neurological: <u>Confusion (seen with hypoxia)</u>

   Neck: Positive jugular vein distention; bruits (carotid stenosis)

   Cardiovascular: Tachycardia; HTN, **normal S_1/S_2 with S_4 gallop; laterally displaced point of maximal impulse**; orthopnea

   Pulmonary: *Inspection:* **Labored respirations; dyspnea; tachypnea; hypoxemia, use of accessory muscles;** cough (**<u>pink frothy sputum</u>**)

   Palpation: Tactile fremitus; egophony; chest expansion and respiratory excursion bilaterally

   Percussion: Dull

   Auscultation: **Rales**; diminished (pleural effusion); **wheezing; coarse rhonchi**

   Gastrointestinal: Distended; **<u>ascites</u>; <u>hepatomegaly</u>**

   Palpation: Tenderness with deep palpation; deep liver palpation

   Percussion: Liver upper and lower borders to assess for hepatomegaly due to volume overload

   Genitourinary: Nocturia

   Integumentary: Cool; **<u>clammy</u>; <u>cyanosis</u>**; pallor

   Extremities: Edema (pitting) worse in lower extremities bilaterally; **nail clubbing**; cyanosis; delayed capillary refill (>3 seconds); pulses weak (radial, posterior tibialis, dorsalis pedis)

   Psychiatric: Anxious

   (Ball et al., 2023; Dains et al., 2024; Goolsby & Grubbs, 2019; Harrington et al. 2023; Heidenreich et al., 2022; Rogers, 2023)

Evaluation and Differential Diagnoses

DIAGNOSTICS

- Labs
  - BNP and NT-proBNP
  - Troponin
  - D-dimer
  - Complete blood count
  - Complete metabolic panel (including sodium, potassium, calcium, magnesium, and glucose; blood urea nitrogen and serum creatinine)
  - Lipid panel
  - Thyroid-stimulating hormone

*****Hallmark signs are bolded** and <u>**Red flags are bolded and underlined**</u>. *Italics are for assessment techniques.*

- Urinalysis
- Liver function tests
- Iron studies (serum iron, ferritin, transferrin saturation
- Diagnostic imaging
  - Cardiac imaging tests, including repeat tests, are performed only when the results have a meaningful impact on clinical care.
  - Electrocardiogram
  - Comprehensive transthoracic echocardiogram/2D echocardiogram (assesses cardiac structure and function; identifies abnormalities of myocardium, heart valves, and pericardium):
    - The determination of LVEF is a fundamental step to classify HF and to guide evidence-based pharmacologic and device-based therapy.
  - Cardiac ultrasound
  - Chest radiograph (assesses cardiomegaly, pulmonary venous congestion, and interstitial or alveolar edema)
  - Coronary angiography (presence of significant CAD)
  - Cardiac magnetic resonance, single-photon emission computed tomography, or radionuclide ventriculography; positron emission tomography or cardiac computed tomography scan (detection of myocardial ischemia to help guide coronary revascularization decisions)
  - Stress test
  - Spirometry
  - Bilateral lower extremity doppler (rule out deep vein thrombosis)
  - Cardiopulmonary exercise testing and the 6-minute walk test (quantify functional capacity)
- Additional diagnostic studies required to diagnose specific causes
  - Ischemic cardiomyopathy, cardiac amyloidosis, sarcoidosis, hemochromatosis, infection (HIV, COVID-19, Chagas), thyroid dysfunction, acromegaly, connective tissue disorders, tachycardia-induced cardiomyopathy, Takotsubo cardiomyopathy, peripartum cardiomyopathy, cardiotoxicity with cancer therapies, or substance abuse
- There are biomarkers for monitoring diagnosis, course, and prognosis in HFrEF, but none for HFpEF (Eidizadeh et al., 2023). There are established pharmacologic agents and devices that have improved symptoms and prognosis in HFrEF. However, only inhibition of the sodium-glucose cotransporter 2 (SGLT2) inhibitor has improved symptoms in HFpEF (Eidizadeh et al., 2023).
(Goolsby & Grubbs, 2019; Heidenreich et al., 2022)

DIFFERENTIAL DIAGNOSIS

- Chronic obstructive pulmonary disease
- Pulmonary hypertension
- Lung cancer

Plan

The New York Heart Association (NYHA) developed a functional classification system that delineates classes I through IV of HF based on subjective symptoms with exertional activity and classes A through D of HF based on objective findings with physical activity. The NYHA HF class assessment defines candidates for certain treatments (https://heart.org/en/health-topics/heart-failure/what-is-heart-failure/classes-of-heart-failure).

Guideline Resources

- Heidenreich, P. A., Bozkurt, B., Aguilar, D., Allen, L. A., Byun, J. J., Colvin, M. M., Deswal, A., Drazner, M. H., Dunlay, S. M., Evers, L. R., Fang, J. C., Fedson, S. E., Fonarow, G.

C., Hayek, S. S., Hernandez, A. F., Khazanie, P., Kittleson, M. M., Lee, C. S., Link, M. S., … Yancy, C. W. (2022). 2022 AHA/ACC/HFSA guideline for the management of heart failure: Executive summary: A report of the American College of Cardiology/American Heart Association Joint Committee on Clinical Practice Guidelines. *Circulation, 145*(18), e876–e894. https://doi.org/10.1161/cir.0000000000001062.

Pharmacotherapy

- Medications
    - See Table 18.1.
    - Stage B:
        - ACE inhibitor
        - ARB if ACE inhibitor intolerant
        - Beta-blocker
    - HFpEF stages C and D
        - Diuretic as needed
        - SGLT2
        - ARNi
        - MRA
        - ARB
    - HFrEF stages C and D
        - ARNi (NYHA II and III)
        - ACE inhibitor or ARB (NYHA II–IV)
        - Beta–blocker (MI or acute coronary syndrome)
        - MRA
        - SGLT2
        - Diuretic
        - Hydral nitrates (NYHA III and IV for Black patients)
        - Ivabradine
        - Vericiguat
        - Digoxin
        - PUFA
        - Potassium binders
        - Statin
    - HFmEF/HFimpEF stages C and D:
        - Diuretic
        - SGLT2
        - ACE inhibitor
        - ARB
        - ARNi
        - MRA
        - Beta-blocker
        - Algorithm 18.1
    - Medications and treatment for comorbid conditions (Table 18.2)
- Smoking cessation aids should be offered to any person currently smoking tobacco.
- Vaccines: Influenza annually, pneumococcal, COVID-19, and zoster according to CDC guidelines and recommendations

ANRi, Angiotensin receptor-neprilysin inhibitor (ARB + sacubitril or Entresto); *ARB*, angiotensin receptor blocker; *MRA*, mineralocorticoid receptor antagonists.

(Heidenreich et al., 2022)

TABLE 18.2 ■ **Comorbid Conditions and Treatment**

Comorbid Condition	Treatment		
Anemia Iron deficiency	Ferritin <100 mcg/L	IV repletion of iron	Erythropoietin stimulating agents are *not recommended*, because they are associated with worse long-term outcomes for patients with HF who have anemia.
Hypertension	Guidelines recommend BP goal of <130/80 mm Hg	Antihypertensives: Titrate medications prescribed for HF to reach goal	Risk of incident HF significantly decreases with a systolic blood pressure target of <120 mm Hg.
Sleep disorders CSA OSA		CPAP can be used to treat OSA and CSA and is associated with improved sleep quality and nocturnal oxygenation.	ASV treatment is *not recommended*, because it is associated with increased mortality rates in those with HFrEF.
Cardiac amyloidosis	Presence of monoclonal light chains Absence of monoclonal light chains and presence of abnormal technetium-99 m pyrophosphate imaging study Individualize treatment based on whether the patient has HFrEF.	Refer the patient to hematology and oncology specialists. Gene sequencing is recommended and genetic counseling and screening is recommended for family members. Tafamidis for patients with NYHA I–III symptoms (class I symptoms, no physical activity limitations; class II, slight limitation; class III, marked limitation)	
Atrial fibrillation	CHA2DS2-VASc risk assessment in males with score of ≥1 or in females with score of ≥2	Anticoagulation	
Cardiomyopathy	Family history that includes at least three generations with weak, enlarged, or thick heart; history of HF, muscular dystrophy, pacemaker or defibrillator use; or sudden death. Identify family members currently on a transplant list.		

TABLE 18.2 ■ Comorbid Conditions and Treatment—cont'd

Comorbid Condition	Treatment	
Malignancy	An interprofessional team should evaluate risk–benefit ratio to determine whether chemotherapy should be continued or temporarily or permanently discontinued	Before initiating chemotherapy, patients at risk for CVD or with known CVD should have cardiac function evaluated and monitored at regular intervals throughout treatment.
		Use of an ACEi, ARB, or beta-blocker benefits in preventing drug-induced cardiomyopathy.
		These medications also help prevent the progression of HF and improve cardiac function in patients with cancer-related cardiomyopathy whose EF is <50%.

ACEi, Angiotensin-converting enzyme inhibitor; *ASV*, adaptive sero-ventilation; CHA2DS2-VASc scoring system: C: Congestive heart failure, H: Hypertension, A: Age ≥75 (double score), D: Diabetes, S2: Prior stroke or transient ischemic attack (TIA), V: Vascular disease, S: Sex category (female); *CPAP*, continuous positive airway pressure; *CVD*, cardiovascular disease; *CSA*, central sleep apnea; EF, ejection fraction; *HF*, heart failure; *HFrEF*, heart failure with reduced ejection fraction; *IV*, intravenous; *NYHA*, New York Heart Association; *OSA*, obstructive sleep apnea (Harrington et al., 2023; Heidenreich et al., 2022).

NONPHARMACOTHERAPY

- Primary prevention lifestyle and behavioral modifications
  - Stages A and B (see Table 18.1)
  - Maintain normal blood pressure. Goal is <130/80 with a CVD risk of ≥10%.
  - Maintain normal glucose:
    - SGLT2 type 2 diabetes mellitus
  - Heart healthy diet: Dietary Approaches to Stop Hypertension diet
  - Limit sodium intake to <1500 mg daily.
  - Limit saturated fats, trans fats, cholesterol, red meat, sweets, and sugary beverages (AHA, 2024a).
  - Limit fluid intake (recommendation per health care provider).
  - Regular physical activity
  - Maintain normal body mass index.
  - Screen at-risk individuals with BNP and calculate risk scores.
  - Smoking cessation
  - Limit alcohol consumption to 1 to 2 drinks daily for males and 1 drink daily for females.
  - Screen for and address social determinants of health (socioeconomic status, food insecurity, homelessness or housing insecurity, abuse, limited English proficiency, low health literacy, social isolation, and limited transportation).
  - Evaluate for medical barriers such as cognitive impairment, depression, substance misuse, and frailty that might affect ability to perform appropriate self-care

(Harrington et al., 2023; Heidenreich et al., 2022)

- Educate
  - Disease process and progression
  - Take medications as prescribed; side effects; importance of compliance
  - Monitor for signs and symptoms of worsening HF.
  - Daily weight
  - Eliminate environmental and occupational irritants, triggers, and/or stressors.
  - Importance of receiving vaccines
  - Self-management/care treatment adherence and health maintenance behaviors
- Estimates of survival
  - Chronic HF:
    - Seattle Heart Failure Model
    - Heart Failure Survival score
    - MAGGIC score
  - Chronic HFrEF:
    - Exercise capacity
    - Natriuretic peptide levels
  - Chronic HFpEF
  - Acute HF short-term survival predictor
- Complementary treatment
  - Psychosocial rehabilitation
  - Physical therapy and occupational therapy
  - Complementary and alternative therapies with natural medicines and supplements may interact with prescription medications. Obtain a complete medication history.
- Referral (identify and refer for treatment of comorbid conditions*)
  - Cardiologist
  - Interventional cardiologist* (cardiac catheterization, percutaneous coronary intervention)
  - Cardiovascular surgeon* (coronary artery bypass graft)
  - Cardiac rehabilitation
  - Transplant center
  - Pulmonologist*(COPD, pulmonary hypertension)
  - Hematologist*(anemia)
  - Dietitian
  - Mental health clinicians* (anxiety, depression)
  - Social workers
  - Palliative care:
    - Patient- and family-centered care with shared decision making about medically reasonable treatment options
    - Advance care planning anticipatory guidance
    - Other supportive needs include home and case management assistance, transportation, and care coordination.
    - Start early and continue across the stages of HF, intensifying in end-stage disease and extending into caregiver bereavement.
- Follow-up
  - Patients at risk for HF screened with BNP or NT-proBNP followed by collaborative care, diagnostic evaluation, and treatment
  - Follow-up appointment within 1 to 2 weeks if recently diagnosed with HF or change in symptoms
  - Follow-up appointment every 1 to 2 months if patient experiencing frequent exacerbations or severe heart failure
  - Follow-up appointment every 3 to 6 months if stable

(Heidenreich, P. A., et al. 2022)

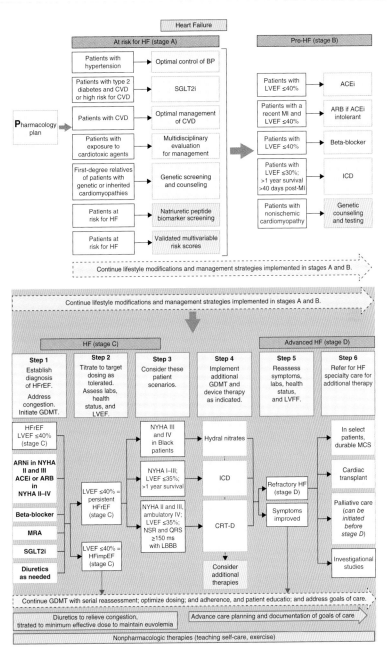

Algorithm 18.1   Heart Failure. (A) At risk for heart failure (HF) (stage A) and pre-HF (stage B). (B) HF (stage C) and advanced HF (stage D). *ACEi*, Angiotensin-converting enzyme inhibitor; *ARB*, angiotensin receptor blocker; *ARNi*, angiotensin receptor neprilysin inhibitor; *BP*, blood pressure; *CRT-D*, cardiac resynchronization therapy with defibrillator; *CVD*, cardiovascular disease; *GDMT*, guideline-directed medical therapy; *HF*, heart failure; *HFimpEF*, heart failure with improved ejection fraction; *HFrEF*, heart failure with reduced ejection fraction; *ICD*, implantable cardiac device; *LBBB*, left bundle branch block; *LVEF*, left ventricular ejection fraction; *MCS*, mechanical circulatory support; *MI*, myocardial infarction; *MRA*, mineralocorticoid receptor antagonist; *NSR*, normal sinus rhythm; *NYHA*, New York Heart Association; *SGLT2i*, sodium-glucose co-transporter-2 inhibitor; *QRS*. (Reprinted with permission Circulation. 2022;145:e895-e1032 ©2022 American Heart Association, Inc. 2022 AHA/ACC/HFSA Guideline for the Management of Heart Failure.)

References

American Heart Association. (2024a). *Heart failure tools and resources.* Retrieved May 9, 2024, from https://www.heart.org/en/health-topics/heart-failure/heart-failure-tools-resources.</bib>

American Heart Association. (2024b). *What is heart failure?* Retrieved May 9, 2024, from https://www.heart.org/en/health-topics/heart-failure/what-is-heart-failure.

Ball, J. W., Dains, J. E., Flynn, J. A., Solomon, B. S., & Stewart, R. W. (2023). *Seidel's guide to physical examination* (10th ed.). Elsevier.

Bhatnagar, A. (2017). Environmental determinants of cardiovascular disease. *Circulation Research, 121*(2), 162–180. https://doi.org/10.1161/circresaha.117.306458.

Brashers, V. (2023a). Alterations of cardiovascular function. In J. L. Rogers (Ed.), *McCance & Huether's pathophysiology: The biological basis for disease in adults and children* (9th ed.). Elsevier.

Brashers, V. L. (2023c). Alterations of pulmonary function. In J. L. Rogers (Ed.), *McCance and Huether's pathophysiology: The biologic basis for disease in adults and children* (9th ed., pp. 1153–1190). Elsevier.

Centers for Disease Control and Prevention. (2024). *Family health history and heart disease.* https://www.cdc.gov/heart-disease-family-history/risk-factors/?CDC_AAref_Val=https://www.cdc.gov/genomics/disease/fh/history_heart_disease.htm.

Czepluch, F. S., Wollnik, B., & Hasenfub, G. (2018). Genetic determinants of heart failure: Facts and numbers. *ESC Heart Failure, 5*(3), 211–217. https://doi.org/10.1002/ehf2.12267.

Dixon, B. M., & Rich, M. W. (2022). Heart failure. In G. A. Warsaw, J. F. Potter, E. Flaherty, M. T. Heflin, M. K. McNabney, & R. J. Ham (Eds.), *Ham's primary care geriatrics* (7th ed.,, pp. 373–378). Elsevier.

Dains, J. E., Baumann, L. C., & Scheibel, P. (2024). *Advanced health assessment & clinical diagnosis in primary care* (7th ed.). Elsevier.

Ellinas, H. (2019). Disorders of cardiac function, and heart failure and circulatory shock. In T. L. Norris (Ed.), *Porth's pathophysiology: Concepts of altered health states* (10th ed., pp. 753–835). Wolters Kluwer.

Eidizadeh, A., Schnelle, M., Leha, A., Edelmann, F., Nolte, K., Werhahn, S. M., Binder, L., & Wachter, R. (2023). Biomarker profiles in heart failure with preserved vs. reduced ejection fraction: Results from the DIAST-CHF study. *ESC Heart Failure, 10*(1), 200–210.

Goolsby, M. J., & Grubbs, L. (2019). Assessment and clinical decision making: An overview. In M. J. Goolsby, & L. Grubbs (Eds.), *Advanced assessment: Interpreting findings and formulating differential diagnoses* (4th ed.). F. A. Davis.

Harrington, D., McDonald Lenahan, C., & Beacom, R. (2023). Heart failure management: Updated guidelines. Understand your role in patient centered care. *American Nurse, 18*(5), 6–11.

Heidenreich, P. A., Bozkurt, B., Aguilar, D., Allen, L. A., Byun, J. J., Colvin, M. M., Deswal, A., Drazner, M. H., Dunlay, S. M., Evers, L. R., Fang, J. C., Fedson, S. E., Fonarow, G. C., Hayek, S. S., Hernandez, A. F., Khazanie, P., Kittleson, M. M., Lee, C. S., Link, M. S., ... Yancy, C. W. (2022). 2022 AHA/ACC/HFSA guideline for the management of heart failure: Executive summary: A report of the American College of Cardiology/American Heart Association Joint Committee on Clinical Practice Guidelines. *Circulation, 145*(18), e876–e894. https://doi.org/10.1161/cir.0000000000001062.

McDonagh, T., Metra, M., Adamo, M., Gardner, R. S., Baumbach, A., Böhm, M., Burri, H., Januzzi, J. L., Čelutkienė, J., Chioncel, O., Cleland, J. G., Coats, A. J., Crespo-Leiro, M. G., Farmakis, D., Gilard, M., Heymans, S., Hoes, A. W., Jaarsma, T., Jankowska, E. A., & Skibelund, A. K. (2022). 2021 ESC guidelines for the diagnosis and treatment of acute and chronic heart failure. *European Journal of Heart Failure, 24*(1), 4–131. https://doi.org/10.1002/ejhf.2333.

Nayak, A., Hicks, A. J., & Morris, A. A. (2020). Understanding the complexity of heart failure risk and treatment in black patients. *Circulation: Heart Failure, 13*(8), e007264.

Njoroge, J. N., & Teerlink, J. R. (2021). Pathophysiology and therapeutic approaches to acute decompensated heart failure. *Circulation Research, 128*(10), 1468–1486.

Rogers, J. L. (2023). *McCance and Huether's pathophysiology: The biologic basis for disease in adults and children* (9th ed.). Elsevier.

Simmonds, S. J., Cuijpers, I., Heymans, S., & Jones, E. A. V. (2020). Cellular and molecular differences between HFpEF and HFrEF: A step ahead in an improved pathological understanding. *Cells, 9*(1), 242. https://doi.org/10.3390/cells9010242.

Tsao, C. W., Aday, A. W., Almarzooq, Z. I., Anderson, C. A., Arora, P., Avery, C. L., Baker-Smith, C. M., Beaton, A. Z., Boehme, A. K., Buxton, A. E., Commodore-Mensah, Y., Elkind, M. S. V., Evenson, K. R., Eze-Nliam, C., Fugar, S., Generoso, G., Heard, D. G., Hiremath, S., & Ho, J. E., ... American Heart Association Council on Epidemiology and Prevention Statistics Committee and Stroke Statistics Subcommittee. (2023). Heart disease and stroke statistics—2023 update: A report from the American Heart Association. *Circulation, 147*(8), e93–e621.

CHAPTER 19

Hyperlipidemia

Julia L. Rogers ▓ Marianne Schallmo

Atherosclerosis

Hyperlipidemia and Atherosclerosis

Atherosclerotic cardiovascular disease (ASCVD) is the buildup of plaque within the arterial walls. Plaque is an accumulation of cells, cholesterol, fatty substances, and other waste products that can develop in any artery of the body (Fig. 19.1). ASCVD is the leading cause of mortality in the United States, causing 1 of every 5 deaths at a cost of greater than $230 billion per year (Grundy et al., 2019; Tsao et al., 2023). Hyperlipidemia is a contributing factor in the development of plaques and ASCVD. Hyperlipidemia is categorized as primary or secondary. Primary hyperlipidemia is a genetic defect that inhibits lipid metabolism and secondary hyperlipidemia is caused by comorbid conditions or medications. The contributing disease processes include diabetes, obesity, chronic kidney disease, hypothyroidism, Cushing's disease, pancreatitis, and excessive alcohol use (Rogers & Baker, 2020a). Medication classes implicated in secondary hyperlipidemia are diuretics, beta-blockers, progestins, steroids, and antiretrovirals (Goolsby & Grubbs, 2019; Rogers & Baker, 2020b). Social determinants of health (SDoH) play a major role in patient outcomes with ASCVD. SDoH are associated with failure to control risk factors, low uptake of prevention implementation strategies, medication nonadherence, and loss to follow-up care (Arnett et al., 2019; Valero-Elizondo et al., 2022) (Box 19.1). ASCVD primary prevention is aimed at individual risk factor assessment and promoting a healthy lifestyle (Tables 19.1 and 19.2). Modifiable risk factors include body mass index (BMI) greater than 30, sedentary lifestyle, high-fat diet, and alcohol and tobacco use; nonmodifiable risk factors include positive family history of ASCVD, age, and gender.

Pathophysiology

HYPERLIPIDEMIA

Hyperlipidemia is an elevated level of any of the serum lipoproteins (i.e., high-density lipoprotein [HDL], low-density lipoprotein [LDL], and very-low-density lipoprotein [VLDL]). Cholesterol and triglycerides are the two primary types of lipids found in lipoproteins. There are two genetic disorders associated with hyperlipidemia: familial hypercholesterolemia and hyperchylomicronemia. Familial hypercholesterolemia leads to ASCVD in childhood and progresses to coronary artery disease (CAD) between the third and fourth decades of life. Hyperchylomicronemia, also seen in childhood, leads to the development of recurrent pancreatitis and hepatosplenomegaly (Goolsby & Grubbs, 2019).

Lipids assist in maintaining daily bodily functions, providing and storing cell energy, producing steroid hormones, and eliminating cells. Lipids enter the body from ingestion of dietary fats and are absorbed in the small intestine (Brashers, 2023). Chylomicrons, the largest lipoproteins,

BOX 19.1 ■ Diversity Considerations

Social determinants of health: Consideration must be given to multiple dimensions of social determinants of health that affect individuals with atherosclerotic cardiovascular disease (ASCVD), including neighborhood environment, community and social context, food poverty, education, and access to health care (Valero-Elizondo et al., 2022).

Ethnic: Since certain ethnic profiles increase ASCVD risk, it is reasonable to obtain a history of identified ethnic groups and adjust treatment, including statin therapy, based on an identified ethnic group (Grundy et al., 2019).

Gender: Conditions specific to females, such as early menopause or conditions that occur during pregnancy (hypertension, preeclampsia, gestational diabetes, preterm delivery, or small for gestational age infant), may increase cardiovascular disease risk. Because statins are contraindicated during pregnancy, females of childbearing age on statin therapy need to use reliable contraceptive methods.

Pregnancy: Because triglycerides and low-density lipoprotein levels rise during pregnancy, there may be a concern in females who have hyperlipidemia before pregnancy. All females regardless of pregnancy status should follow lifestyle modifications to lower cholesterol levels. Most pharmacotherapy is contraindicated during pregnancy; therefore females are advised to stop taking statin therapy, proprotein convertase subtilisin/kexin type 9 inhibitors, fenofibrate, and ezetimibe 1 to 2 months prior to attempting pregnancy or immediately upon positive pregnancy confirmation. Bile acid sequestrants are the only hyperlipidemia medication approved during pregnancy. Females with genetic lipid disorders or severe hypertriglyceridemia should be referred to a lipid specialist prior to pregnancy (Grundy et al., 2019).

---

are formed in the intestine and provide the transportation needed for lipids to move. A carrier protein is required because the lipids are insoluble in water. The chylomicrons primarily contain triglycerides, some of which are extracted and used as an energy source for adipose tissue and muscle, and the remaining components (i.e., cholesterol) are processed in the liver and result in the production of LDL, HDL, and VLDL (Rogers & Baker, 2020b). The liver is the primary regulator of the amount of LDL in the bloodstream. Hepatic receptors bind with LDL molecules and initiate enzymatic degradation, decreasing LDL production. A diet high in fat and cholesterol and/or impairment of the hepatic receptors (i.e., genetic predisposition) leads to increased levels of serum LDL (Brashers, 2023; Rogers & Baker, 2020b).

There are two important enzymes that play a vital role in reducing LDL. The enzyme 3-hydroxy-3-methylglutaryl coenzyme A reductase is a catalyst that produces cholesterol. Therefore inhibitors of this enzyme, also known as statins, are widely used as treatment for hyperlipidemia (Brashers, 2023; Rogers & Baker, 2020b). The proprotein convertase subtilisin/kexin type 9 (PCSK9) is a proteolytic enzyme that is expressed predominantly in the liver and plays a vital role in cholesterol metabolism. The PCSK9-inhibitors prevent LDL receptor degradation, reduce LDL hepatic synthesis, increase LDL clearance, and regulate overall LDL receptor levels (Brashers, 2023; Rogers & Baker, 2020b). Scavenger cells such as monocytes aid the liver in eliminating LDL by attaching to oxidized LDL, penetrating the endothelium, and differentiating into macrophages, which are phagocytic cells that digest excess cholesterol. Macrophages transition into foam cells when the macrophage ingests excessive LDL and becomes oversaturated with LDL, leading to macrophage cell death. The dysfunction of macrophages to metabolize the excess LDL leads to release of cytokines, inflammation within the vascular endothelium, and the formation of foam cells (Brashers, 2023) (Fig. 19.1).

HDL is responsible for removing excess cholesterol from tissues and transporting it to the liver for elimination, a process known as reverse cholesterol transport. Low HDL levels contribute to hyperlipidemia due to the inability to remove the excess cholesterol (Brashers, 2023; Rogers & Baker, 2020b). VLDL is a triglyceride-enriched particle synthesized by the liver. VLDL mainly carries triglycerides, which is how it differentiates from LDL that carries cholesterol (Brashers,

TABLE 19.1 ■ Primary Prevention Strategies Based on Age

	0–19 Years of Age	20–39 Years of Age	40–75 Years of Age	≥76 Years of Age
ASCVD risk assessment	Complete ASCVD risk assessment			
Lifestyle modifications	Discuss lifestyle modifications to reduce lifetime ASCVD risk. Recommendations: ■ Smoking cessation ■ Get at least 150 minutes of moderate-intensity aerobic exercise weekly. ■ Reduce saturated fat to less than 6% of daily calories and limit trans-fat intake. ■ Consume a heart-healthy diet that emphasizes fruits, vegetables, whole grains, poultry, fish, nuts, and nontropical vegetable oils. ■ Limit red and processed meats, sodium, dairy products made with whole milk, and sugar-sweetened foods and beverages. (American Heart Association, 2024)			
Lab work	If LDL ≥190 mg/dL: Start high-intensity statin.			
Other	If history of familial hypercholesterolemia: Start statin.	If LDL 189–160 mg/dL and family history of premature ASCVD and LDL: Consider statin.	If diabetic: Start moderate-intensity statin (or high-intensity statin if multiple ASCVD risk factors). If nondiabetic and LDL 70–189 mg/dL: Treatment plan is based on ASCVD risk assessment. See Table 19.2 for primary prevention strategies based on ASCVD risk score.	

ASCVD, Atherosclerotic cardiovascular disease; *LDL*, low-density lipoprotein.

2023; Rogers & Baker, 2020b). Triglycerides serve as a primary source of fuel for the body. Any nonessential calories consumed are converted into triglycerides and stored in fat cells. Hormones are able to trigger the release of triglycerides for energy needed between meals. Consumption of more calories than the body requires, particularly calories from high-carbohydrate foods, may cause hypertriglyceridemia.

Atherosclerosis

Atherosclerosis is the buildup of plaque in the cardiovascular arterial vessel wall (Fig. 19.1). Atherosclerotic plaques can occur due to any chronic disease process causing endothelial injury, including hypertension, diabetes, smoking, and hyperlipidemia (Brashers, 2023; Rogers & Baker, 2020b). Endothelial damage causes inflammation in the vessel, adherence of monocytes to the arterial walls, and LDL trapping in the subintima, leading to oxidation (Brashers, 2023; Rogers & Baker, 2020b). After consuming the lipids, macrophages form foam cells, which build up and

TABLE 19.2 ■ Primary Prevention Strategies Based on ASCVD Risk Score

ASCVD Risk Score	<5% Low Risk	5%–7.4% Borderline Risk	7.5%–19% Intermediate Risk	≥20% High Risk
Risk discussion	Discuss ASCVD risk and lifestyle modification, heart healthy diet, and exercise.			
Risk enhancers[a]	N/A	If risk enhancers present, consider moderate-intensity statin.	If risk enhancers present, start moderate-intensity statin to lower LDL by 30%–49%.	Start moderate-intensity statin to lower LDL by ≥50%.
Risk decision uncertain	CAC in selected adults to determine treatment			
	CAC = 0, consider statin only if diabetic, current smoker, or family history of coronary heart disease			
	CAC = 1–99, consider statin, especially if ≥55 years of age			
	CAC = ≥100 and/or ≥75th percentile, start statin			

[a]Risk enhancers: Family history of premature ASCVD, persistent elevated LDL ≥160, chronic kidney disease, metabolic syndrome, conditions specific to females (preeclampsia, premature menopause), inflammatory diseases, and ethnicity (South Asian ancestry).

ASCVD, Atherosclerotic cardiovascular disease; *CAC*, coronary artery calcium; *LDL*, low-density lipoprotein.

develop a fatty streak. Growth factors are released and smooth muscle cell proliferation in the vessel triggers expansion of the fatty streak (Brashers, 2023; Rogers & Baker, 2020b). Collagen then develops over the fatty streak, resulting in the formation of a fibrous plaque. The plaque can calcify, expand into the lumen of the vessel, and limit or obstruct blood flow, leading to coronary artery disease, which can lead to acute coronary syndrome (Brashers, 2023; Rogers & Baker, 2020b). Algorithm 17.1 shows the pathophysiologic processes involved in atherosclerosis. Atherosclerotic plaques that form are considered unstable because of the possibility of rupture before fully adhering to the vessel. T lymphocytes are recruited in the same way as monocytes into the intima and are implicated in the formation of atherosclerotic plaques. T cells play a role in triggering inflammation, which is a contributable factor in atherosclerosis. The inflammatory cascade is the reason the high-sensitivity C-reactive protein (hs-CRP) has emerged as a leading biomarker of cardiovascular disease (CVD) risk prediction (Brashers, 2023; Rogers & Baker, 2020b). Atherosclerotic plaques are responsible for an array of CVDs, including acute coronary syndrome, which can include angina and myocardial infarction, cerebral vascular accident, transient ischemic attack, and peripheral arterial disease (Brashers, 2023; Rogers & Baker, 2020b).

Physical Clinical Presentation

SUBJECTIVE

The onset of hyperlipidemia and ASCVD is often subtle and individuals may remain asymptomatic until they experience decreased blood flow to surrounding tissues or organs. The history of present illness documentation should include the onset of chest pain, angina, back pain, or leg pain symptoms. Ask if there were any precipitating events that may have led to the symptoms. Document the location, intensity, and quality of pain (e.g., dull, crushing, stabbing). Ask if the pain radiates anywhere else, such as the arms, neck, back, leg, or buttocks, and ask about other symptoms (shortness of breath, wheezing, cough, edema). Document whether the symptoms have progressed, if there are any alleviating or aggravating factors, previous episodes, and associated symptoms. The medical record should contain information on whether the symptoms worsen with

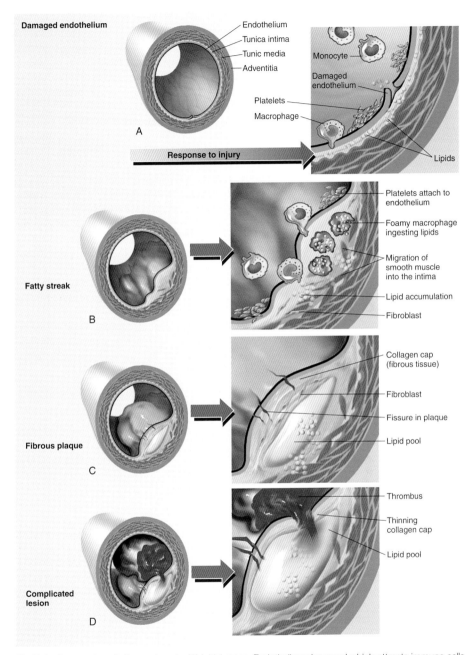

Fig. 19.1 Progression of atherosclerosis. (A) Initial stage: Endothelium damaged which attracts immune cells (i.e. monocytes & macrophages) (B) Fatty streak: Lipids accumulate within smooth muscle cells and macrophages, forming a visible fatty streak in the artery (C) Fibrous plaque: Collagen covers the fatty streak, and smooth muscle cells form a cap over the lipid core, creating a more stable but still problematic plaque (D) Complicated lesion: Advanced stage with severe arterial damage, including thrombosis over a ruptured plaque, foam cells, lipid pools, calcification, and hemorrhage. (From Rogers, J. L. (2024). McCance & Huether's pathophysiology: The biologic basis for disease in adults and children (9th ed.). Elsevier.)

activity and/or are relieved with rest. Pain or shortness of breath may increase when tissue oxygen demand exceeds blood flow capacity, such as during exercise, stress, and cold environments. Partial vessel lumen obstruction can cause inadequate tissue perfusion, which leads to transient signs and symptoms during increased oxygen demand (e.g., exercise). The clinical presentation of atherosclerosis is related to tissue infarction caused by decreased blood flow and supply from narrowing of the vessel lumen. Sudden vessel occlusion may occur due to plaque rupture or thrombosis and is a medical emergency.

Document allergies, current and past medications, and medical, social, and family histories. Medications that may elevate LDL include diuretics, cyclosporin, glucocorticoids, and amiodarone. Medications that may elevate triglycerides include oral estrogen, glucocorticoids, protease inhibitors, and bile acid sequestrants. Past medical history should include disorders that elevate lipid levels, such as hypothyroidism, nephrotic disorder, liver disease, and obesity. Document ASCVD risk factors such as metabolic syndrome, hypertension, diabetes, chronic kidney disease, hyperlipidemia, conditions specific to females (preeclampsia, premature menopause), and inflammatory diseases. Social history should include any habits or lifestyle behaviors that increase the risk for heart disease, such as smoking, as well as secondhand smoke, sedentary lifestyle, high-fat diet, alcohol and drug abuse, and environmental and occupational stress. There are multiple familial associations with dyslipidemia along with CVD and hypertension. Family history is important to document as familial dyslipidemia is an autosomal dominant genetic disorder. Ask about any family history of sudden cardiac death or other CVD-associated deaths and age of event. Document any family dysrhythmias or congenital heart conditions such as Marfan syndrome or prolonged QT syndrome. This is especially important for school-age children when performing sports physicals (Box 19.2). Document any family history of hypercholesterolemia, premature ASCVD, type 2 diabetes, hypertension, or obesity because they are secondary risk factors (increased risks come with young mortality).

OBJECTIVE*

The physical exam is done to determine ASCVD risk factors, any secondary causes for hyperlipidemia, and signs of tissue ischemia or infarction.

Vital signs: *Bradycardia*; **elevated blood pressure**; **increased BMI waist-to-hip measurement ratio**

Generalized: Obesity, *fever*; fatigue

Neurological: <u>Confusion; paresthesia</u>

HEENT: Arcus senilis (hyperlipidemia)

Neck: Bruits; *jugular vein distention (JVD) (right ventricular pressure; right heart failure)*; *thyromegaly; thyroid nodules*

Cardiovascular: Ankle-brachial index; bruits of the carotid artery, renal artery, and abdominal artery; chest pain, tachycardia; *pulsus paradoxes (left ventricular failure)*; *heave or lift (ventricular hypertrophy)*; *splitting first/second heart sounds (right bundle branch block [RBBB], left bundle branch block [LBBB], premature ventricular contraction [PVC])*

Pulmonary: *Inspection: Labored respirations; tachypnea; use of accessory muscles*
Auscultation: Wheezing; coarse rhonchi; rales; diminished (pulmonary disease or congestive heart failure [CHF])

Musculoskeletal: Xanthomas of tendons (hyperlipidemia); *short or tall stature (Turner syndrome or Marfan syndrome causing congenital heart defects)*

Integumentary: Xanthomas/xanthelasma of the skin (hyperlipidemia); **<u>diaphoresis</u>**; **<u>pallor</u>**; **<u>coolness</u>**; hyperpigmentation (arterial/venous insufficiency)

---

*Hallmark signs are bolded and <u>Red flags are bolded and underlined</u>. *Italics represent noncardiac conditions.*

> ### BOX 19.2 ■ Pediatric Considerations
>
> It is prudent to screen all children and adolescents for hyperlipidemia between the ages of 9 and 11 and again between the ages of 17 and 21 (Grundy et al., 2019). Regardless of lipid values, all children and adolescents benefit from therapeutic lifestyle modifications such as exercise, diet, weight management, and smoking cessation (de Ferranti et al., 2019). It is prudent to screen starting at the age of 2 if there is a family history of premature CVD or severe hyperlipidemia (Grundy et al., 2019). Children aged 10 years and older who have a history of familial hypercholesterolemia and despite 6 months of lifestyle changes continue to have an LDL >190 mg/dL may begin statin therapy (de Ferranti et al., 2019). In children or adolescents with severe hyperlipidemia, first-, second-, and possibly third-degree family members may be screened for familial hypercholesterolemia (Grundy et al., 2019).
>
> Children with underlying structural or functional cardiac conditions have elevated premature CVD risk. These individuals may be more susceptible to the adverse effects of traditional cardiovascular risk factors (de Ferranti et al., 2019). In this population, the goal is early risk factor identification and treatment. These risk factors include heterozygous or homozygous familial hypercholesterolemia, hypertension, obesity, and type 2 diabetes. Other potential risk factors include type 1 diabetes, chronic renal disease, childhood cancer treatment, and chronic inflammatory diseases. Specific treatment for each condition is outside the scope of this chapter, but overall management includes lipid screening along with pharmacotherapy and nonpharmacotherapy management of blood pressure, serum LDL and triglycerides, and blood glucose (de Ferranti et al., 2019).

Extremities: Edema; weak/diminished pulses (radial, posterior tibialis, dorsalis pedis); **cyanosis**
Psychiatric: *Anxiety*

Refer to Algorithm 19.1 (Ball et al., 2023; Dains et al., 2024; Goolsby & Grubbs, 2019; Brashers, 2023)

Evaluation and Differential Diagnoses

DIAGNOSTICS

- Labs
  - Complete blood count
  - Complete metabolic panel
  - Magnesium
  - Lipid profile
  - Thyroid-stimulating hormone
- American College of Cardiology/American Heart Association ASCVD risk estimator
- 12-lead electrocardiogram (atherosclerosis)
- Diagnostic imaging
  - Coronary artery calcium scan in selected adults if risk decision is uncertain
  - Stress testing (atherosclerosis)
  - Echocardiogram (atherosclerosis)

DIFFERENTIAL DIAGNOSIS

- Metabolic syndrome—Presence of three or more of the following: Elevated fasting blood glucose or current treatment for hyperglycemia, elevated blood pressure or current treatment for hypertension, increased waist circumference with abdominal fat, or dyslipidemia with increased triglycerides and/or decreased HDL
- Hypothyroidism—May elevate cholesterol. The exam will reveal weight gain, fatigue, and elevated thyroid stimulating hormone with low free T4.

■ Drug or alcohol induced—Medications may elevate LDL or triglycerides and alcohol may elevate triglycerides.

■ Chronic kidney disease—Elevated blood urea nitrogen and creatinine with a decreased estimated glomerular filtration rate <60

Plan

Guideline Resources

■ Arnett, D. K., Blumenthal, R. S., Albert, M. A., Buroker, A. B., Goldberger, Z. D., Hahn E. J., Dennison Himmelfarb, C., Khera, A., Lloyd-Jones, D., McEvoy, J. W., Michos, E. D., Miedema, M. D., Muñoz, D., Smith, S. C. Jr, Virani, S. S., Williams, K. A. Sr, Yeboah, J., & Ziaeian, B. (2019). 2019 ACC/AHA guideline on the primary prevention of cardiovascular disease: A report of the American College of Cardiology/American Heart Association task force on clinical practice guidelines. *Circulation*, *140*(11), e596–e646. https://doi.org/10.1161/cir.0000000000000678.

■ American College of Cardiology and American Heart Association. (2023). *ASCVD risk estimator.* https://tools.acc.org/ldl/ascvd_risk_estimator/index.html#!/calulate/estimator.

■ Grundy, S. M., Stone, N. J., Bailey, A. L., Beam, C., Birtcher, K. K., Blumenthal, R. S., Braun, L. T., de Ferranti, S., Faiella-Tommasino, J., Forman, D. E., Goldberg, R., Heidenreich, P. A., Hlatky, M. A., Jones, D. W., Lloyd-Jones, D., Lopez-Pajares, N., Ndumele, C. E., Orringer, C. E., Peralta, C. A., … Yeboah, J. (2019). 2018 AHA/ACC/AACVPR/AAPA/ABC/ACPM/ADA/AGS/APhA/ASPC/NLA/PCNA guideline on the management of blood cholesterol. *Journal of the American College of Cardiology*, *73*(24), e285–e350. https://doi.org/10.1016/j.jacc.2018.11.003.

Pharmacotherapy

The initiation of medication therapy is complex and involves a combination of patient preferences, lifestyle choices, and comorbidities. Specific pharmacotherapy guidelines for hyperlipidemia stages are discussed below.

■ Medications

　■ Statin therapy is the first-line treatment for ASCVD risk reduction for those with elevated LDL. Statin therapy is divided into high-intensity, moderate-intensity, and low-intensity (Algorithm 19.1). Lowering LDL level with a statin by 1% equals approximately 1% ASCVD reduction (Arnett et al., 2019):

　　■ High-intensity statin therapy lowers LDL by ≥ 50% (average LDL lowering) (See guideline for medication and dosages: https://doi.org/10.1016/j.jacc.2018.11.003)

　　■ Moderate-intensity statin therapy usually lowers LDL by 30% to 49% (average LDL lowering) (See guideline for medication and dosages: https://doi.org/10.1016/j.jacc.2018.11.003).

　　■ Low-intensity statin therapy usually lowers LDL by <30% (average LDL lowering) (See guideline for medication and dosages: https://doi.org/10.1016/j.jacc.2018.11.003).

　■ Nonstatin therapy may be used in specific situations along with statin therapy to lower LDL level. Ezetimibe, bile acid sequestrants, and PCSK9 augment LDL lowering when used with a statin. Niacin and fibrates should not be given with a statin (Arnett et al., 2019):

　　■ Ezetimibe lowers LDL by 13% to 20%.

　　■ Bile acid sequestrants lower LDL by 15% to 30%.

　　■ PCSK9 inhibitors lower LDL by 43% to 64%.

- Pharmacologic treatment of fasting triglycerides <500 mg/dL is not recommended for the primary prevention of ASCVD (Grundy et al., 2019).
- See Tables 19.1 and 19.2:
  - Triglyceride lowering pharmacotherapy:
    - Niacin
    - Fibrates
- Smoking cessation aids should be offered to any person currently smoking tobacco.
- In adults with ASCVD risk of ≥10% and average systolic blood pressure (BP) of ≥130 mm Hg or average diastolic BP of ≥80 mm Hg, use of anti-hypertensive medication is recommended (see Chapter 20, Hypertension, for recommendations) (Whelton et al., 2018).
- Review medications prescribed and possible side effects.

NONPHARMACOTHERAPY

- Educate
  - Primary prevention of ASCVD includes risk assessment and strategies aimed at lowering lifetime risk factors (see Tables 19.1 and 19.2).
    - Primary prevention: Keep LDL <130 mg/dL, HDL >40 mg/dL, and triglycerides <200 mg/dL.
  - Successful ASCVD management includes a patient-centered approach aimed at atherosclerosis risk factor reduction including the shared decision making of a cholesterol management treatment plan (Arnett et al., 2019).
  - The CDC has developed several patient education pamphlets on cholesterol management (see https://www.cdc.gov/cholesterol/php/toolkit/).
  - Disease and disease progression
  - Self-management
  - Review medications and side effects.
  - Importance of vaccines
- Lifestyle and behavioral modifications (see Table 19.1)
  - Lifestyle modification should be introduced at the first office visit and reassessed during every subsequent office visit (Grundy et al., 2019).
  - See Box 19.3.
  - Diet:
    - Dietary Approaches to Stop Hypertension (DASH) diet
    - Increase consumption of vegetables, fruits, legumes, nuts, whole grains, and fish.
    - Replace saturated fats with monounsaturated and polyunsaturated fats.
    - Reduce cholesterol, processed meat, simple carbohydrates, sodium, and sweetened beverages.

BOX 19.3 ■ Older Adult Considerations

All adults aged 75 years and older benefit from therapeutic lifestyle management. Those individuals with a low-density lipoprotein of 70 to 189 mg/dL may benefit from starting a statin. In individuals with cognitive or physical functional decline, multiple comorbidities, or reduced life expectancy, the risks of statin therapy may outweigh the benefits and it may be prudent to stop statin therapy. For those with a low-density lipoprotein of 70 to 189 mg/dL with a coronary artery calcium score of 0, it may be prudent to not initiate statin therapy (Grundy et al., 2019).

> **BOX 19.4 ■ Acute Care Considerations**
>
> Individuals with elevated triglycerides (>500–999 mg/dL) are at increased risk of acute triglyceridemic pancreatitis. Most cases involve a genetic factor but there may be secondary contributing factors. Reduction of triglyceride levels is achieved by consuming a very low-fat diet and initiating fibrates and omega-3 fatty acids (Grundy et al., 2019).

- Hypertriglyceridemia management: Low-carbohydrate, low-fat diet (reduce simple, refined sugar) and increase intake of omega-3 fatty acids and protein (Grundy et al., 2019; Oh et al., 2020)
- Exercise: Physical activity at moderate intensity for 150 minutes or 75 minutes of vigorous activity weekly
- Weight loss (target BMI <22 kg/m² for females and <27 kg/m² for males) (waist-to-hip ratio >0.85 for females and >0.95 for males increases risk for heart disease)
- Smoking cessation
- Limit daily alcohol intake to 1 drink for females and 2 drinks for males.
- Decrease/eliminate modifiable risk factors.
- Limit/eliminate environmental and occupational stressors.
- Complementary treatment
  - Psychosocial therapy
  - Complementary and alternative therapies with natural medicines and supplements may interact with prescription medications. Obtain a complete medication history.
- Referral (identify and refer for treatment of comorbid conditions*)
  - Cardiologist:
    - Individuals not meeting LDL goals despite therapeutic lifestyle and pharmacologic treatment should be referred to a cardiologist.
  - Cardiology interventionalist
  - Nephrologist* (acute kidney injury, chronic kidney disease)
  - Pulmonologist* (pulmonary hypertension, chronic obstructive pulmonary disease)
  - Gastroenterologist* (gastroesophageal reflux; pancreatitis):
    - Individuals with severely elevated triglycerides should be treated to prevent acute pancreatitis (Box 19.4).
  - Hematologist* (coagulopathy, anemia)
- Follow-up
  - Frequency of labs and follow up including ASCVD risk assessment is a mutually developed plan between the provider and patient:
    - 1 month after starting new medication with follow-up lipid profile
  - If lipids are improving, follow-up in 3 months with lipid profile.
  - Office visit every 3 to 6 months depending on changes in medication or lipid profile results
  - An ASCVD risk analysis should be completed on every patient to assess for 10-year ASCVD risk.

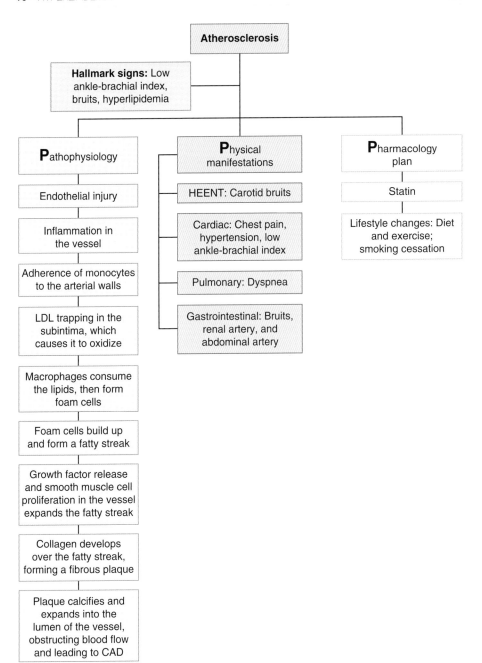

Algorithm 19.1 Atherosclerosis. *CAD*, Coronary artery disease; *LDL*, low-density lipoprotein.

References

American Heart Association. (2024). AHA diet and lifestyle recommendations. Retrieved September 2, 2024, from https://www.heart.org/en/healthy-living/healthy-eating/eat-smart/nutrition-basics/aha-diet-and-lifestyle-recommendations.

Arnett, D. K., Blumenthal, R. S., Albert, M. A., Buroker, A. B., Goldberger, Z. D., Hahn, E. J., Himmelfarb, C. D., Khera, A., Lloyd-Jones, D., McEvoy, J. W., Michos, E. D., Miedema, M. D., Muñoz, D., Smith, S. C. Jr, Virani, S. S., Williams, K. A. Sr, Yeboah, J., & Ziaeian, B (2019). 2019 ACC/AHA guideline on the primary prevention of cardiovascular disease: Executive summary: A report of the American College of Cardiology/American Heart Association task force on clinical practice guidelines. *Circulation, 140*, e563–e595. http://doi.org/10.1161/CIR.0000000000000677.

Ball, J. W., Dains, J. E., Flynn, J. A., Solomon, B. S., & Stewart, R. W. (2023). *Seidel's guide to physical examination* (10th ed.). Elsevier.

Brashers, V. L. (2023). Alterations in cardiovascular function. In J. L. Rogers (Ed.), *McCance & Huether's pathophysiology: The biologic basis for disease in adults and children (9th ed., pp. 1059–1108)*. Elsevier.

Dains, J. E., Baumann, L. C., & Scheibel, P. (2024). *Advanced health assessment & clinical diagnosis in primary care* (7th ed.). Elsevier.

de Ferranti, S. D., Steinberger, J., Ameduri, R., Baker, A., Gooding, H., Kelly, A. S., Mietus-Snyder, M., Mitsnefes, M. M., Peterson, A. L., St-Pierre, J., Urbina, E. M, Zachariah, J. P., & Zaidi, A. N. (2019). Cardiovascular risk reduction in high-risk pediatric patients: A scientific statement from the American Heart Association. *Circulation, 139*(13), e603–e634. https://doi.org/10.1161/CIR.0000000000000618.

Goolsby, M. J., & Grubbs, G. L. (2019). *Advanced assessment interpreting findings and formulating differential diagnoses* (4th ed.). F. A. Davis Company.

Grundy, S. M., Stone, N. J., Bailey, A. L., Beam, C., Birtcher, K. K., Blumenthal, R. S., Braun, L. T., de Ferranti, S., Faiella-Tommasino, J., Forman, D. E., Goldberg, R., Heidenreich, P. A., Hlatky, M. A., Jones, D. W., Lloyd-Jones, D., Lopez-Pajares, N., Ndumele, C. E., Orringer, C. E., Peralta, C. A., ... Yeboah, J. (2019). 2018 AHA/ACC/AACVPR/AAPA/ABC/ACPM/ADA/AGS/APhA/ASPC/NLA/PCNA guideline on the management of blood cholesterol: A report of the American College of Cardiology/American Heart Association task force on clinical practice guidelines. *Circulation, 139*(25), e1082–e1143. https://www.ahajournals.org/doi/10.1161/CIR.0000000000000625.

Oh, R. C., Trivette, E. T., & Westerfield, K. L. (2020). Management of hypertriglyceridemia: Common questions and answers. *American Family Physician, 102*(6), 347–354.

Rogers, J., & Baker, M. (2020a). Understanding the most commonly billed diagnoses in primary care: Atherosclerotic cardiovascular disease. *Nurse Practitioner, 45*(7), 35–41.

Rogers, J., & Baker, M. (2020b). Understanding the most commonly billed diagnoses in primary care: Hyperlipidemia. *Nurse Practitioner, 45*(8), 42–48.

Tsao, C. W., Aday, A. W., Almarzooq, Z. I., Anderson, C. A. M., Arora, P., Avery, C. L., Baker-Smith, C. M., Beaton, A. Z., Boehme, A. K., Buxton, A. E., Commodore-Mensah, Y., Elkind, M. S. V., Evenson, K. R., Eze-Nliam, C., Fugar, S., Generoso, G., Heard, D. G., Hiremath, S., & Ho, J. E., ... American Heart Association Council on Epidemiology and Prevention Statistics Committee and Stroke Statistics Subcommittee. (2023). Heart disease and stroke statistics—2023 update: A report from the American Heart Association. *Circulation, 147*(8), e93–e621.

Valero-Elizondo, J., Javed, Z., Khera, R., Tano, M. E., Dudum, R., Acquah, I., & Nasir, K. (2022). Unfavorable social determinants of health are associated with higher burden of financial toxicity among patients with atherosclerotic cardiovascular disease in the US: Findings from the National Health Interview Survey. *Archives of Public Health, 80*(1), 1–12.

Whelton, P. K., Carey, R. M., Aronow, W. S., Casey, D. E. Jr, Collins, K. J., Himmelfarb, Dennison, C., DePalma, S., M., Gidding, S., Jamerson, K. A., Jones, D. W., MacLaughlin, E. J., Muntner, P., Ovbiagele, B., Smith, S. C. Jr, Spencer, C. C., Stafford, R. S., Taler, S. J., Thomas, R. J., Williams, K. A. Sr, ..., Wright Jr, J. T. (2018). 2017 ACC/AHA/AAPA/ABC/ACPM/AGS/APhA/ASH/ASPC/NMA/PCNA guideline for the prevention, detection, evaluation, and management of high blood pressure in adults: A report of the American College of Cardiology/American Heart Association task force on clinical practice guidelines. *Hypertension, 71*(6), e13–e115. https://doi.org/10.1161/HYP.0000000000000065.

CHAPTER 20

Hypertension

Julia L. Rogers ▓ Marianne Schallmo

Hypertension

Hypertension (HTN) is a common diagnosis with high morbidity, high mortality, and a financial burden of approximately $198 billion per year (Centers for Disease Control and Prevention [CDC], 2021a; Ostchega et al., 2020; Tsao et al., 2022; Virani et al., 2020). In the United States, HTN affects nearly 46% of all adults aged 20 years and older and up to 60% of all adults aged 60 years and older (CDC, 2021a; Ostchega et al., 2020). Elevated blood pressure (BP) is a major risk factor for cardiovascular disease, with uncontrolled HTN increasing the risk of angina, myocardial infarction, heart failure, cerebral vascular disease, and kidney disease (Virani et al., 2020). HTN is a preventable and treatable disease. Risk factors associated with HTN include smoking, diabetes (see Chapter 14), obesity, dyslipidemia (see Chapter 19), sedentary lifestyle, stress, males older than age 55 years, and postmenopausal females older than age 45 years (Goolsby & Grubbs, 2019). The current American College of Cardiology and American Heart Association guidelines recommend that BP remain below 130/80 mm Hg (Whelton et al., 2018). HTN is diagnosed when the average of two or more BP readings exceeds 130/80 mm Hg on two or more occasions (Whelton et al., 2018). Patients diagnosed with HTN are often poorly controlled, with the majority of those on medication not meeting current BP guidelines (CDC, 2021b). Successful HTN management encompasses an interdisciplinary approach that includes the patient and healthcare provider nurse, dietitian, and pharmacist (Box 20.1).

Pathophysiology

HTN is the result of various genetic and environmental factors mediated by neurohormonal effects (Fig. 20.1). The primary intermediaries involved in BP regulation are the sympathetic nervous system (SNS), the renin-angiotensin-aldosterone system (RAAS), and natriuretic peptides (Algorithm 20.1) (Brashers, 2023). A shift in the pressure–natriuresis relationship between vascular volume, which is increased, and renal salt excretion, which is decreased, occurs from a disturbance in one or more of the intrinsic mechanisms (Brashers, 2023). BP reacts to changes in the environment to maintain accurate perfusion. The SNS plays an important role in regulating arterial blood pressure (ABP). A product of cardiac output and systemic vascular resistance, ABP is essential for organ perfusion; therefore HTN that is left untreated or uncontrolled can negatively affect the stru3cture and function of multiple organ systems (retinol changes, renal disorders, cardiovascular disease, and neurologic conditions).

Overactivity of the RAAS ultimately leads to HTN secondary to increased blood volume and vascular resistance. First, renin reacts with angiotensinogen, converting it to angiotensin I, which then transforms to the potent vasoconstrictor angiotensin II. Angiotensin II targets the arterioles and stimulates the adrenal cortex to secrete aldosterone (Brashers, 2023). This release of aldosterone leads to vasoconstriction and increases blood volume through the retention of sodium and water. Natriuretic hormonal modulation of renal sodium excretion maintains a homeostatic

BOX 20.1 ■ Diversity Considerations

Ethnic: Hypertension (HTN) prevalence is higher among the non-Hispanic Black population than the Hispanic and non-Hispanic White population (Ostchega et al., 2020). In Black patients, blood pressure (BP) control rates are lower, HTN is more severe, and certain anti-hypertensive medications are less effective at achieving BP control (Whelton et al., 2018). First-line agents should include a thiazide diuretic or calcium channel blocker (CCB), as these are found to be more effective in lowering BP than angiotensin converting enzyme (ACE) inhibitors, angiotensin II reception blockers (ARBs), or beta-blockers (BBs). Thiazide diuretics and CCBs are also more effective than ACE inhibitors, ARBs, direct renin inhibitors, and alpha-blockers at reducing cardiovascular events among the Black population (Whelton et al., 2018). ACE inhibitors or ARBs are appropriate for Black patients with diabetes and nephropathy or heart failure (Whelton et al., 2018).

Gender: HTN prevalence among those younger than 60 years is higher in males than in females but is similar in both genders after age 60 (Ostchega et al., 2020). BP goals and treatment plans, including lifestyle modifications and medications, are the same for males and females (Whelton et al., 2018).

Pregnancy: The management of HTN during pregnancy is beyond the scope of this chapter and pregnant females with HTN should be referred to a specialist for care. ACE inhibitors, ARBs, direct renin inhibitors, and mineralocorticoid blockers are fetotoxic and are not approved for use during pregnancy (Castro & Hobel, 2016). Medication for females who are pregnant or planning to become pregnant must be changed to methyldopa, nifedipine, and/or labetalol (Castro & Hobel, 2016).

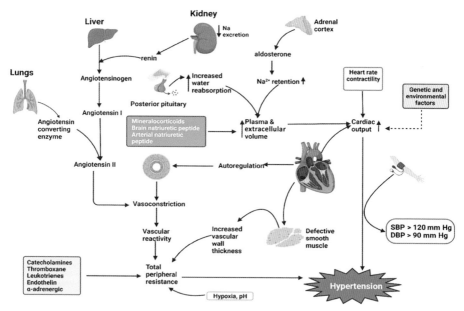

Fig. 20.1 The multiple factors involved in the regulation of blood pressure (BP). BP is the product of cardiac output and peripheral vascular resistance. Peripheral resistance can be influenced by local factors such as pH, hypoxia, and humoral factors (angiotensin II, catecholamines, thromboxanes), and cardiac output is influenced by blood volume, atrial and brain natriuretic peptides, and cardiac factors (heart rate and contractility). In response to decreased systemic BP, renin is produced by the juxtaglomerular cells of the kidney, which stimulates the activation of angiotensinogen in the liver to angiotensin I. Angiotensin I is converted to angiotensin II by angiotensin converting enzymes from the lungs. Angiotensin II constricts blood vessels and promotes the release of aldosterone from the adrenal glands, which subsequently triggers sodium reabsorption. Antidiuretic hormones from the pituitary glands are also released to cause water reabsorption. Combined, this leads to increased blood volume and BP. From Adua, E. (2023). Decoding the mechanism of hypertension through multiomics profiling. *Journal of Human Hypertension, 37*(4), 253–264. https://doi.org/10.1038/s41371-022-00769-8.

pressure–natriuretic relationship. The most common natriuretic hormone is the B-type natriuretic peptide (BNP), which is released in response to volume and pressure overload. Other natriuretic hormones include the atrial natriuretic peptide (ANP), C-type natriuretic peptide (CNP), and urodilatin. The main function of the peptides is to decrease BP and control electrolyte homeostasis by inducing diuresis, increasing systemic vasodilation, boosting renal blood flow, suppressing aldosterone, and inhibiting the SNS (Brashers, 2023). These natriuretic hormones regulate renal sodium excretion and require adequate electrolyte consumption to function properly. This is the significance behind maintaining sufficient intake of potassium, calcium, and magnesium. A deficiency in these electrolytes induces the body to retain sodium, which causes increased volume. The reabsorption of water by the kidneys occurs with the release of antidiuretic hormone, a compensatory response related to detection of increased blood osmolality or decreased blood volume (Brashers, 2023). As water is reabsorbed, the blood plasma volume increases, which elevates the BP. The immune system, inflammation, and obesity all play a pivotal role in HTN. Activation of the immune response system results in a cascade of events causing chronic inflammation. This eventually leads to endothelial cell damage, weakened production of vasodilators, vascular alteration, and smooth muscle contraction (Brashers, 2023). The chronic inflammation contributes to insulin resistance, reduced natriuresis, autonomic dysfunction, and renal dysfunction. Obesity, which is linked to chronic inflammation, is associated with HTN beginning in adolescence. Obesity not only is a risk factor for HTN but also contributes to the neurohormonal, metabolic, renal, and cardiovascular complications associated with the disease. Obesity causes changes in the adipokines (leptin, resistin, adiponectin) and leads to vascular remodeling, insulin resistance, increased RAAS action, and heightened SNS activity (Brashers, 2023).

Physical Clinical Presentation

SUBJECTIVE

Individuals may not have any presenting symptoms and only discover that they have HTN after vital signs are taken at a routine visit. During the focused history, documentation should include the onset of any associated symptoms (e.g., headache or chest pain); precipitating events; location, intensity, and quality of pain; progression of symptoms; alleviating and aggravating factors; and previous episodes. Individuals may report throbbing or bounding headaches or palpitations with or without dull chest pain/angina. Crushing chest pain may also be described with sweating, dizziness, or back pain. Document whether the pain radiates elsewhere in the body and if symptoms worsen with caffeine, stimulants, or alcohol. Use a 0-to-10 pain scale for a description of headache and chest pain. Verify if headaches or other symptoms occur daily, weekly, or monthly. Ask what the patient was doing or eating before the pain started; whether symptoms come in the morning, afternoon, or night; and whether the symptoms awaken the patient from sleep. Ask open-ended questions about which activities aggravate or relieve symptoms, such as stress, exercise or rest. Determine if the patient has a home BP monitor and, if so, what their BP is at home and at what time of day. Asking about being around ill contacts is important because some viral and bacterial infections can affect the heart. Obtain a current medication list and any recent changes. Document any complaints that may lead to secondary causes of HTN such as a report of anxiety, diaphoresis, palpitations, dyspnea, tremor muscle weakness, polyuria, nocturia, nausea, or vomiting.

Document allergies, medications, and medical, social, and family histories. Many medications are implicated in elevating BP; therefore ask if the patient is taking or has recently taken contraception, steroids, nonsteroidal antiinflammatory drugs, decongestants, appetite suppressants, recreational/illegal drugs, tricyclic antidepressants, cyclosporin, or monoamine oxidase inhibitors. Medical history should include previous diagnoses and/or treatment for anxiety, obesity, dyslipidemia (see Chapter 19), type II diabetes (see Chapter 14), dysrhythmia (e.g., atrial fibrillation) (see Chapter 17), congenital heart disease, murmur, palpitation, abnormal electrocardiogram, or obstructive sleep apnea (Goolsby & Grubbs, 2019). Surgical history should include any angiography, angioplasty, stent placement, or coronary artery bypass graft. Social history should include occupation and associated stress; home or environmental stress; vaping and/or tobacco use, past or present, and type; consumption of alcohol including both type and amount; illegal substance or drug abuse; and if consuming a high-fat/high-sodium diet. Capture any family history of HTN, cardiovascular disease, early sudden cardiac death, myocardial infarction, or substance abuse.

OBJECTIVE*

Vital signs: Elevated BP (measured after resting for 5 minutes in both arms while sitting in a chair with both feet on the floor and back supported, empty bladder, without talking, and no caffeine, exercise, or smoking at least 30 minutes prior); temperature, pulse, respirations, and oxygen saturations should be taken (see Algorithm 20.1).

Generalized: Obesity; fatigue

Neurological: *Migraine with aura; tremor*

HEENT: Headache; retinopathy, retina hemorrhage, **A-V nicking**, retina exudates; copper or silver wire appearance; *exophthalmos;* **papilledema**

Neck: *Thyromegaly; thyroid nodules; bruits; jugular vein distention (JVD)*

Cardiovascular: <u>S_3 or S_4 **(decreased left ventricular, ventricular hypertrophy);**</u> *palpitations* or **bounding pulse, chest pain, tachycardia;** <u>**systolic murmur (aortic stenosis); diastolic murmur (aortic insufficiency)**</u>

Pulmonary: *Inspection: Labored respirations; dyspnea; tachypnea; use of accessory muscles Auscultation: Wheezing; rales; diminished*

Gastrointestinal: <u>**Aortic bruit**</u>

Genitourinary: <u>**Renal artery bruit;**</u> *hesitancy; polyuria; nocturia*

Musculoskeletal: *Muscle weakness*

Integumentary: *Diaphoresis;* hyperemic or ruddy

Extremities: *Edema; pulses irregular,* <u>**upper and lower extremity pulses unequal (coarctation);**</u> *cyanosis*

Psychiatric: *Anxious, nervousness*

(Ball, 2023; Brashers, 2023; Dains et al., 2024; Goolsby & Grubbs, 2019)

Evaluation and Differential Diagnoses

DIAGNOSTICS

- Blood pressure log from home monitoring
- Labs
  - Complete blood count
  - Fasting blood glucose
  - Lipid profile
  - Serum renin and aldosterone (rule out hyperaldosteronism)
  - Serum creatinine with estimated glomerular filtration rate (kidney disease)
  - Electrolytes: Serum sodium, potassium, calcium (kidney disease)
  - Thyroid-stimulating hormone (thyroid disease)
  - Uric acid
  - Urinalysis; ratio of urinary albumin to creatinine
- Diagnostic imaging
  - 12-lead electrocardiogram (ventricular hypertrophy or valvular disease)
  - Echocardiogram (structural or functional abnormality)

****Hallmark signs are bolded** and <u>**Red flags are bolded and underlined**</u>. *Findings associated more with noncardiac conditions or secondary causes are in italics.*

- Renal doppler ultrasound (rule out renal vascular disease)
- Chest X-ray (rule out cortication and pulmonary disease)

(Goolsby & Grubbs, 2019; Shimbo et al., 2020; Whelton et al., 2018)

DIFFERENTIAL DIAGNOSIS

- Hyperaldosteronism—Resistant HTN with hypokalemia and muscle weakness or cramps
- Hyperthyroidism—Exam will reveal weight loss, nervousness, exophthalmos, tremors, fatigue, and palpitations
- Obstructive sleep apnea—Resistant HTN with snoring or respiratory pauses during sleep
- Drug or alcohol induced—Has a history of alcohol or drug use
- Chronic kidney disease—Elevated blood urea nitrogen and creatinine with an estimated glomerular filtration rate <60

Plan

Guideline Resources

- American College of Cardiology and American Heart Association. (2023). *ASCVD risk estimator*. https://tools.acc.org/ldl/ascvd_risk_estimator/index.html#!/calulate/estimator
- Whelton, P. K., Carey, R. M., Aronow, W. S., Casey, D. E. Jr, Collins, K. J., Dennison Himmelfarb, C., DePalma, S. M., Gidding, S., Jamerson, K. A., Jones, D. W., MacLaughlin, E. J., Muntner, P., Ovbiagele, B., Smith, S. C. Jr, Spencer, C. C., Stafford, R. S., Taler, S. J., Thomas, R. J., Williams, K. A., Sr, & Wright, J. T. Jr. (2018). 2017 ACC/AHA/AAPA/ABC/ACPM/AGS/APhA/ASH/ASPC/NMA/PCNA guideline for the prevention, detection, evaluation, and management of high blood pressure in adults: A report of the American College of Cardiology/American Heart Association Task Force on Clinical Practice Guidelines. *Hypertension*, 71(6), e13–e115. https://doi.org/10.1161/hyp.0000000000000065
- Mancia, G., Kreutz, R., Brunström, M., Burnier, M., Grassi, G., Januszewicz, A., Kahan, T., Mahfoud, F., Redon, J., Ruilope, L., Volpe, M., Williams, B., Tsioufis, K., & Lurbe, E. (2023). 2023 ESH guidelines for the management of arterial hypertension: The Task Force for the management of arterial hypertension of the European Society of Hypertension: Endorsed by the International Society of Hypertension (ISH) and the European Renal Association (ERA). *Journal of Hypertension*, 41(10), 1874-2071. https://doi.org/10.1097/HJH.0000000000003540

Pharmacotherapy

- Medications
    - The initiation of medication therapy is complex and involves a combination of patient preference, lifestyle choices, and comorbidities. See Table 20.1 for specific pharmacotherapy guidelines for each stage of HTN. Refer to Algorithm 20.1.
    - First-line agents used in the initiation of pharmacologic treatment for HTN include (Whelton et al., 2018):
        - Thiazide diuretics
        - Calcium channel blockers (dihydropyridines and nondihydropyridines)
        - Angiotensin converting enzyme inhibitors
        - Angiotensin receptor blockers
    - Second-line agents are recommended for patients unable to attain BP goal with monotherapy and lifestyle modifications. Second-line agents are added to the first-line agents already prescribed but may not be in the same class as the first-line agents (Whelton et al., 2018):
        - Other diuretics (loop, potassium-sparing, aldosterone antagonists)

TABLE 20.1 ■ Hypertension Pharmacotherapy and Nonpharmacotherapy Decision Guide

BP Reading	Initial Office Visit	Follow-up Office Visits
Normal BP <120/80 mm Hg	Promote healthy lifestyle habits.	Reassess yearly.
Elevated BP 120–129/<80 mm Hg	Nonpharmacotherapy treatment	Reassess every 3–6 months.

Stage 1 BP 130–139/80–89 mm Hg and ASCVD <10%	Nonpharmacotherapy treatment	Reassess every 3–6 months.
		• If BP goal met:
		  a. Continue therapy.
		  b. Reassess every 3–6 months.
		• If BP goal not met after 6 months:
		  a. Consider initiating treatment with a first-line agent (Jones et al., 2021).
		  b. Reassess in 1 month.

Stage 1 BP 130–139/80–89 mm Hg and ASCVD ≥10%	Nonpharmacotherapy and BP-lowering medication:
	• Initiate treatment with a first-line agent.
	• Reassess in 1 month.
		At 1-month follow-up:
		• If BP goal met:
		  a. Continue therapy.
		  b. Reassess every 3–6 months.
		• If BP goal not met:
		  a. Assess adherence to therapy.
		  b. Consider intensifying therapy by either titrating the first-line agent, adding another first-line agent, or adding a second-line agent.
		  c. Reassess 1 month after initiating or titrating agent.

Stage 2: BP ≥140/90 mm Hg	Nonpharmacotherapy and BP-lowering medication:
	• Initiate treatment with a first-line agent.
	• Reassess in 1 month.
	• May consider initial treatment with two agents from two different drug classes.
	• Reassess in 1 month.
	• BP >160/100 mm Hg should be promptly treated and monitored.
		At 1-month follow-up:
		• If BP goal met:
		  a. Continue therapy.
		  b. Reassess every 3–6 months.
		• If BP goal not met:
		  a. Assess adherence to therapy.
		  b. Consider intensifying therapy by either titrating the first-line agent, adding another first-line agent, or adding a second-line agent.
		  c. Reassess 1 month after initiating or titrating agent.

Stage 2 with hypertensive emergency: BP ≥180/120 mm Hg	Immediate emergency room referral. See Box 20.4.	

ASCVD, Atherosclerotic cardiovascular disease; BP, blood pressure.
(Jones et al., 2021; Whelton et al., 2018)

- ▨ Beta-blockers (cardioselective and vasodilatory, noncardioselective, intrinsic sympathomimetics activity, and combined alpha- and beta-receptors)
- ▨ Direct renin inhibitor
- ▨ Alpha-1 blocker
- ▨ Central alpha-2-agonist and other centrally acting drugs
- ■ Concurrent ACE inhibitor, ARB, and direct renin inhibitor combinations are not recommended. For renin-angiotensin system (RAS) inhibitor or diuretic therapy, monitor electrolytes and renal function 2 to 4 weeks after initiating or titrating therapy.

- Smoking cessation aids should be offered to any person currently smoking tobacco.
- Vaccines: Influenza annually, pneumococcal, COVID-19, and zoster according to CDC guidelines and recommendations

(Whelton et al., 2018)

NONPHARMACOTHERAPY

- HTN management and optimal cardiovascular health are achieved by developing a comprehensive plan including patient participation, interdisciplinary care, and telehealth strategies (Tsao et al., 2022). Considerations should be given to specific populations (e.g., pediatrics and older adults) (Boxes 20.2 and 20.3).
- An atherosclerotic cardiovascular disease (ASCVD) risk analysis should be completed on every patient to assess for 10-year ASCVD risk as this assists the practitioner in determining pharmacotherapy.
  - Educate
  - Disease process and progression
  - Prescribed medication purpose and side effects
  - Nonpharmacotherapy treatment and importance

BOX 20.2 ■ Pediatric Considerations

Beginning at age 1, blood pressure (BP) is categorized as normal, prehypertension (90th–94th percentile); stage 1 (95th–99th percentile; or stage 2 (above stage 1) based on age, gender, and height tables (Whelton et al., 2018). Starting at age 14, hypertension (HTN) is classified according to JNC 7 thresholds (Whelton et al., 2018). BP needs to be taken on three separate occasions before an HTN diagnosis can be assigned. As with all diagnoses, the provider must determine whether HTN is primary or secondary to other causes. Diagnostic evaluation of stages 1 and 2 includes evaluating for causes of secondary HTN and any target organ damage (Newcombe, 2020). After secondary causes are ruled out, treatment will focus on primary HTN, including comorbidities and target organ damage (Newcombe, 2020; Whelton et al., 2018).

Nonpharmacologic treatment should be discussed at every visit and include diet, exercise, weight management, and avoidance of smoking, caffeine, alcohol, and illicit drugs (Newcombe, 2020). Those with prehypertension should follow up for repeat BP in 6 months. Those with stage 1 should follow up for repeat BP in 1 to 2 weeks. If stage 1 BP persists despite nonpharmacologic methods, a referral to a pediatric cardiologist or nephrologist is necessary for antihypertensive medications. An immediate referral is necessitated when BP is greater than the 99th percentile (Newcombe, 2020).

BOX 20.3 ■ Older Adult Considerations

Approximately 80% of older adults have high blood pressure (Egan, 2022). Isolated systolic hypertension (HTN), caused by a decrease in arterial compliance, is the predominant form of HTN in older adults (Egan, 2022). According to 2017 American College of Cardiology/American Heart Association guidelines, adults aged 65 and older (described as noninstitutionalized ambulatory community-dwelling adults) have the same treatment guidelines as younger adults, with a systolic blood pressure (SBP) goal <130 mm Hg (Whelton et al., 2018).

Nonpharmacologic treatment should be discussed at every visit, with an added emphasis on dietary salt restrictions and weight reduction (Egan, 2022). If blood pressure goal is not met with lifestyle changes, antihypertensive medication should be initiated (Helton, 2022) but at a lower initial dose and over a more gradual titration period of 2 to 4 months. A gradual titration is to avoid orthostatic hypotension (Egan, 2022). Diuretics and calcium channel blockers (CCB) are a more effective and appropriate first-line therapy (Helton, 2022). Angiotensin converting enzyme (ACE) inhibitors and angiotensin II reception blockers (ARB) can be prescribed but may be less effective as older adults have a less active renin angiotensin-aldosterone system (RAAS) (Egan, 2022; Helton, 2022; Whelton et al., 2018).

BOX 20.4 ■ Acute Care Considerations

Hypertensive emergency occurs when a severe blood pressure (BP) elevation (>180/120 mm Hg) is associated with new, progressing, or worsening target organ damage. Examples of target organ damage include hypertensive encephalopathy, intracerebral brain hemorrhage, acute ischemic stroke, acute myocardial infarction, acute left ventricular failure with pulmonary edema, unstable angina pectoris, dissecting aortic aneurysm, acute renal failure, and eclampsia. The actual BP may not be as important as the rate of BP rise because patients with chronic hypertension may tolerate a higher BP than previously normotensive patients. Patients experiencing a hypertensive emergency will need immediate emergency room referral for evaluation and treatment. Hypertensive urgency occurs with a severe BP elevation in otherwise stable patients and without new, progressing, or worsening target organ damage. These patients do not require emergency room referral and should be evaluated for antihypertensive medication adherence. Treatment includes reinstituting or intensifying antihypertensive medication therapy and close follow-up visits (Whelton et al., 2018).

- ■ AHA Blood Pressure Toolkit for patients based on American College of Cardiology/ American Heart Association clinical practice guidelines
- ■ Self-management
- ■ Reduce/eliminate environmental and occupational stress.
- ■ Importance of vaccines
- ■ Lifestyle and behavioral modifications
  - ■ Diet: Heart-healthy Dietary Approaches to Stop Hypertension diet
  - ■ Salt restriction: 1500 mg/day is optimal but at least 1000 mg reduction daily
  - ■ Dietary potassium supplementation: 3500–500 mg/day
  - ■ Limit daily alcohol intake to 1 drink for females and 2 drinks for males.
  - ■ Get 90–150 minutes of aerobic activity and dynamic resistance training or physical activity/ muscle strengthening three times weekly.
  - ■ Smoking cessation
- ■ Complementary treatment
  - ■ Psychosocial counseling
  - ■ Spiritual and/or mindfulness meditation
  - ■ Yoga
  - ■ Tai chi
  - ■ Guided imagery meditation
  - ■ Complementary and alternative therapies with natural medicines and supplements may interact with prescription medications. Obtain a complete medication history.

(Unger et al., 2020; Whelton et al., 2018)
- ■ Referral (identify and refer for treatment of comorbid conditions*)
  - ■ Emergency department for hypertensive crisis (Box 20.4)
  - ■ Cardiologist: Secondary HTN; BP uncontrolled after 6 months of medication and lifestyle modification; resistant HTN
  - ■ Nephrologist* (acute kidney injury, chronic kidney disease, kidney involvement)
  - ■ Pulmonologist* (pulmonary HTN)

(Whelton et al., 2018)
- ■ Follow-up
  - ■ Monthly until BP <130/85 mm Hg; every follow-up visit should reinforce the importance of adherence and treatment
    - ■ Then, office visit every 3 months until BP is stable; lifestyle modification should be reassessed during every office visit.
  - ■ Then, office visit every 6 months

(Whelton et al., 2018)

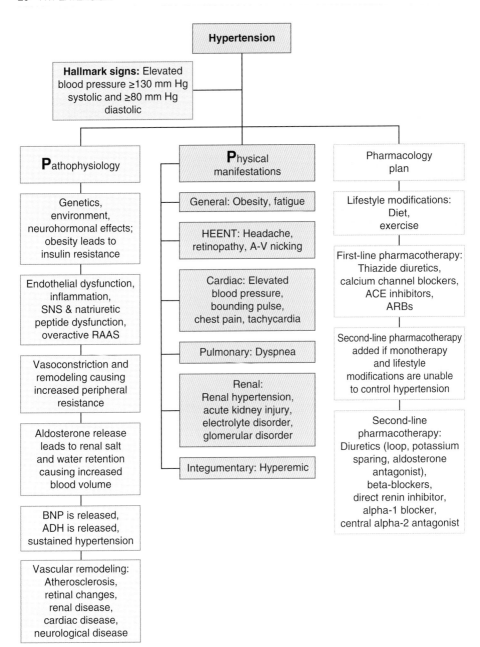

Algorithm 20.1   Hypertension

ACE, Angiotensin converting enzyme; *ADH*, antidiuretic hormone; *ARBs*, angiotensin II reception blockers; *BNP*, brain natriuretic peptide; *RAAS*, renin angiotensin aldosterone system; *SNS*, sympathetic nervous system.

References

Ball, J. W., Dains, J. E., Flynn, J. A., Solomon, B. S., & Stewart, R. W. (2023). *Seidel's guide to physical examination* (10th ed.). Elsevier.

Brashers, V. L. (2023). Alterations in cardiovascular function. In J. L. Rogers (Ed), *McCance & Huether's pathophysiology: The biologic basis for disease in adults and children* (9th ed., pp. 1061–1067). Elsevier.

Castro, L. C., & Hobel, C. J. (2016). Hypertensive disorders of pregnancy. In N. F. Hacker, J. C. Gambone, & C. J. Hobel (Eds.), *Hacker & Moore's essentials of obstetrics & gynecology* (6th ed., pp. 183–193). Elsevier.

Centers for Disease Control and Prevention. (2021a). Polaris health topics—High blood pressure. https://www.cdc.gov/policy/polaris/healthtopics/highbloodpressure/index.html.

Centers for Disease Control and Prevention. (2021b). Hypertension cascade: Hypertension prevalence, treatment, and control estimates among U.S. adults 18 years and older applying the criteria from the American College of Cardiology and American Heart Association's 2017 hypertension guideline—NHANES 2015–2018. https://millionhearts.hhs.gov/data-reports/hypertension-prevalence.html.

Dains, J. E., Baumann, L. C., & Scheibel, P. (2024). *Advanced health assessment & clinical diagnosis in primary care* (7th ed.). Elsevier.

Egan, B. M. (2022). *Initial evaluation of the hypertensive adult.* UpToDate. Retrieved September 2, 2024, from https://www.uptodate.com/contents/overview-of-hypertension-in-adults?.

Goolsby, M. J., & Grubbs, G. L. (2019). *Advanced assessment interpreting findings and formulating differential diagnoses* (4th ed.). F. A. Davis Company.

Helton, M. R. (2022). Hypertension. In G. A. Warshaw, J. F. Potter, E. Flaherty, M. T. Heflin, M. K. McNabney, & R. J. Ham (Eds.), *Ham's primary care geriatrics: A case-based approach* (7th ed., pp. 349–372). Elsevier.

Jones, D. W., Whelton, P. K., Allen, N., Clark, D., 3rd, Gidding, S. S., Muntner, P., Nesbitt, S., Mitchell, N. S., Townsend, R., Falkner, B., American Heart Association Council on Hypertension, Council on the Kidney in Cardiovascular Disease, Council on Arteriosclerosis, Thrombosis and Vascular Biology, Council on Cardiovascular Radiology and Intervention, Council on Lifelong Congenital Heart Disease and Heart Health in the Young, & Stroke Council. (2021). Management of stage 1 hypertension in adults with a low 10-year risk for cardiovascular disease: Filling a guidance gap: A scientific statement from the American Heart Association. *Hypertension,, 77*, e58–e67.

Newcombe, J. (2020). Cardiovascular disorders. In D. L. Garzon Maaks, N. B. Starr, M. A. Brady, N. M. Gaylord, M. Driessnack, & K. G. Duderstadt (Eds.), *Burns' pediatric primary care* (7th ed., pp. 700–737). Elsevier.

Ostchega, Y., Fryar, C. D., Nwankwo, T., & Nguyen, D. T. (2020). *Hypertension prevalence among adults aged 18 and over: United States 2017–2018. NCHS data brief no. 364, April 2020.* National Center for Health Statistics. https://www.cdc.gov/nchs/data/databriefs/db364-h.pdf.

Shimbo, D., Artinian, N. T., Basile, J. N., Krakoff, L. R., Margolis, K. L., Rakotz, M. K., & Wozniak, G. (2020). Self-measured blood pressure monitoring at home: A joint policy statement from the American Heart Association and American Medical Association. *Circulation, 142*, e42–e63. https://doi.org/10.1161/CIR.0000000000000803.

Tsao, C. W., Aday, A. W., Almarzooq, Z. I., Alonso, A., Beaton, A. Z., Bittencourt, M. S., Boehme, A. K., Buxton, A. E., Carson, A. P., Commodore-Mensah, Y., Elkind, M., Evenson, K. R., Eze-Nliam, C., Ferguson, J. F., Generoso, G., Ho, J. E., Kalani, R., Khan, S. S., Kissela, B. M., American Heart Association Council on Epidemiology and Prevention Statistics Committee and Stroke Statistics Subcommittee, (2022). Heart disease and stroke statistics—2022 update: A report from the American Heart Association. *Circulation, 145*(8), e153–e639. https://doi.org/10.1161/CIR.0000000000001052.

Unger, T., Borghi, C., Charchar, F., Khan, N. A., Poulter, N. R., Prabhakaran, D., Ramirez, A., Schlaich, M., Stergiou, G. S., Tomaszewski, M., Wainford, R. D., Williams, B., & Schutte, A. E. (2020). 2020 International Society of Hypertension global hypertension practice guidelines. *Journal of Hypertension, 38*(6), 982–1004. https://doi.org/10.1097/HJH.0000000000002453.

Virani, S. S., Alonso, A., Benjamin, E. J., Bittencourt, M. S., Callaway, C. W., Carson, A. M., Chamberlain, A. M., Chang, A. R., Cheng, S., Delling, F. N., Djousse, L., Elkind, M. S. V., Ferguson, J. F., Fornage, M., Khan, S. S., Kissela, B. M., Knutson, K. L., Kwan, T. W., & Lackland, D. T., … American Heart Association Council on Epidemiology and Prevention Statistics Committee and Stroke Statistics Subcommittee. (2020). Heart disease and stroke statistics—2020 update: A report from the American Heart Association. *Circulation, 141*(9), e139–e596. https://www.ahajournals.org/doi/10.1161/CIR.0000000000000757.

Whelton, P. K., Carey, R. M., Aronow, W. S., Casey, D. E., Jr, Collins, K. J., Dennison Himmelfarb, C., De Palma, S. M., Gidding, S., Jamerson, K. A., Jones, D. W., MacLaughlin, E. J., Muntner, P., Ovbiagele, B., Smith, S. C., Jr, Spencer, C. C., Stafford, R. S., Taler, S. J., Thomas, R. J., Williams, K. A., Sr, & Wright, J. T., Jr. (2018). 2017 ACC/AHA/AAPA/ABC/ACPM/AGS/APhA/ASH/ASPC/NMA/PCNA guideline for the prevention, detection, evaluation, and management of high blood pressure in adults: A report of the American College of Cardiology/American Heart Association task force on clinical practice guidelines. *Hypertension, 71*(6), e13–e115. https://doi.org/10.1161/HYP.0000000000000065.

Respiratory System

SECTION OUTLINE

21 Pneumonia

22 Chronic Obstructive Pulmonary Disease

23 Restrictive Lung Disease

24 Pharyngitis

CHAPTER 21

Pneumonia

Julia L. Rogers

Community Acquired

Viral and Bacterial Pneumonia Lung Infections

Pneumonia is a lower respiratory tract infection characterized by inflammation of lung parenchyma, typically caused by infectious agents such as bacteria, viruses, fungi, protozoa, or parasites (Brashers, 2023). The microbes cause alveola consolidation, interstitial inflammation, and impaired gas exchange. Bacterial pneumonia is broadly categorized by whether it occurs outside the hospital (community-acquired pneumonia [CAP]) or within the hospital (nosocomial or hospital-acquired pneumonia) (Box 21.1), which includes ventilator-associated pneumonia. For the purposes of this chapter only bacterial and viral CAP are discussed. Individuals at the highest risk for pneumonia are children younger than 5 years of age (Box 21.2), adults older than 65 years of age (Box 21.3), and individuals with dysphagia, chronic medical conditions, immobility, or alcoholism; those who smoke cigarettes; or those who use gastric acid suppressive medications (Brashers, 2023; Centers for Disease Control and Prevention [CDC], 2022). Social determinants of health also play a role in the risk factors associated with pneumonia (Box 21.4).

Typical bacteria, atypical bacteria, and respiratory viruses are the three major categories of pathogens causing CAP. Typical pathogens have been detected in up to 56% of the cases in different studies (Cavallazzi & Ramirez, 2022). The most common bacterial-related cause of CAP is *Streptococcus pneumoniae*. Other common typical pathogens causing CAP include *Haemophilus influenzae*, *Moraxella catarrhalis*, and *Enterobacteriaceae* (e.g., *Klebsiella* spp., *Escherichia coli*, *Enterobacter* spp., *Serratia marcescens*, *Proteus mirabilis*, and *Morganella morganii*) (Cavallazzi & Ramirez, 2022). Atypical pathogens have been identified in 22% to 31% of patients with CAP treated in the outpatient setting (Cavallazzi & Ramirez, 2022). Common atypical microorganisms causing CAP include *Mycoplasma pneumoniae*, *Chlamydophila pneumoniae*, and *Legionella* (Cavallazzi & Ramirez, 2022).

Novel diagnostic technologies have improved the identification of viral respiratory pathogens. Therefore viruses are increasingly being identified as frequent etiologies of CAP. The prevalence of viral infection detected by polymerase chain reaction in the outpatient population with CAP has been reported to be 12.1%. However, a metaanalysis of studies that included a mix of inpatient and outpatient populations with CAP showed a prevalence of viral infection of 22.4% (Metlay et al., 2019). The most common viral pathogens are influenza, rhinovirus, and COVID-19.

The most common etiologic microorganisms of hospital-acquired pneumonia (HAP) are *P. aeruginosa* and MRSA, likely due to the increase in antibiotic-resistant organisms (see Box 21.1). Individuals who are severely immunocompromised (e.g., HIV infection) may have CAP caused by a fungi, such as *Pneumocystis jirovecii*, *Aspergillus*, or *Cryptococcus* (Brashers, 2023).

BOX 21.1 ■ Acute Care Considerations

The most common pathogens causing hospital-acquired pneumonia are methicillin-resistant *Staphylococcus aureus* (MRSA), *Pseudomonas aeruginosa* (*P. aeruginosa*), *Enterobacteriaceae*, *Acinetobacter*, *Klebsiella pneumoniae*, and *Escherichia coli*.

For adult patients in the acute care setting with nonsevere community-acquired pneumonia who do not have risk factors for MRSA or *P. aeruginosa*, the following empiric treatment regimen should be followed (shown here in no order of preference):

- Combination therapy with a beta-lactam (ampicillin plus sulbactam 1.5–3 g every 6 hours, or cefotaxime 1–2 g every 8 hours, or ceftriaxone 1–2 g daily, or ceftaroline 600 mg every 12 hours) *and* a macrolide (azithromycin 500 mg daily or clarithromycin 500 mg twice daily) *OR*
- Respiratory fluoroquinolone as monotherapy (levofloxacin 750 mg daily, or moxifloxacin 400 mg daily) (CDC, 2023)

For adult patients with severe community-acquired pneumonia who *do not have risk factors* for MRSA or *P. aeruginosa*, the following treatment regimen should be followed (shown here in no order of preference):

- Beta-lactam *plus* a macrolide *OR*
- Beta-lactam *plus* a respiratory fluoroquinolone

Adult patients who *have risk factors* for MRSA or *P. aeruginosa* should be empirically covered if locally validated risk factors for either pathogen are present.

Empiric treatment options for MRSA include:

- Vancomycin (15 mg/kg every 12 hours; adjust based on levels) *OR*
- Linezolid (600 mg every 12 hours)

Empiric treatment options for *P. aeruginosa* include:

- Piperacillin-tazobactam (4.5 g every 6 hours) *OR*
- Cefepime (2 g every 8 hours) *OR*
- Ceftazidime (2 g every 8 hours) *OR*
- Aztreonam (2 g every 8 hours) *OR*
- Meropenem (1 g every 8 hours) *OR*
- Imipenem (500 mg every 6 hours)

(Reprinted with permission of the American Thoracic Society. Copyright © 2024 American Thoracic Society. All rights reserved.)

Duration of antibiotic therapy should be guided by a validated measure of clinical stability (resolution of vital sign abnormalities, ability to eat, and normal mentation). Antibiotic therapy should be continued until the patient achieves stability and for no less than a total of 5 days.

BOX 21.2 ■ Pediatric Considerations

Pneumonia is the single largest infectious cause of death in children worldwide, accounting for 14% of all deaths of children under 5 years of age and 22% of all deaths in children aged 1 to 5 years. Environmental factors such as indoor air pollution caused by cooking and heating with biomass fuels (i.e., wood or dung), living in crowded homes, and parental smoking increase a child's susceptibility to pneumonia. *Streptococcus pneumoniae* is the most common bacterial pathogen causing pneumonia in children and *Haemophilus influenzae* type b is the second most common. The most common viral cause of pneumonia in children is the respiratory syncytial virus (RSV). Pneumonia in children under 5 years of age is diagnosed by the presence of fast breathing or lower chest wall indrawing where the chest moves in or retracts during inhalation, with symptoms of cough and/or difficulty breathing and with or without fever. Wheezing is associated with viral infections more than bacterial infections. Ill infants and children may not drink or feed, which can lead to severe dehydration rather quickly. Providers need to educate parents on the importance of vaccinations. Immunization against pneumococcus, *Haemophilus influenzae* type b, measles, and whooping cough (pertussis) is the most effective way to prevent pneumonia (World Health Organization [WHO], 2022).

BOX 21.3 ■ Older Adult Considerations

Older adults may present with atypical symptoms of pneumonia, which may contribute to the high mortality rates in this population. The presence of concomitant illness and delays in diagnosis contribute to significant mortality from this disease in the elderly. Providers should be highly suspicious of pneumonia in an older adult presenting with an exacerbation of underlying illness along with atypical symptoms such as confusion, headache, and being afebrile. The usual symptoms of fever, chills, rigors, and sputum production that are present in younger adults, but may be absent in older adults. Even consolidation on a chest X-ray can be difficult to distinguish pneumonia from other diseases of the elderly such as congestive heart failure (see Chapter 18). The other factor contributing to higher mortality is increased risk factors for multidrug-resistant organisms, particularly for individuals residing in long-term care facilities. Providers need to consider this when making empiric treatment decisions as well as any underlying comorbid conditions. It is important to review medication history to avoid any potential drug–drug interactions and drug-related adverse events in elderly patients (Henig & Kaye, 2017).

BOX 21.4 ■ Diversity Considerations

Community-acquired pneumonia is linked to numerous social determinants of health factors and represents a public health challenge. Factors that play a role in poor outcomes for individuals with pneumonia include socioeconomic status, race, smoking habits or exposure to tobacco, air pollution, crowding, educational status, age, and nutrition. Higher mortality rates are linked to poverty-related factors such as malnourishment, lack of safe water and sanitation, indoor air pollution, and inadequate access to health care. Multiple studies have documented racial differences in access to treatment and prevention services (i.e., vaccines). One study revealed that mortality rates from pneumonia were higher for Black patients than White patients treated in the same hospital because of a difference in treatment options such as receiving antibiotics and oxygenation within the recommended time (Bazie et al., 2020; Lippert et al., 2022).

Pathophysiology

Pneumonia is characterized by inflammation of lung parenchyma, alveoli, and terminal airspaces in response to invasion by an infectious agent introduced into the lungs through inhalation or hematogenous spread (Algorithm 21.1). Transmission can occur through direct or indirect contact via droplets, aerosols, or blood (Boehmer et al., 2021). Infection occurs when host defenses are impaired, allowing microorganisms to enter the lower airways. Aspiration, which is seen more in elderly adults, accounts for 5% to 15% of CAP (Mandell & Niederman, 2019). Invading pathogens ensure infection by synthesizing and secreting microbial enzymes, proteins, toxic lipids, and toxins that cause direct damage to the host cell membranes, organelles, and extracellular matrix. Endotoxin, leukocidin, and toxic shock syndrome toxin-1 are toxins that provide certain microbes with increased virulence. These toxins are capable of destroying the body's immune cells (e.g., leukocytes, T lymphocytes, natural killer cells) and mediate indirect injury by causing interference with oxygen and nutrient delivery, altering vasomotor tone and integrity, and interrupting removal of waste products from local tissues. Alveolar macrophages respond to lower airway bacteria invasion by releasing TNF alpha and interleukin-1, along with chemokines and chemotactic factors from mast cells and fibroblasts, which contribute to widespread inflammation and the recruitment of neutrophils from the capillaries into the alveoli. Neutrophil extracellular traps are released by neutrophils to assist in removing the invading microorganism; however, they also cause damage to lung tissue (Grudzinska et al., 2020). Airway smooth muscle tone and resistance are increased by the activation of the inflammatory cascade. Inflammatory mediators, immune complexes, and toxins damage alveolocapillary membranes and bronchial mucus membranes. The injuries cause overstimulation to goblet cells, increasing mucus secretion and leading to partial or complete obstruction of airways, air trapping, atelectatic or hyperexpanded alveoli, ventilatory dead space, and shunting.

Many of the physical manifestations present in pneumonia are linked to this response. For example, crackles are heard from atelectatic alveoli and small airways attempting to open, and from hyperexpanded alveoli collapsing from fluid or exudate, diminished breath sounds from air trapping, wheezing from increased mucus and narrowed airways, and dyspnea and cough related to airway resistance, obstruction, and poor gas exchange. Hypoxemia may result from the ventilation–perfusion mismatch (Brashers, 2023), and fever is part of the inflammatory response. Secondary complications may potentially occur with pneumonia. Exudative effusions, called parapneumonic effusions, may occur and often resolve with treatment of bacterial pneumonia but can progress to empyema. A spontaneous pneumothorax may occur in individuals with pneumonia because the integrity of the visceral pleura is compromised (Brashers, 2023).

VIRAL PNEUMONIA

Viral pneumonia is typically associated with interstitial inflammation and diffuse alveolar damage (Torres et al., 2021). The inflammatory response triggers the leakage of plasma and the loss of surfactant, resulting in air loss and consolidation. Disease progresses when the alveolar type II cells lose their structural integrity and surfactant production is diminished. Alveolar damage follows an organized pattern and resolution similar to the intraalveolar inflammation in bacterial pneumonia (Torres et al., 2021). Viral pneumonias caused by influenza and COVID-19 initiate a cytokine storm, which causes epithelial and endothelial damage, hypercoagulability, and increased vascular permeability leading to alveolar edema and acute respiratory distress disorder (Brashers, 2023). Respiratory viruses may lead to a secondary bacterial infection. This occurs due to the virus damaging the normally protectant ciliated epithelial cells, which prevent pathogens from reaching the lower airways (Brashers, 2023).

BACTERIAL PNEUMONIA

Pathogenic bacteria colonization of the upper respiratory tract followed by aspiration of oropharyngeal secretions is the most common route of lower respiratory tract infection. However, infection may also ensue following inhalation of certain microorganisms, or hematogenously from infection elsewhere in the body or intravenous drug use (Torres et al., 2021). In bacterial infections, the alveoli fill with proteinaceous fluid, triggering an influx of red blood cells and polymorphonuclear cells (red hepatization) followed by the deposition of fibrin and the degradation of inflammatory cells (gray hepatization). During resolution, intraalveolar debris is ingested and removed by the alveolar macrophages. This consolidation leads to decreased air entry and dullness to percussion (Waseem & Lominy, 2023).

Bronchopneumonia, a patchy consolidation involving one or more lobes, usually involves the dependent lung zones, a pattern attributable to aspiration of oropharyngeal contents. The neutrophilic exudate is centered in the bronchi and bronchioles, with centrifugal spread to the adjacent alveoli. In interstitial pneumonia, patchy or diffuse inflammation involving the interstitium is characterized by infiltration of lymphocytes and macrophages. The alveoli do not contain a significant exudate, but protein-rich hyaline membranes similar to those found in adult acute respiratory distress disorder may line the alveolar spaces. Bacterial superinfection of viral pneumonia can also produce a mixed pattern of interstitial and alveolar airspace inflammation. *Miliary pneumonia* is a term applied to multiple discrete lesions resulting from the spread of the pathogen to the lungs hematogenously (Waseem & Lominy, 2023).

Physical Clinical Presentation

SUBJECTIVE

The subjective clinical manifestations associated with bacterial pneumonia include a sudden onset of cough, pleuritic chest pain, dyspnea, and chills or rigors. The cough may be productive with purulent, yellow, green, or rust-colored sputum or the patient may report hemoptysis. Individuals may also complain of nonspecific abdominal symptoms of pain, nausea and vomiting, or right lower quadrant pain. The pain likely represents involvement of the right lower lobe because that area can stimulate the 10th and 11th thoracic nerves to cause and simulate an abdominal process. The onset of symptoms is more insidious with mycobacterial, fungal, or atypical lung infections.

During the focused history, documentation should include the onset of symptoms; precipitating events; location, intensity, and quality of pain; progression of symptoms; alleviating and aggravating factors; previous episodes; and associated symptoms. Document allergies, ill contacts, autoimmune diseases, and medical, social, and family histories. (Ball et al., 2023; Dains et al., 2024)

OBJECTIVE*

Generalized: Fatigue; **fever; chills or rigor**
Neurological: Confusion
HHENT: Halitosis
Cardiovascular: Tachycardia; **pleuritic chest pain**
Pulmonary: *Inspection:* Rapid shallow respirations; **dyspnea**; tachypnea; **cough productive**; **use of accessary muscles; nasal flaring**; splinting side of consolidation
Palpation: **Increased fremitus in presence of consolidation**; decreased fremitus in presence of a concomitant empyema or pleural effusion; **increased egophony; decreased respiratory excursion and chest wall motion unilaterally**
Percussion: Dullness or flatness over consolidation
Auscultation: **Crackles inspiratory**; rhonchi; bronchial breath sounds; pleural rub; **bronchophony**; egophony; whispered pectoriloquy
Integumentary: Cyanosis peripheral
(Ball et al., 2023; Dains et al., 2024) (Algorithm 21.1)

Evaluation and Differential Diagnoses

DIAGNOSTICS

- Complete the Pneumonia Severity Index (Fine et al., 1997; Metlay et al., 2019), a validated clinical prediction rule for prognosis, to determine the need for hospitalization in adults diagnosed with CAP.
- Chest radiograph posterior-anterior and lateral when consolidation or infiltrate is present (Fig. 21.1)
- Rapid influenza molecular assay when influenza viruses are circulating in the community (influenza A/influenza B)
- Recommendation not to obtain sputum Gram stain and culture or blood cultures routinely in adults with CAP managed in the outpatient setting
(Metlay et al., 2019)

---

*Hallmark signs are bolded and <u>Red flags are bolded and underlined</u>.

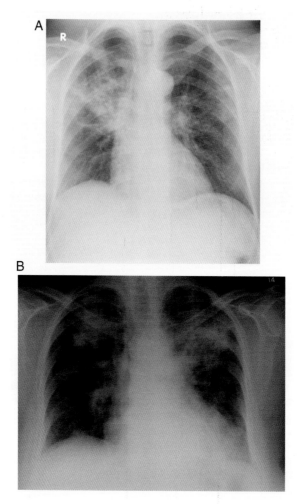

Fig. 21.1 Pneumonia. Consolidation on chest X-ray. (**A**) Right upper lobe pneumonia. (**B**) Multilobar pneumonia. (From Loebinger, M. R., & Wilson, R. G. (2012). Pneumonia. *Medicine*, *40*(6), 329–334. https://doi.org/10.1016/j.mpmed.2012.03.005).

DIFFERENTIAL DIAGNOSIS

- Acute bronchitis
- Exacerbation of chronic obstructive pulmonary disease
- Atelectasis
- Heart failure
- Bronchiectasis

Plan

Guideline Resources

- Metlay, J. P., Waterer, G., Long, A., Anzueto, A., Brozek, J., Crothers, K., Cooley, L. A., Dean, N. C., Fine, M. J., Flanders, S. A., Griffin, M. R., Metersky, M. L., Musher, D. M., Restrepo, M. I., Whitney, C. G., & on behalf of the American Thoracic Society and Infectious Diseases Society of America. (2019). Diagnosis and treatment of adults with community-acquired pneumonia. An official clinical practice guideline of the American Thoracic Society and Infectious Diseases Society of America. *American Journal of Respiratory and Critical Care Medicine*, *200*(7), e45–e67. https://doi.org/10.1164/rccm.201908-1581st.

Pharmacotherapy

- Bacterial community acquired pneumonia
  - Antibiotics** (Algorithm 21.1)
    - Empiric antibiotic therapy initiated in adults with clinically suspected and radiographically confirmed CAP:
      - Amoxicillin 1 g three times daily *OR*
      - Doxycycline 100 mg twice daily *OR*
      - Macrolide only in areas with pneumococcal resistance to macrolides <25%:
        - Azithromycin 500 mg on day 1, then 250 mg daily for 4 days *OR*
        - Clarithromycin 500 mg twice daily *OR*
        - Clarithromycin extended release 1000 mg daily
    - Outpatient adults with comorbidities such as chronic heart, lung, liver, or renal disease; diabetes mellitus; alcoholism; malignancy; or asplenia:
      - Amoxicillin/clavulanate 500 mg/125 mg three times daily, or amoxicillin/clavulanate 875 mg/125 mg twice daily, or 2000 mg/125 mg twice daily, or a cephalosporin *AND*
      - Macrolide (azithromycin 500 mg on day 1, then 250 mg daily, or clarithromycin 500 mg twice daily or extended release 1000 mg once daily), or doxycycline 100 mg twice daily *OR*
      - Fluoroquinolone as monotherapy (levofloxacin 750 mg daily, or moxifloxacin 400 mg daily, or gemifloxacin 320 mg daily)
  - Oxygen for SpO_2 <90%
- Viral pneumonia
  - Antiinfluenza treatment (e.g., oseltamivir) for adults with CAP who test positive for influenza
  - Supportive care for bacterial and viral pneumonia
  - Supportive care: Rest; aspirin, nonsteroidal antiinflammatory drugs, or acetaminophen for fever and body aches; fluids
  - Smoking cessation aids if current tobacco use
  - Vaccines (two pneumococcal vaccines available in the United States)
    - Pneumococcal conjugate vaccines (PCV13, PCV15, and PCV20)

**Duration of antibiotic therapy should be guided by a validated measure of clinical stability (resolution of vital sign abnormalities, ability to eat, and normal mentation). Antibiotic therapy should be continued until the patient achieves stability and for no less than a total of 5 days.

- PCV13 or PCV15 for children younger than 5 years of age and those 5 to 18 years of age with medical conditions that increase risk of pneumococcal disease
- PCV15 or PCV20 for adults aged 65 years and older who have never received a pneumococcal conjugate vaccine. If PCV15 is used, this should be followed by a dose of PPSV23.**
- PCV20 can be given to adults aged 65 years and older who have already received PCV13 (but not PCV15 or PCV20) at any age and PPSV23 at or after age 65.
- PCV15 or PCV20 for adults 19 to 64 years of age with medical conditions or risk factors. If PCV15 is used, this should be followed by a dose of PPSV23.**
- Pneumococcal polysaccharide vaccine (PPSV23)
  - PPSV23 for children 2 to 18 years of age with medical conditions that increase risk of pneumococcal disease
  - PPSV23 for adults aged 19 years and older who previously received PCV15**

(CDC, 2023; Metlay et al., 2019)

NONPHARMACOTHERAPY

- Educate
  - Good hand hygiene
  - Respiratory etiquette
  - Avoid environmental and occupational irritants.
  - Importance of vaccines
- Lifestyle and behavioral modifications
  - Smoking cessation
  - Wearing a cold weather mask
  - Maintain hydration with oral water intake
- Complementary treatment
  - Vitamin C
  - Complementary and alternative therapies with natural medicines and supplements may interact with prescription medications. Obtain a complete medication history.
- Referral
  - Consult pulmonologist
- Follow-up
  - Follow up if symptoms do not improve within 72 hours of initiating antibiotics.
  - Follow-up chest X-ray only if symptoms have resolved in 5 to 7 days

(CDC, 2023; Metlay et al., 2019)

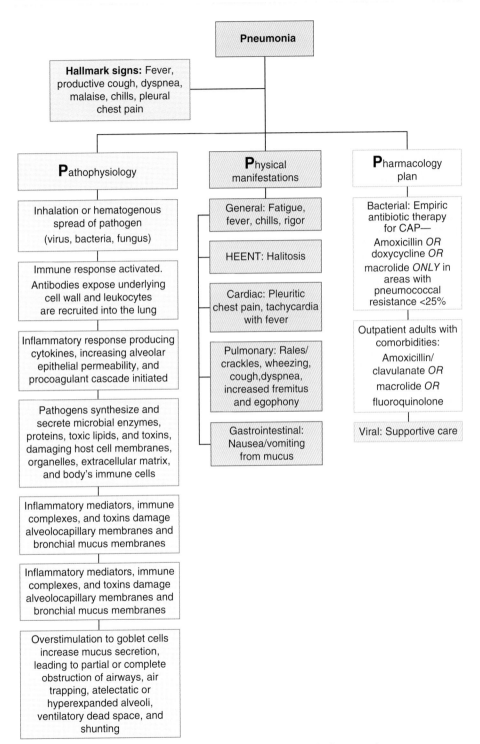

Pneumonia

Hallmark signs: Fever, productive cough, dyspnea, malaise, chills, pleural chest pain

Pathophysiology

Inhalation or hematogenous spread of pathogen (virus, bacteria, fungus)

Immune response activated. Antibodies expose underlying cell wall and leukocytes are recruited into the lung

Inflammatory response producing cytokines, increasing alveolar epithelial permeability, and procoagulant cascade initiated

Pathogens synthesize and secrete microbial enzymes, proteins, toxic lipids, and toxins, damaging host cell membranes, organelles, extracellular matrix, and body's immune cells

Inflammatory mediators, immune complexes, and toxins damage alveolocapillary membranes and bronchial mucus membranes

Inflammatory mediators, immune complexes, and toxins damage alveolocapillary membranes and bronchial mucus membranes

Overstimulation to goblet cells increase mucus secretion, leading to partial or complete obstruction of airways, air trapping, atelectatic or hyperexpanded alveoli, ventilatory dead space, and shunting

Physical manifestations

General: Fatigue, fever, chills, rigor

HEENT: Halitosis

Cardiac: Pleuritic chest pain, tachycardia with fever

Pulmonary: Rales/crackles, wheezing, cough,dyspnea, increased fremitus and egophony

Gastrointestinal: Nausea/vomiting from mucus

Pharmacology plan

Bacterial: Empiric antibiotic therapy for CAP—
Amoxicillin *OR* doxycycline *OR* macrolide *ONLY* in areas with pneumococcal resistance <25%

Outpatient adults with comorbidities:
Amoxicillin/clavulanate *OR* macrolide *OR* fluoroquinolone

Viral: Supportive care

Algorithm 21.1 Pneumonia. *CAP*, Community-acquired pneumonia

References

Ball, J. W., Dains, J. E., Flynn, J. A., Solomon, B. S., & Stewart, R. W. (2023). *Seidel's guide to physical examination* (10th ed.). Elsevier.

Bazie, G. W., Seid, N., & Admassu, B. (2020). Determinants of community acquired pneumonia among 2 to 59 months of age children in northeast Ethiopia: A case-control study. *Pneumonia, 12*(1), 14. https://doi.org/10.1186/s41479-020-00077-0.

Boehmer, T. K., Kompaniyets, L., Lavery, A. M., Hsu, J., Ko, J. Y., Yusuf, H., Romano, S. D., Gundlapalli, A. V., Oster, M. E., & Harris, A. M. (2021). Association between COVID-19 and myocarditis using hospital-based administrative data—United States, March 2020–January 2021. *Morbidity and Mortality Weekly Report, 70*(35), 1228–1232.

Brashers, V. (2023). *Alterations of pulmonary function.* In J. L. Rogers (Ed.) *McCance & Huether's pathophysiology: The biologic basis for disease in adults and children.* (9th ed. pp. 1153–1157). Elsevier.

Cavallazzi, R., & Ramirez, J. A. (2022). How and when to manage respiratory infections out of hospital. *European Respiratory Review, 31*(166), 220092. http://doi.org/10.1183/16000617.0092-2022.

Centers for Disease Control and Prevention. (2022). Risk factors for pneumonia. Retrieved December 19, 2022, from https://www.cdc.gov/pneumonia/riskfactors.html.

Centers for Disease Control and Prevention. (2023). Pneumococcal vaccination. Retrieved March 22, 2023, from https://www.cdc.gov/vaccines/vpd/pneumo/index.html.

Dains, J. E., Baumann, L. C., & Scheibel, P. (2024). *Advanced health assessment & clinical diagnosis in primary care* (7th ed.). Elsevier.

Fine, M. J., Auble, T. E., Yealy, D. M., Hanusa, B. H., Weissfeld, L. A., Singer, D. E., Coley, C. M., Marrie, T. J., & Kapoor, W. N. (1997). A prediction rule to identify low-risk patients with community-acquired pneumonia. *New England Journal of Medicine, 336*(4), 243–250. http://doi.org/10.1056/NEJM199701233360402.

Grudzinska, F. S., Brodlie, M., Scholefield, B. R., Jackson, T., Scott, A., Thickett, D. R., & Sapey, E. (2020). Neutrophils in community-acquired pneumonia: Parallels in dysfunction at the extremes of age. *Thorax, 75*(2), 164–171.

Henig, O., & Kaye, K. S. (2017). Bacterial pneumonia in older adults. *Infectious Disease Clinics of North America, 31*(4), 89–713. http://doi.org/10.1016/j.idc.2017.07.015.

Lippert, J. F., Buscemi, J., Saiyed, N., Silva, A., & Benjamins, M. R. (2022). Influenza and pneumonia mortality across the 30 biggest U.S. cities: Assessment of overall trends and racial inequities. *Journal of Racial and Ethnic Health Disparities, 9*(4), 1152–1160. https://doi.org/10.1007/s40615-021-01056-x.

Mandell, L. A., & Niederman, M. S. (2019). Aspiration pneumonia. *New England Journal of Medicine, 380*(7), 651–663.

Metlay, J. P., Waterer, G. W., Long, A. C., Anzueto, A., Brozek, J., Crothers, K., Cooley, L. A., Dean, N. C., Fine, M. J., Flanders, S. A., Griffin, M. R., Metersky, M. L., Musher, D. M., Restrepo, M. I., & Whitney, C. G. (2019). Diagnosis and treatment of adults with community-acquired pneumonia. An official clinical practice guideline of the American Thoracic Society and Infectious Diseases Society of America. *American Journal of Respiratory and Critical Care Medicine, 200*(7), e45–e67. https://www.atsjournals.org/doi/full/10.1164/rccm.201908-1581ST.

Torres, A., Cilloniz, C., Niederman, M. S., Menendez, R., Chalmers, J. D., Wunderink, R. G., & van der Poll, T. (2021). Pneumonia. *Nature Reviews Disease Primers, 7*(1), 25. https://doi.org/10.1038/s41572-021-00259-0.

Waseem, M., & Lominy, M. M. (2023). *Pediatric pneumonia.* Medscape, Retrieved September 7, 2024, https://emedicine.medscape.com/article/967822-overview#a3.

World Health Organization. (2022). Pneumonia in children. Retrieved December 19, 2022, from https://www.who.int/news-room/fact-sheets/detail/pneumonia.

CHAPTER 22

Chronic Obstructive Pulmonary Disease

Julia L. Rogers

Emphysema and Bronchitis

Chronic Obstructive Pulmonary Disease

Chronic obstructive pulmonary disease (COPD) is characterized by air flow limitation and persistent respiratory symptoms due to airway and/or alveolar abnormalities usually caused by exposure to noxious particles or gases. COPD is the most common chronic lung disease in the world and the sixth leading cause of death in the United States (Syamlal et al., 2022). Risk factors for COPD include tobacco smoke (cigarette, pipe, cigar), occupational dust and chemical vapors (irritants and fumes), indoor air pollution from biomass fuel used for cooking and heating (in poorly ventilated dwellings), outdoor air pollution, factors that affect lung growth during gestation, and certain infections such as tuberculosis. There is emerging evidence that the use of electronic cigarettes for vaping may also lead to an increased risk for COPD (Brashers, 2023). The most common cause of COPD is smoking. Approximately 80% of deaths related to COPD are associated with the history of smoking (Global Initiative for Chronic Obstructive Lung Disease [GOLD], 2024). A second, less common factor is a hereditary deficiency in alpha-1 antitrypsin (AAT). The two most common phenotypes are emphysema and chronic bronchitis (Brashers, 2023). Emphysema is defined as abnormal permanent enlargement of gas exchange airways accompanied by destruction of alveolar walls without obvious fibrosis, while chronic bronchitis is defined as hypersecretion of mucus and chronic productive cough that continues for at least 3 months of the year (usually the winter months) for at least 2 consecutive years.

Pathophysiology

The main characteristics of the pathophysiologic process of COPD are inflammation, excessive mucus secretion, incomplete reversible airflow limitation, and bronchial mucosal epithelial lesions (Algorithm 22.1) (Guo et al., 2022). The pathologic mechanisms of COPD are the result of environmental and genetic interactions. Alpha-1-antitrypsin deficiency (A1ATD) is the primary genetic factor and smoking tobacco is the primary environmental factor. Lung growth and development plays a significant role in a person's susceptibility to COPD and may have a link to genetics (Guo et al., 2022).

The innate and adaptive immune systems have been implicated in the pathogenesis of COPD (Fig. 22.1). Sustained activation of the innate immune response causes increased aggregation of neutrophils, triggering inflammatory mediators, which produce large amounts of reactive oxygen species (ROS) and provoke the oxidative stress response (Guo et al., 2022). The severity of airflow obstruction is associated with the number of activated immune cell accumulations (e.g.,

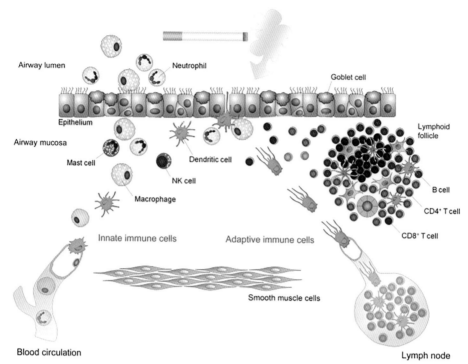

Fig. 22.1 Cells of the innate and adaptive immune systems in the pathogenesis of chronic obstructive pulmonary disease (COPD). Epithelial cells and cells of the innate immune system become activated upon cigarette smoke exposure. Dendritic cells initiate an adaptive immune response, including CD8+ cytotoxic T cells and CD4+ T helper cells. In patients with severe COPD there is organization of B and T cells in lymphoid follicles. *NK,* Natural killer. (From Wedzicha, J. A., & Hurst, J. R. (2006). Chronic obstructive pulmonary disease: Acute exacerbations. In G. J. Laurent & S. D. Shapiro (Eds.), *Encyclopedia of Respiratory Medicine* (pp. 439–443). Academic Press. https://doi.org/10.1016/b0-12-370879-6/00498-1.)

neutrophils, macrophages, and lymphocytes) within the airway mucosa (Linden et al., 2019). Goblet cells are also increased, causing excessive mucus secretion. The chronic inflammation and irreversible airway remodeling may be due in part to the dysregulation of adaptive immune mechanisms (Linden et al., 2019).

EMPHYSEMA

Emphysema is characterized by a loss of lung elasticity from the breakdown of elastin and abnormal enlargement of the airspaces distal to the terminal bronchioles. There is destruction of the alveolar walls and capillary beds by enzymes called proteases, which digest proteins. Structural changes include narrowing and luminal exudates in the small airways and destruction of the lung parenchyma, which contribute to airflow obstruction and mucociliary dysfunction (GOLD, 2024). Enlargement of the air spaces leads to trapping of gas and hyperinflation of the lungs and produces an increase in total lung capacity, decreases the volume of air in the first second of forced expiration (FEV1), and decreases the ratio of FEV1 to forced vital capacity (FVC), which is the volume of air forcibly exhaled from the point of maximal inspiration (GOLD, 2024). Two of the recognized causes of emphysema are smoking, which incites lung injury, and an inherited genetic deficiency of AAT, an antiprotease enzyme that normally protects the lung from injury. Cigarette smoke and other irritants stimulate the movement of inflammatory cells into the lungs, resulting in increased release of elastase and other proteases. In smokers who develop COPD, antiprotease production and release appears to be inadequate to neutralize the excess protease production, leading to elastic tissue destruction.

A1ATD is an autosomal recessive disorder resulting in early-onset emphysema and liver disease. A mutation in the SERPINA 1 gene can cause A1ATD (GOLD, 2024). A1ATD deficiency affects 1% to 2% of patients with COPD and approximately 1 in 2500 individuals. Consider diagnosis in adults with emphysema with onset at ≤40 years of age and without risk factors (no history of smoking or occupational dust exposure). Diagnosis should be made through serum AAT levels and confirmed with genetic testing.

CHRONIC BRONCHITIS

Chronic bronchitis represents airway obstruction of the major and small airways. The condition is seen most in middle-aged males and is associated with chronic irritation from smoking and recurrent infections. A clinical diagnosis of chronic bronchitis requires the history of a chronic productive cough for at least 3 consecutive months for at least 2 consecutive years. Typically the cough has been present for many years, with a gradual increase in acute exacerbations that produce purulent sputum.

The earliest feature of chronic bronchitis is hypersecretion of mucus in the large airways associated with hypertrophy of the submucosal glands in the trachea and bronchi. Accompanying histologic changes in the small airways (small bronchi and bronchioles) are physiologically important in the airway obstruction that develops in chronic bronchitis. These changes include a marked increase in goblet cells and excess mucus production with plugging of the airway lumen, inflammatory infiltration, and fibrosis of the bronchiolar wall. It is thought that both the submucosal hypertrophy in the larger airways and the increase in goblet cells in the smaller airways are a protective reaction against tobacco smoke and other pollutants (Higham et al., 2019). Viral and bacterial infections (see Chapter 21) are common in people with chronic bronchitis and are thought to be the result rather than the cause of the problem.

Physical Clinical Presentation

SUBJECTIVE

The clinical presentation of COPD usually has an insidious onset, with complaints of progressive dyspnea, exertional dyspnea, fatigue, exercise intolerance, and chronic cough with or without sputum production (GOLD, 2024). Complaints are often described as air hunger or gasping for air. A productive cough usually occurs in the morning and is associated with chronic bronchitis but can be seen less frequently with emphysema. Dyspnea on exertion that progresses to marked dyspnea even at rest is the most common symptom of COPD and becomes more severe as the disease progresses. During the focused history, documentation should include the onset of symptoms; intensity and quality of symptoms (e.g., severe shortness of breath with wheezing and coughing worse in the morning); precipitating events; progression of symptoms; alleviating and aggravating factors (e.g., exacerbated by exertion and alleviated or improved with rest); previous episodes; and associated symptoms including pain. Document allergies, ill contacts, and medical, social, and family histories. Medical history should include hospitalizations related to exacerbation since the last visit and history of recurrent lower respiratory tract infections. Frequent exacerbations of infection and respiratory insufficiency are common and may progress to chronic respiratory failure (GOLD, 2024). Document any past contributory medical history such as developmental abnormalities, premature birth, or childhood respiratory illness (Box 22.1). Document all current medical conditions and concomitant chronic diseases including cardiovascular disease

> **BOX 22.1 ■ Pediatric Considerations**
>
> Congenital lobar emphysema (CLE) is a developmental anomaly of the lower respiratory tract in the pediatric population. Males are three times more likely to be affected than females and it is observed mainly in the White population. The most common cause of CLE is obstruction of the developing airway caused by defects in the bronchial wall, such as a deficiency of bronchial cartilage. Infants may present with persistent hypoxemia, irritability, and decreased air movement over the affected area. Diagnostic imaging with chest X-ray and subsequent computed tomography (CT) scan would likely reveal hyperinflation of the affected lung with mediastinal shift. In cases of CLE, the infant will undergo a lobectomy of the affected lung (Scott et al., 2023).

(CVD) (see Cardiovascular System section), skeletal muscle dysfunction, metabolic syndrome (see Chapter 9), osteoporosis, depression (see Chapter 6), anxiety (see Chapter 5), obstructive sleep apnea, and lung cancer, which occur frequently in patients with COPD. Any history of exposure to risk factors for COPD should be documented. Social history must contain any history of smoking (tobacco or cannabis) or being around secondhand smoke and environmental and/or occupational exposures. Include any inhalation of toxic particles or exposure to noxious stimuli, and indoor or outdoor air pollution. Any family history of A1ATD should be documented. A formal assessment of the symptoms experienced by the individual can be done using a validated questionnaire (Ball et al., 2023; Brashers, 2023; Dains et al., 2024; GOLD, 2024).

OBJECTIVE*

Generalized: Fatigue; restless
    Neurological: <u>Confusion (with respiratory acidosis)</u>
    HEENT: Postnasal drip
    Cardiovascular: Chest tightness; **<u>jugular venous distention and peripheral edema</u>** (if concomitant right-sided heart failure due to pulmonary hypertension); muffled heart sounds (due to lung hyperinflation); tachycardia; orthopnea (if concomitant heart failure)
    Pulmonary: *Inspection:* **Dyspnea** (**<u>worsening</u>**); labored respirations; **prolonged expiration**; tachypnea; **use of accessary muscles**; **pursed lip breathing**; **cough** (same or **<u>worsening</u>**; nonproductive or productive; color of sputum and amount [clear to yellow, **<u>increased purulent sputum</u>**]); **increased anterior-posterior chest diameter (barrel-shaped chest)**
    Palpation: Decreased fremitus; decreased egophony; decreased respiratory excursion bilaterally
    Percussion: Hyperresonance
    Auscultation: **Prolonged expiration**; **wheezing**; coarse rhonchi; early inspiratory crackles (scattered); **diminished** (Box 22.2)
    Integumentary: Ecchymosis
    Extremities: Nail clubbing; central **<u>cyanosis</u>**; peripheral edema
    Psychiatric: Anxious
    (Ball et al., 2023; Brashers, 2023; Dains et al., 2024) (Algorithm 22.1)

Evaluation and Differential Diagnoses
DIAGNOSTICS

- Spirometry postbronchodilator/complete pulmonary function test with diffusing capacity of the lungs for carbon monoxide

---

*Hallmark signs are bolded and <u>Red flags are bolded and underlined.</u>

BOX 22.2 ■ Older Adult Considerations

Aspects of a standard physical exam may need to be modified for diagnostic utility in elderly patients. Older adults generally have loss of muscle strength, which may decrease chest expansion. There are also skeletal changes, with dorsal curve of the thoracic spine possibly causing difficulty taking in deep breaths. In an elderly adult who has chronic obstructive pulmonary disease (COPD), there are changes inside the body as well, such as loss of elastic recoil, fibrous alveoli, and decreased alveoli surface for gas exchange. All of these confounding elements may make it difficult for elderly individuals to take in and hold deep breaths. However, this can be an important factor when differentiating diagnoses. It is not uncommon to auscultate crackles in a geriatric patient's lungs, but to reach a diagnosis, it's important to hear when and where the crackles occur during the breathing process. Older adults also have decreased sensation of dyspnea and diminished ventilatory response to hypoxia and hypercapnia, making them more vulnerable to respiratory failure. For these reasons, it is vital that providers adapt the respiratory exam appropriately for a geriatric individual with COPD (Sharma & Goodwin, 2006; Zeng et al., 2018).

BOX 22.3 ■ Diversity Considerations

Skin pigmentation has been shown to affect pulse oximetry readings. Black patients have been shown to have occult hypoxemia that was not detected by pulse oximetry at nearly three times the frequency as White patients. Black patients have had an ABG-Co of less than 88% despite a pulse oximetry reading of 92% to 96% compared with White patients (12%–17% versus 4%–6%). These findings suggest that only relying on pulse oximetry to make clinical decisions may place Black individuals at an increased risk for occult hypoxemia. This could be detrimental if a Black patient has an inaccurate 6-minute walk test using a pulse oximeter. It may not reveal that the patient has hypoxia. Providers should be aware of this discrepancy and have a low threshold to perform arterial blood gas analysis, particularly in Black patients (Sjoding et al., 2020).

- ■ FEV1/FVC <0.7 to designate COPD diagnosis
- ■ Stages 1 through 4 based on percentage of predicted value for FEV1 (GOLD, 2024)
- ■ Chest radiograph (x-ray) posterior-anterior and lateral
- ■ Computed tomography (CT) (if criteria met)**
- ■ Hemoglobin (erythrocytosis can indicate chronic hypoxia)
- ■ Pulse oximetry with 6-minute walk test (Box 22.3)
- ■ Arterial blood gas
- ■ A1ATD screening (Riley et al., 2023)
- ■ Blood eosinophil count

(GOLD, 2024)

DIFFERENTIAL DIAGNOSIS

- ■ Asthma
- ■ Restrictive lung disease
- ■ Heart failure
- ■ Pneumonia
- ■ Lung cancer

**Persistent exacerbations, symptoms not proportional to disease severity on lung function testing, FEV1 less than 45% predicted with significant hyperinflation, and gas trapping, or for those who meet criteria for lung cancer screening.

Plan

GUIDELINE RESOURCES

- Global Initiative for Chronic Obstructive Lung Disease. (2024). *2024 Gold Report*. https://goldcopd.org/2024-gold-report/.
- Jacobs, S. S., Krishnan, J. A., Lederer, D. J., Ghazipura, M., Hossain, T., Tan, A-Y. M., Carlin, B., Drummond, M. B., Ekström, M., Garvey, C., Graney, B. A., Jackson, B., Kallstrom, T., Knight, S. L., Lindell, K., Prieto-Centurion, V., Renzoni, E. A., Ryerson, C. J., Schneidman, A., … Holland, A. E. (2020). Home oxygen therapy for adults with chronic lung disease. An official American Thoracic Society clinical practice guideline. *American Journal of Respiratory and Critical Care Medicine, 202*(10), e121–e141. https://doi.org/10.1164/rccm.202009-3608st.
- Nici, L., Mammen, M. J., Charbek, E., Alexander, P. E., Au, D. H., Boyd, C. M., Criner, G. J., Donaldson, G. C., Dreher, M., Fan, V. S., Gershon, A. S., Han, M. K., Krishnan, J. A., Martinez, F. J., Meek, P. M., Morgan, M., Polkey, M. I., Puhan, M. A., Sadatsafavi, M., … Aaron, S. D. (2020). Pharmacologic management of chronic obstructive pulmonary disease. An official American Thoracic Society clinical practice guideline. *American Journal of Respiratory and Critical Care Medicine, 201*(9), e56–e69. https://doi.org/10.1164/rccm.202003-0625st.

Pharmacotherapy

- Medication (Algorithm 22.1)
- Inhalers: Pharmacologic treatment based on results of dyspnea scale and number of moderate exacerbations and hospitalizations. Refer to guideline links.
  - Bronchodilators: Duration 4–12 hours
    - Inhaled beta-2 agonist: Relax smooth airway muscle; bronchoconstriction antagonists
      - Short acting (SABA)
      - Long acting (LABA)
    - Inhaled antimuscarinic (anticholinergic): Blocks bronchoconstrictor effects of acetylcholine: Duration 4–24 hours
      - Short acting (SAMA)
      - Long acting (LAMA)
    - Combination SABA + SAMA
    - Combination LABA + LAMA
  - Inhaled corticosteroid (ICS): Duration 12–24 hours
    - Combination LABA + ICS (based on blood eosinophil count, 1 or more moderate exacerbations per year, hospitalizations for exacerbation, and concomitant asthma)
  - Triple-therapy combination LABA + LAMA + ICS: Duration 24 hours
- Oral glucocorticoids for acute exacerbations only
- Antibiotics
  - Exacerbation: Duration of ≤5 days of antibiotic treatment for outpatient treatment of exacerbations. Choice of antibiotic should be based on local bacterial resistance pattern. Empirical treatment is an aminopenicillin with clavulanic acid, or macrolide, or tetracycline.
  - Long-term azithromycin (250 mg/day or 500 mg three times/week) or erythromycin (250 mg twice daily) for 1 year. Use for patients prone to exacerbations.
- Methylxanthines
- Phosphodiasterase-4 inhibitors (use if prior hospitalization for exacerbation)
- Mucolytic agents

> **BOX 22.4 ■ Acute Care Considerations**
>
> Acute exacerbations of chronic obstructive pulmonary disease (AECOPD) requiring hospitalization are common. Close to 20% of patients are readmitted within 30 days after hospital discharge, and approximately 25% of patients hospitalized for AECOPD die within 1 year and 65% die within 5 years. Importantly, close to 70% of readmissions after an AECOPD hospitalization result from decompensation of comorbidities, such as cardiovascular disease (CVD), chronic kidney disease, obstructive sleep apnea, anxiety, depression, and lung cancer. Therefore all patients with COPD who are hospitalized with worsening dyspnea or respiratory symptoms, but without evidence of an active infection, should be assessed for any comorbidities that may be the underlying cause or driver of the AECOPD (Celli et al., 2023).

- Oxygen: If PaO_2 <55 mm Hg or SpO_2 <88% at rest or with exercise to maintain a saturation of at least 90% at rest, with sleep, and with exertion
- Nicotine replacement/smoking cessation aids (bupropion, nortriptyline, nicotine gum or patch)
- Vaccines: Influenza annually; pneumococcal***; SARS-CoV-2 (COVID-19); Tdap (dTRaP/dTPa); and zoster according to guideline recommendations.
- AAT augmentation therapy intravenously
- Comorbidities should be actively treated appropriately when present, because they influence health status, hospitalizations, and mortality independent of the severity of airflow obstruction due to COPD (Box 22.4).

(GOLD, 2024)

NONPHARMACOTHERAPY

- Educate
  - Avoid environmental and occupational irritants.
  - Correct and appropriate use of inhaler(s)/spacer if provided
  - Action plan for self-management
  - Importance of vaccines
  - Pursed lip breathing techniques
  - Resuscitation, advance directives, and end-of-life care
- Lifestyle and behavioral modifications
  - Strategies for smoking cessation: Ask, Advise, Assess, Assist, and Arrange
  - Active lifestyle and exercise
  - Nutrition
  - Wearing a cold-weather mask
- Complementary treatment
  - Psychosocial rehabilitation: Concomitant depression, anxiety
  - Nutritional supplementation
  - Complementary and alternative therapies with natural medicines and supplements may interact with prescription medications. Obtain a complete medication history.
- Referral
  - Consult a pulmonologist in cases of COPD, lung cancer, obstructive sleep apnea, lung volume reduction surgery, or lung transplant.
  - Pulmonary rehabilitation
  - Cardiologist: Concomitant CVD
  - Endocrinologist: Concomitant metabolic syndrome
  - Orthopedist: Concomitant osteoporosis, skeletal muscle dysfunction

---

***See Chapter 21, Pneumonia, for guidelines on pneumococcal vaccines.

- Palliative care
- Hospice care
- Follow-up
- Office visit every 3 months or if symptoms worsen
- Annual spirometry

(GOLD, 2024)

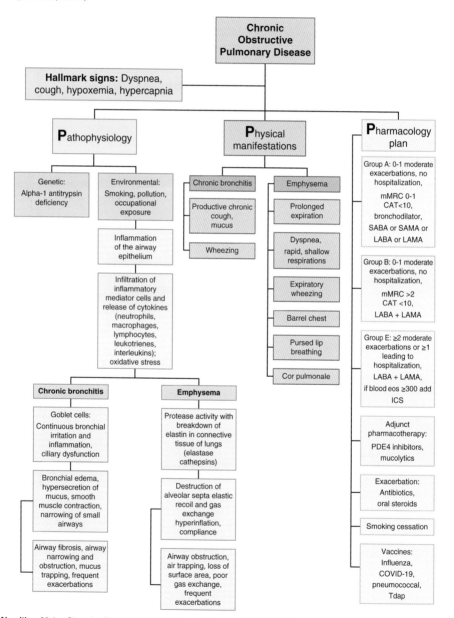

Algorithm 22.1 Chronic Obstructive Pulmonary Disease. *CAT*, COPD assessment test; *eos*, eosinophils; *ICS*, inhaled corticosteroid; *LABA*, long-acting beta agonist; *LAMA*, long-acting muscarinic; *mMRC*, modified Medical Research Council; *PDE*, phosphodiesterase; *SABA*, short-acting beta agonist; *SAMA*, short-acting muscarinic; *Tdap*, tetanus, diphtheria, pertussis.

References

Ball, J. W., Dains, J. E., Flynn, J. A., Solomon, B. S., & Stewart, R. W. (2023). *Seidel's guide to physical examination* (10th ed.). Elsevier.

Brashers, V. (2023). Alterations of pulmonary function. In J. L. Rogers (Ed.), *McCance & Huether's pathophysiology: The biological basis for disease in adults and children*, (9th ed., pp. 1167–1175). Elsevier.

Celli, B. R., Fabbri, L. M., Aaron, S. D., Agusti, A., Brook, R. D., Criner, G. J., Franssen, F. M. E., Humbert, M., Hurst, J. R., Montes de Oca, M., Pantoni, L., Papi, A., Rodriguez-Roisin, R., Sethi, S., Stolz, D., Torres, A., Vogelmeier, C. F., & Wedzicha, J. A. (2023). Differential diagnosis of suspected chronic obstructive pulmonary disease exacerbations in the acute care setting: Best practice. *American Journal of Respiratory and Critical Care Medicine, 207*(9), 1134–1144. https://doi.org/10.1164/rccm.202209-1795CI.

Dains, J. E., Baumann, L. C., & Scheibel, P. (2024). *Advanced health assessment & clinical diagnosis in primary care* (7th ed.). Elsevier. https://pageburstls.elsevier.com/books/9780323832083.

Global Initiative for Chronic Obstructive Lung Disease. (2024). *2024 Gold Report*. https://goldcopd.org/2024-gold-report-2.

Guo, P., Li, R., Piao, T. H., Wang, C. L., Wu, X. L., & Cai, H. Y. (2022). Pathological mechanism and targeted drugs of COPD. *International Journal of Chronic Obstructive Pulmonary Disease, 17*, 1565–1575. https://doi.org/10.2147/COPD.S366126.

Higham, A., Quinn, A. M., Cançado, J. E. D., & Singh, D. (2019). The pathology of small airways disease in COPD: Historical aspects and future directions. *Respiratory Research, 20*(1), 49. https://doi.org/10.1186/s12931-019-1017-y.

Linden, D., Guo-Parke, H., Coyle, P. V., Fairley, D., McAuley, D. F., Taggart, C. C., & Kidney, J. (2019). Respiratory viral infection: A potential "missing link" in the pathogenesis of COPD. *European Respiratory Review, 28*(151), 180063. https://doi.org/10.1183/16000617.0063-20.

Riley, L., Sriram, A., Brantly, M., & Lascano, J. (2023). Testing patterns and disparities for alpha-1 antitrypsin deficiency. *The American Journal of Medicine, 136*(10), 1011–1017.

Scott, Z., Zhou, C., Tracy, E., ElMallah, M. K., & Yousef, S. (2023). Congenital lobar emphysea in monozygotic twins. *Respiratory Medicine Case Reports, 43*, 101842. https://doi.org/10.1016/j.rmcr.2023.101842.

Sharma, G., & Goodwin, J. (2006). Effect of aging on respiratory system physiology and immunology. *Clinical Interventions in Aging, 1*(3), 253–260. https://doi.org/10.2147/ciia.2006.1.3.253.

Sjoding, M. W., Dickson, R. P., Iwashyna, T. J., Gay, S. E., & Valley, T. S. (2020). Racial bias in pulse oximetry measurement. *New England Journal of Medicine, 383*(25), 2477–2478. https://doi.org/10.1056/NEJMc2029240.

Syamlal, G., Kurth, L. M., Dodd, K. E., Blackley, D. J., Hall, N. B., & Mazurek, J. M. (2022)). Chronic obstructive pulmonary disease mortality by industry and occupation—United States, 2020. *Morbidity and Mortality Weekly Report, 71*(49), 1550–1554. https://doi.org/10.15585/mmwr.mm7149a3.

Zeng, Y., Jiang, F., Chen, Y., Chen, P., & Cai, S. (2018). Exercise assessments and trainings of pulmonary rehabilitation in COPD: A literature review. *International Journal of Chronic Obstructive Pulmonary Disease, 13*, 2013–2023. https://doi.org/10.2147/COPD.S167098.

CHAPTER 23

Restrictive Lung Disease

Julia L. Rogers

Pulmonary Fibrosis

Pulmonary Fibrosis

Pulmonary fibrosis (PF) is a progressive inflammatory pattern that causes fibrotic (or scarring) lung tissue. *Pulmonary fibrosis* is a general term that refers to any interstitial lung disease (ILD) in which fibrosis is present. ILDs comprise a family of over 200 related conditions characterized by inflammation, fibrosis, or other abnormalities in the alveolar walls or interstitium. ILDs are divided into two groups: (1) those in which a cause can be identified and (2) those in which the cause is unknown. There are four types of PF that are most common, three of which are identifiable conditions and risk factors associated with the disease. Disease-related PF includes different illnesses such as viruses or autoimmune and connective tissue disorders (CTDs) such as rheumatoid arthritis (see Chapter 8) or lupus. There is exposure-related PF, which results from being exposed to asbestos, silica, or other hazardous materials. Cigarette smoking, medications, and prolonged exposure to radiation also cause this type. Finally, there is familial PF. This is a rare genetic type of PF wherein two or more members of the family have PF ILD. However, the most common cause in the majority of cases is idiopathic, meaning undetermined. Idiopathic PF (IPF) is a specific form of chronic, progressive, fibrosing interstitial pneumonia of unknown etiology, occurring primarily in older adults and limited to the lungs. PF can affect anyone—males, females, and children (Box 23.1)—but it is much more common in older adults and seems to be slightly more common in males than females (Mortimer et al., 2020) (Box 23.2). IPF accounts for 17% to 37% of all ILD diagnoses (Sauleda et al., 2018), with the global incidence and prevalence of IPF in the range of 0.09 to 1.30 per 10,000 people and increasing year by year (Maher et al., 2021; Mortimer et al., 2020; Schäfer et al., 2020). Compared with other countries studied, the United States, South Korea, and Canada have the highest incidence. Environmental factors such as smoking, viral infections, gastroesophageal reflux disease (GERD), inhalational injuries, and associated aberrant DNA methylation patterns are felt to be a critical component of risk for IPF. PF has a high mortality rate, with life expectancy of 2 to 4 years after diagnosis (Richeldi et al., 2017; Mei et al., 2022). Therefore it is important for healthcare providers to identify the disease to provide a timely diagnosis.

Pathophysiology

The complex pathophysiology of PF includes chronic inflammation that affects the spongy parts of the lung and causes abnormalities in the alveolar walls and interstitium. It eventually leads to fibrosis, making the lung stiff and difficult for oxygen to diffuse into the bloodstream. There appears to be an interaction between genetic predisposition and injurious environmental agents that involves repeated microinjuries to the aging alveolar epithelium (Richeldi et al., 2017).

BOX 23.1 ■ Pediatric Considerations

A concern for pediatric patients is related to a form of fibrosis known as cystic fibrosis (CF). CF is an autosomal recessive trait caused by mutations of cystic fibrosis transmembrane conductance regulator. Every newborn in the United States is screened for CF with an assay for the pancreatic enzyme immunoreactive trypsinogen or immunoreactive trypsinogen with DNA, or with a sweat test that checks for high levels of chloride in the sweat. Healthcare providers should monitor the chest in pediatric patients at every visit, and if the roundness of the chest persists past the second year of life, they should be concerned about the possibility of a chronic pulmonary problem such as cystic fibrosis. A constant productive cough with mucus is the hallmark sign in children younger than 5 years of age. Another distinctive feature is the parent or caregiver reporting that the child's skin tastes unusually salty. This is due to salt loss in the sweat. There may also be a history of malabsorption leading to large bulky stools, constipation, poor weight gain, meconium ileus, or intestinal obstruction. Triple therapy was introduced in 2019 and has shown to improve pulmonary function, reduce exacerbations, and enhance the quality of life of CF patients (Dawood et al., 2022; Mall et al., 2022; National Institutes of Health, 2022).

BOX 23.2 ■ Diversity Considerations

Recent studies demonstrate substantial racial and ethnic minority disparities in pulmonary fibrosis (PF)–related outcomes. Black patients are significantly younger than Hispanic and White patients at the time of initial hospitalization, lung transplant, and mortality. This may be contributable to White patients being diagnosed with PF between the median ages of 60 and 70 years and Black patients are being diagnosed with PF between the ages of 50 and 60 years. Black patients also experience delays in being diagnosed with PF; therefore there is concern that the median age may actually be earlier in Black patients. Because of the earlier onset, the number of hospitalizations related to PF was also found to be higher among Black patients than Hispanic and White patients. These studies reported lower lung transplant rates and disproportionately higher hospitalization rates among Black and Hispanic patients with PF compared with White patients, further underscoring the impact of healthcare disparities on these racial and ethnic minority populations (Adegunsoye et al., 2023).

Epithelial damage along with innate and adaptive immune responses involving neutrophils, macrophages, fibrocytes, and T lymphocytes trigger the secretion of inflammatory cytokines, growth factors, and coagulants. Oxidative stress associated with activation of inflammatory and epithelial cells contributes to DNA damage, alveolar epithelial cell apoptosis, and the release of profibrotic cytokines. This initiates miscommunications between the epithelium and the body's network of fibroblasts, causing excess myofibroblasts to be produced (Brashers, 2023; Richeldi et al., 2017). It is this fibrotic process that leads to extracellular matrices that accumulate to the point that there is abnormal remodeling of the interstitium of the lungs. The interstitial and alveolar fibrin deposition, scarring, and remodeling are what give the appearance in diagnostic imaging of "honeycombing" along the lung parenchyma. Dysfunctional surfactant production and alveolar collapse also occur. Fibrosis of the interstitial lung tissue around the alveoli causes decreased oxygen diffusion across the alveolocapillary membrane and hypoxemia (Brashers, 2023). As the disease progresses, decreased lung compliance leads to increased work to breathe, a disordered gas exchange, a decreased tidal volume, and resultant hypoventilation with hypercapnia, hypoxemia, and potentially life-threatening respiratory failure. Mechanical stress from fibrotic tissue pulling apart the small airways may contribute to cough in PF by sensitizing rapidly adapting receptors within the peripheral airways, thereby lowering the cough threshold (Vega-Olivo & Criner, 2018). Another possibility is due to the matrix stiffening, which is a prominent feature of lung fibrosis.

BOX 23.3 ■ Acute Care Considerations

There are conflicting studies on whether delaying mechanical intubation and keeping patients with pulmonary fibrosis on high-flow oxygen is associated with an increased or a decreased risk of mortality in the intensive care unit as compared to early intubation. However, considering life expectancy with pulmonary fibrosis, complications of mechanical ventilation, need for lung transplant, and palliative or end-of-life care decisions, being placed on mechanical ventilation should be planned cautiously with the patient, family, and provider (Bae et al., 2022; Lee et al., 2020).

Disease progression is highly variable, with some individuals demonstrating a slow decline and others progressing to death within a few years. Diffuse PF has a poor prognosis. Acute exacerbation may occur without clear provocation and accelerate decline (Box 23.3).

DISEASE-RELATED PULMONARY FIBROSIS

Autoimmune diseases such as rheumatoid arthritis, scleroderma, Sjogren's syndrome, and dermatomyositis/polymyositis can damage the lungs and cause CTD-associated ILD. Sometimes ILD is the first manifestation of a CTD.

Microorganisms (viruses, bacteria, and fungi) play a potential role in the pathogenesis of PF (Lipinski et al., 2020). Patients with PF as compared to patients without PF have an imbalance in the composition of the lung microbiota, which can serve as a persistent stimulus for repetitive alveolar injury. The inflammatory and fibrotic mediators and immune disorders in the lungs of IPF patients are related to bacterial load. While the evidence that viral infection in general may elevate a patient's risk for PF is mixed and inconclusive, there appears to be an association with chronic viral infections. Epstein–Barr virus, cytomegalovirus, and herpes virus are detected within alveolar epithelial cells of patients with IPF, suggesting a link between viral infection and increased risk of IPF (Mei et al., 2022). In addition, it is thought to occur secondary to viral pneumonia, especially COVID-19 infection. This is because PF can occur following acute respiratory distress syndrome, which occurs in a subset of patients with COVID-19 (Lai et al., 2019). The highly atypical inflammatory responses seen in COVID-19 have complicated analysis of the relationship of this viral infection to IPF (Lai et al., 2019; McDonald, 2021).

EXPOSURE-RELATED PULMONARY FIBROSIS

Currently PF is regarded as a disease caused by repeated subclinical injury leading to epithelial damage and subsequent destruction of the alveolar-capillary basement membrane. In exposure-related fibrosis, this is caused by chronic exposure to environmental stresses, occupational toxins, medications, radiation, and microorganisms.

Environmental stresses such as smoke, dust (metal and wood), air pollution, agriculture and farming, viruses, and stone and silica can cause PF (Brashers, 2023; Richeldi et al., 2017). Inhaled mold spores or bird proteins can lead to hypersensitivity pneumonitis, which triggers inflammation and subsequent fibrosis. While smoking does not directly cause fibrosis, it is a risk factor. Smoking and environmental exposures to lung epithelium contain the strongest risk factors for IPF. Cigarette smoke can cause a variety of cellular changes through epigenetic mechanisms and also induces miRNA imbalance and endoplasmic reticulum stress, promoting spontaneous lung injury and differentiation from fibroblast to myofibroblast. Oxidant stress from smoking may damage alveolar epithelial cells and contribute to the pathogenesis of idiopathic PF (Song et al., 2019).

Occupational exposures include a wide variety of workplace exposures that are toxic to the lungs—for example, exposure to asbestosis and coal dust causing "black lung." These specific toxins cause pneumoconiosis. Other occupational exposures that may cause PF are radiation, chemicals, toxic materials, sandblasting, and inhaled metal dust. Agricultural workers can also be affected; in this case, often referred to as "farmer's lung," exposure to organic and inorganic substances, fumes, or moldy hay causes allergic inflammation and fibrosis.

Medications such as amiodarone, nitrofurantoin, methotrexate, and certain chemotherapy agents can also cause fibrosis.

FAMILIAL-RELATED PULMONARY FIBROSIS

Many gene polymorphisms (mutations) for inflammatory immune and fibrotic responses have been linked to the development of PF. Familial interstitial pneumonia is an autosomal dominant genetic disease with variable penetrance in which rare genetic variants have been identified (Lorenzo-Salazar et al., 2019; Richeldi et al., 2017). In some genetic forms, there is also extrapulmonary disease that manifests as bone marrow failure and liver disease. In some patients, biological members of the family (primary relatives) also have IPF. At least 30% of patients who have sporadic or familial PF have genetic predisposing factors that are known to increase the risk of PF. Genes associated with IPF include MUC5B and telomerase reverse transcriptase or telomerase RNA (Barros et al., 2019; Moore et al., 2019). These gene mutations are a major monogenic cause of PF and are found in approximately 15% of all familial cases. In both sporadic and familial PF, environmental exposures to lung epithelium can increase the risk of IPF (Kropski et al., 2015; Richeldi et al., 2017).

Physical Clinical Presentation

SUBJECTIVE

The most common presenting symptom is progressive exertional dyspnea with an insidious onset and dry cough (Algorithm 23.1). As the disease progresses, individuals may become breathless while taking part in activities of daily living such as showering, getting dressed, speaking on the phone, or even eating (Box 23.4). The dry, hacking, nonproductive cough generally ensues with or slightly after the onset of shortness of breath. Evidence of arthralgia, arthritis, photosensitivity, Raynaud phenomenon, dry eyes, and/or dry mouth on review of systems may indicate the presence of a collagen-vascular disease.

It is imperative to obtain complete present and past histories including medication history and environmental, occupational, social, or recreational exposure. A thorough history should be obtained for present and past medications. Key medications associated with PF are amiodarone, bleomycin, and nitrofurantoin. When gathering current and past environmental histories, consider

---

BOX 23.4 ■ Older Adult Considerations

The aging process is associated with dynapenia or loss of muscle strength. As a person ages, the body changes in several ways; for example, the dorsal curve of the thoracic spine is more prominent (kyphosis) with flattening of the lumbar curve, and the anterior-posterior (AP) diameter of the chest is increased in relation to the lateral diameter. Because pulmonary fibrosis (PF) generally affects adults aged 65 years and older, there is the tendency to also observe some decreased muscle functioning due to aging. This includes muscles that assist in respiration. Another connection to aging and PF was reported in a study conducted by Caporarello et al. (2022). The study shed light on the role of aging pulmonary endothelial cells and transcriptional abnormalities that were suspected in causing vascular dysregulated repair and perpetuating PF. The loss of chromatin homeostasis in the vasculature of the fibrotic aged lungs characteristic of idiopathic PF may contribute to dysfunctional repair leading to PF (Caporarello et al., 2022).

factors that can contribute to PF. Any prior exposure to smoke, pollution, moldy foliage and/or pigeon droppings, asbestos, silica, heavy metals, or contaminated ventilation systems should be investigated.

Occupational history is critical, including any time served in the armed forces, especially naval shipyards. A history to dampness, mold, or bird exposure in the home or workplace should immediately raise suspicion for hypersensitivity pneumonitis. Silica exposure has also been implicated in increasing the expression of DNA methyltransferase 1 in patients with PF, leading to the accumulation of collagen and lung fibrosis. Individuals should be asked if they have ever received radiation therapy or worked around or been exposed to radiation to the chest.

Take the time to carefully question the patient about any symptoms that could indicate underlying disease or CTD such as joint pain, stiffness, or swelling; skin thickening or tightening; rash; dry eyes; dry mouth; Raynaud's phenomenon; diffuse recurrent muscle pain or weakness; and severe heartburn with gastric regurgitation.

Many individuals also present with symptoms and signs of comorbid conditions such as coronary artery disease, emphysema, and/or lung cancer. Individuals with common comorbidities such as GERD, pulmonary hypertension, and CTDs may present with low-grade fevers, fatigue, arthralgias, myalgias, leg edema, and/or weight loss.

OBJECTIVE*

Generalized: Fatigue; weight loss

Neurological: <u>**Confusion (with respiratory acidosis or hypoxia)**</u>

HEENT: **Cough** (dry); trachea deviation (if volume loss from fibrosis pulls the trachea toward the affected lung)

Cardiovascular: If pulmonary hypertension is present: loud P2 component of the second heart sound, fixed split S2, holosystolic tricuspid regurgitation murmur, and pedal edema

Pulmonary: *Inspection:* Tachypnea; labored respirations; use of accessory muscles

Palpation: Increased fremitus; increased egophony; decreased chest expansion and respiratory excursion bilaterally

Percussion: Dull

Auscultation: **Bibasilar crackles**, (fine high-pitched on inspiration); diminished

Extremities: Digital clubbing; **<u>cyanosis</u>**

(Ball et al., 2023; Brashers, 2023; Dains et al., 2024; Raghu et al., 2022; Richeldi et al., 2017)

Evaluation and Differential Diagnoses

DIAGNOSTICS

- Complete pulmonary function test with diffusion capacity of the lung carbon monoxide. Restrictive pattern: Reduced forced vital capacity, reduced forced expiratory volume in 1 second, and reduced diffusion capacity of the lung carbon monoxide. Typically normal is a >70% ratio of reduced forced expiratory volume in 1 second to forced vital capacity.
- Chest radiograph posterior-anterior and lateral may show peripheral reticular opacities at the lung bases. Honeycombing and lower lobe volume loss are also present (Fig. 23.1).
- In high-resolution computed tomography scan without contrast, subpleural honeycombing and patchy, peripheral, subpleural, and bibasilar reticular opacity reticulation are generally present. Areas that are severely involved with reticular markings may also demonstrate traction bronchiectasis.

---

*Hallmark signs are bolded and <u>Red flags are bolded and underlined</u>.

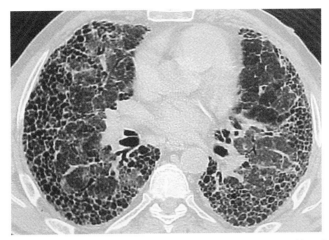

Fig. 23.1 High-resolution computed tomography image of a case of severe idiopathic pulmonary fibrosis. Diffuse honeycombing and traction bronchiectasis are present.

- Pulse oximetry with 6-minute walk test
- Lung biopsy showing usual interstitial pneumonia. Histologic hallmarks include dense fibrosis and microhoneycombing in the subpleural areas.
- In labs, the presence of autoantibodies is suggestive of ILD associated with connective tissue disease (Antinuclear antibody (ANA), rheumatoid factor (RF), C-reactive protein (CRP)); hemoglobin and hematacrit to evaluate oxygenation capability.
- Genetic testing only in persons with a personal or family history of extrapulmonary features associated with a telomeropathy such as aplastic anemia, cryptogenic cirrhosis, or premature graying

(Raghu et al., 2018, 2022; Richeldi et al., 2017)

DIFFERENTIAL DIAGNOSIS

- Connective tissue disease–associated interstitial lung disease
- Drug-induced pulmonary toxicity
- Obstructive lung disease
- Pneumonia
- Heart failure
- Lung cancer

Plan

GUIDELINE RESOURCES

- Raghu, G., Remy-Jardin, M., Richeldi, L., Thomson, C. C., Inoue, Y., Johkoh, T., Kreuter, M., Lynch, D. A., Maher, T. M., Martinez, F. J., Molina-Molina, M., Myers, J. L., Nicholson, A. G., Ryerson, C. J., Strek, M. E., Troy, L. K., Wijsenbeek, M., Mammen, M. J., Hossain, T., ... Wilson, K. C. (2022). Idiopathic pulmonary fibrosis (an update) and progressive pulmonary fibrosis in adults: An official ATS/ERS/JRS/ALAT clinical practice guideline. *American Journal of Respiratory and Critical Care Medicine, 205*(9), e18–e47. https://doi.org/10.1164/rccm.202202-0399st.

- Raghu, G., Remy-Jardin, M., Myers, J. L., Richeldi, L., Ryerson, C. J., Lederer, D. J., Behr, J., Cottin, V., Danoff, S. K., Morell, F., Flaherty, K. R., Wells, A., Martinez, F. J., Azuma, A., Bice, T. J., Bouros, D., Brown, K. K., Collard, H. R., Duggal, A., … American Thoracic Society, European Respiratory Society, Japanese Respiratory Society, and Latin American Thoracic Society. (2018). Diagnosis of idiopathic pulmonary fibrosis. An official ATS/ERS/JRS/ALAT clinical practice guideline. *American Journal of Respiratory and Critical Care Medicine, 198*(5), e44–e68. https://doi.org/10.1164/rccm.201807-1255st.

Pharmacotherapy

- Medication (Algorithm 23.1)
  - Pirfenidone 267-mg capsules or tablets; titrate up to 3 capsules orally three times daily with meals over 14 days. *Must* be taken with full meals. Once on a stable dose, an 801-mg tablet (equivalent to 3 capsules) is available.
  - Nintedanib 150-mg capsules; 1 capsule orally every 12 hours, taken with food
  - Corticosteroids (high dose) for acute exacerbations
  - Oxygen: If PaO_2 <55 mm Hg or SpO_2 <88% at rest or with exercise to maintain a saturation of at least 90% at rest, with sleep, and with exertion
  - Antacid for concomitant GERD
- Smoking cessation aids should be offered to any person currently smoking tobacco.
- Vaccines: Influenza annually, pneumococcal, COVID-19, and zoster according to Centers for Disease Control and Prevention guidelines and recommendations

(Raghu et al., 2018, 2022)

NONPHARMACOTHERAPY

- Educate
  - Eliminate environmental and occupational irritants.
  - Importance of vaccines
  - Self-management
  - Disease progression
- Lifestyle and behavioral modifications
  - Smoking cessation
  - Wearing a cold weather mask
- Complementary treatment
  - Psychosocial rehabilitation
  - Complementary and alternative therapies with natural medicines and supplements may interact with prescription medications. Obtain a complete medication history.
- Referral (identify and refer for treatment of comorbid conditions*)
  - Lung transplant center
  - Palliative care
  - Pulmonary rehabilitation
  - Pulmonologist (*lung cancer, obstructive sleep apnea)
  - Cardiologist (*pulmonary hypertension or cardiac disease)
  - Gastroenterologist (*GERD; *liver disease)
  - Hematologist (*bone marrow failure)
- Follow-up
  - Office visit every 4 to 6 months with 6-minute walk test and pulmonary funtion test (PFT)

(Raghu et al., 2022)

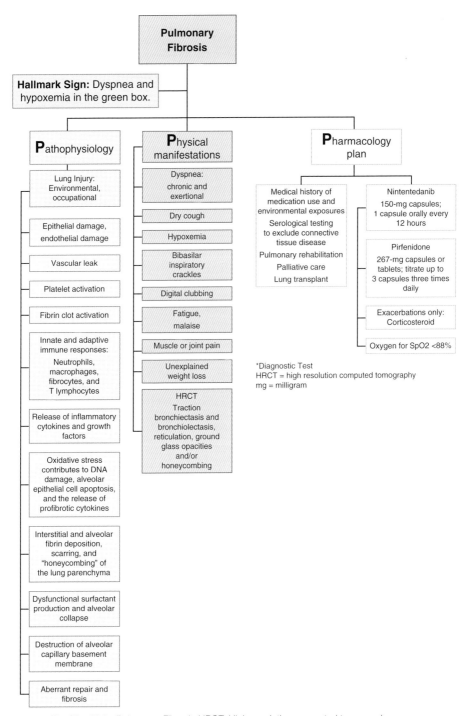

Algorithm 23.1 Pulmonary Fibrosis *HRCT*, High-resolution computed tomography scan.

References

Adegunsoye, A., Freiheit, E., White, E. N., Kaul, B., Newton, C. A., Oldham, J. M., Lee, C. T., Chung, J., Garcia, N., Ghodrati, S., Vij, R., Jablonski, R., Flaherty, K. R., Wolters, P. J., Garcia, C. K., & Strek, M. E. (2023). Evaluation of pulmonary fibrosis outcomes by race and ethnicity in US adults. *JAMA Network Open, 6*(3), e232427. http://doi.org/10.1001/jamanetworkopen.2023.2427.

Bae, E., Park, J., Choi, S. M., Lee, J., Lee, S. M., & Lee, H. Y. (2022). Association between timing of intubation and mortality in patients with idiopathic pulmonary fibrosis. *Acute and Critical Care, 37*(4), 561–570. http://doi.org/10.4266/acc.2022.00444.

Ball, J. W., Dains, J. E., Flynn, J. A., Solomon, B. S., & Stewart, R. W. (2023). *Seidel's guide to physical examination* (10th ed.). Elsevier.

Barros, A., Oldham, J., & Noth, I. (2019). Genetics of idiopathic pulmonary fibrosis. *American Journal of the Medical Sciences, 357*(5), 379–383. http://doi.org/10.1016/j.amjms.2019.02.009.

Brashers, V. (2023). *Alterations of pulmonary function*. In J. L. Rogers (Ed.), *McCance & Huether's pathophysiology: The biologic basis for disease in adults and children* (9th ed., pp. 1163-1167). Elsevier.

Caporarello, N., Lee, J., Pham, T. X., Jones, D. L., Guan, J., Link, P. A., Meridew, J. A., Marden, G., Yamashita, T., Osborne, C. A., Bhagwate, A. V., Huang, S. K., Nicosia, R. F., Tschumperlin, D. J., Trojanowska, M., & Ligresti, G. (2022). Dysfunctional ERG signaling drives pulmonary vascular aging and persistent fibrosis. *Nature Communications, 13*(1), 4170. https://doi.org/10.1038/s41467-022-31890-4.

Dains, J. E., Baumann, L. C., & Scheibel, P. (2024). *Advanced health assessment & clinical diagnosis in primary care* (7th ed.). Elsevier.

Dawood, S. N., Rabih, A. M., Niaj, A., Raman, A., Uprety, M., Calero, M. J., Villanueva, M. R. B., Joshaghani, N., Villa, N., Badla, O., Goit, R., Saddik, S. E., & Mohammed, L. (2022). Newly discovered cutting-edge triple combination cystic fibrosis therapy: A systematic review. *Cureus, 14*(9), e29359. http://doi.org/10.7759/cureus.29359.

Kropski, J. A., Blackwell, T. S., & Loyd, J. E. (2015). The genetic basis of idiopathic pulmonary fibrosis. *European Respiratory Journal, 45*(6), 1717–1727. http://doi.org/10.1183/09031936.00163814.

Lai, C. C., Shih, T. P., Ko, W. C., Tang, H. J., & Hsueh, P. R. (2019). Severe acute respiratory syndrome coronavirus 2 (SARS-CoV-2) and coronavirus disease—2019 (COVID-19): The epidemic and the challenges. *International Journal of Antimicrobial Agents, 55*(3), 105924. http://doi.org/10.1016/j.ijantimicag.2020.105924.

Lee, J. H., Lim, C. M., Koh, Y., Hong, S. B., Song, J. W., & Huh, J. W. (2020). High-flow nasal cannula oxygen therapy in idiopathic pulmonary fibrosis patients with respiratory failure. *Journal of Thoracic Disease, 12*(3), 966–972. http://doi.org/10.21037/jtd.2019.12.48.

Lipinski, J. H., Moore, B. B., & O'Dwyer, D. N (2020). The evolving role of the lung microbiome in pulmonary fibrosis. *American Journal of Physiology—Lung Cellular and Molecular Physiology, 319*(4), L675–L682. http://doi.org/10.1152/ajplung.00258.2020.

Lorenzo-Salazar, J. M., Ma, S. F., Jou, J., Hou, P. C., Guillen-Guio, B., Allen, R. J., Jenkins, R. G., Wain, L. V., Oldham, J. M., Noth, I., & Flores, C. (2019). Novel idiopathic pulmonary fibrosis susceptibility variants revealed by deep sequencing. *ERJ Open Research, 5*(2), 1–11. http://doi.org/10.1183/23120541.00071-2019.

Maher, T. M., Bendstrup, E., Dron, L., Langley, J., Smith, G., & Khalid, J. M. (2021). Global incidence and prevalence of idiopathic pulmonary fibrosis. *Respiratory Research, 22*(1), 197. http://doi.org/10.1186/s12931-021-01791-z.

Mall, M. A., Brugha, R., Gartner, S., Legg, J., Moeller, A., Mondejar-Lopez, P., Prais, D., Pressler, T., Ratjen, F., Reix, P., Robinson, P. D., Selvadurai, H., Stehling, F., Ahluwalia, N., Arteaga-Solis, E., Bruinsma, B. G., Jennings, M., Moskowitz, S. M., Noel, S., … Davies, J. C. (2022). Efficacy and safety of elexacaftor/tezacaftor/ivacaftor in children 6 through 11 years of age with cystic fibrosis heterozygous for F508del and a minimal function mutation: A phase 3b, randomized, placebo-controlled study. *American Journal of Respiratory and Critical Care Medicine, 206*(11), 1361–1369. http://doi.org/10.1164/rccm.202202-0392OC.

McDonald, L. T. (2021). Healing after COVID-19: Are survivors at risk for pulmonary fibrosis? *American Journal of Physiology—Lung Cellular and Molecular Physiology, 320*(2), L257–L265. http://doi.org/10.1152/ajplung.00238.2020.

Mei, Q., Liu, Z., Zuo, H., Yang, Z., & Qu, J. (2022). Idiopathic pulmonary fibrosis: An update on pathogenesis. *Frontiers in Pharmacology, 12*, 797292. http://doi.org/10.3389/fphar.2021.797292.

Moore, C., Blumhagen, R. Z., Yang, I. V., Walts, A., Powers, J., Walker, T., Bishop, M., Russell, P., Vestal, B., Cardwell, J., Markin, C. R., Mathai, S. K., Schwarz, M. I., Steele, M. P., Lee, J., Brown, K. K., Loyd, J. E., Crapo, J. D., Silverman, E. K., … Schwartz, D. A. (2019). Resequencing study confirms that host defense and cell senescence gene variants contribute to the risk of idiopathic pulmonary fibrosis. *American Journal of Respiratory and Critical Care Medicine, 200*(2), 199–208. http://doi.org/10.1164/rccm.201810-1891OC.

Mortimer, K. M., Bartels, D. B., Hartmann, N., Capapey, J., Yang, J., Gately, R., & Enger, C. (2020). Characterizing health outcomes in idiopathic pulmonary fibrosis using US health claims data. *Respiration, 99*(2), 108–118. http://doi.org/10.1159/000504630.

National Institutes of Health. (2022). What is cystic fibrosis? Retrieved September 7, 2024, https://www.nhlbi.nih.gov/health/cystic-fibrosis#:~:text=Cystic%20fibrosis%20(CF)%20is%20a,and%20other%20organs%20and%20tissues.

Raghu, G., Remy-Jardin, M., Myers, J. L., Richeldi, L., Ryerson, C. J., Lederer, D. J., Behr, J., Cottin, V., Danoff, S. K., Morell, F., Flaherty, K. R., Wells, A., Martinez, F. J., Azuma, A., Bice, T. J., Bouros, D., Brown, K. K., Collard, H. R., & Duggal, A., American Thoracic Society, European Respiratory Society, Japanese Respiratory Society, and Latin American Thoracic Society. (2018). Diagnosis of idiopathic pulmonary fibrosis. An official ATS/ERS/JRS/ALAT clinical practice guideline. *American Journal of Respiratory and Critical Care Medicine, 198*(5), e44–e68. https://doi.org/10.1164/rccm.201807-1255ST.

Raghu, G., Remy-Jardin, M., Richeldi, L., Thomson, C. C., Inoue, Y., Johkoh, T., Kreuter, M., Lynch, D. A., Maher, T. M., Martinez, F. J., Molina-Molina, M., Myers, J. L., Nicholson, A. G., Ryerson, C. J., Strek, M. E., Troy, L. K., Wijsenbeek, M., Mammen, M. J., Hossain, T., … Wilson, K. C. (2022). Idiopathic pulmonary fibrosis (an update) and progressive pulmonary fibrosis in adults: An official ATS/ERS/JRS/ALAT clinical practice guideline. *American Journal of Respiratory and Critical Care Medicine, 205*(9), e18–e47. https://doi.org/10.1164/rccm.202202-0399S.

Richeldi, L., Collard, H. R., & Jones, M. G. (2017). Idiopathic pulmonary fibrosis. *Lancet, 389*(10082), 1941–1952. http://doi.org/10.1016/S0140-6736(17)30866-8.

Sauleda, J., Núñez, B., Sala, E., & Soriano, J. B. (2018). Idiopathic pulmonary fibrosis: Epidemiology, natural history, phenotypes. *Medical Sciences, 6*(4), 110. http://doi.org/10.3390/medsci6040110.

Schäfer, S. C., Funke-Chambour, M., & Berezowska, S. (2020). Idiopathic pulmonary fibrosis—Epidemiology, causes, and clinical course. *Der Pathologe, 41*(1), 46–51. http://doi.org/10.1007/s00292-019-00747-x.

Song, M., Peng, H., Guo, W., Luo, M., Duan, W., Chen, P., & Zhou, Y. (2019). Cigarette smoke extract promotes human lung myofibroblast differentiation by the induction of endoplasmic reticulum stress. *Respiration, 98*(4), 347–356.

Vega-Olivo, M., & Criner, G. J. (2018). Idiopathic pulmonary fibrosis: A guide for nurses. *Nurse Practitioner, 43*(5), 48–54. http://doi.org/10.1097/01.NPR.0000531121.07294.36.

CHAPTER 24

Pharyngitis

Julia L. Rogers

Viral and Bacterial

Pharyngitis

Acute pharyngitis can be caused by viral or bacterial infections or sexually transmitted infections (STIs). Viral etiologies include the rhinovirus, adenovirus, coxsackievirus, parainfluenza, coronavirus, and Epstein–Barr virus (Cunha, 2017; Wolford et al., 2023). The most common bacterial cause of acute pharyngitis is group A beta-hemolytic streptococcus (GAS), accounting for approximately 5% to 15% of adult cases (Gottlieb et al., 2018; Ressner, 2020; Shulman et al., 2012). STIs such as herpes simplex virus (HSV) and gonorrhea can cause acute pharyngitis among those with high-risk behaviors (Lee & White, 2018). Other, less common causes of acute pharyngitis include allergies, cancer, gastroesophageal reflux disease (GERD), trauma, and certain toxins (Alzahrani et al., 2018). The most common risk factor is having close contact with a person who has pharyngitis. Adults who are parents of school-age children, are in close contact with children, or work in crowded areas are at increased risk for GAS (Centers for Disease Control and Prevention [CDC], 2024) (Box 24.1).

Pathophysiology

Respiratory transmission of pathogens causing pharyngitis occurs through several interconnected mechanisms. The primary routes include respiratory droplets and direct contact with infectious secretions such as saliva, wound discharge, or nasal secretions from an infected person. The coughing, sneezing, and breathing of an infected individual can produce airborne droplets, which create an infectious mist. The droplets can be inhaled by others, potentially leading to the transmission of microorganisms capable of causing pharyngitis (Rogers, 2023; Rogers & Eastland, 2021). The most common mode of transmission is person-to-person contact, however, pathogens can spread through droplet inhalation, airborne transmission of aerosolized particles, or indirect contact (i.e., contaminated surfaces). Initially, pathogens colonize and adhere to the pharyngeal mucosa. This is followed by invasion, where microorganisms penetrate the epithelial barrier. Once established, the pathogens enter a phase of rapid multiplication within host tissues. Finally, dissemination occurs as the infection spreads to surrounding tissues or, in some cases, systemically.

Viral and bacterial pathogens invade the pharynx after evading the first line of defense provided by the nasopharynx and oropharynx. The nasopharynx is lined with hair and pseudostratified columnar epithelium, which can trap most unwanted organisms. While both the nasopharynx and oropharynx allow air to pass freely, large particles such as bacteria and viruses have difficulty making the 90-degree turn and become stuck to the mucosa near the tonsils, allowing colonization (Rogers, 2023; Rogers & Eastland, 2021). The adenoids and tonsils have immunologic cells that attempt to destroy any undesired pathogens but are not always successful (Rogers, 2023;

Group A streptococcus (GAS) causes 20% to 30% of pharyngitis in the pediatric population and is most common among children aged 5 to 15 years. GAS is rarely seen in children younger than 3 years of age. Pediatric patients may become dehydrated quickly with GAS because with a sore throat, they are reluctant to drink or eat due to pain. Parents should be educated to monitor for signs of dehydration. The most prevalent manifestations include dry mouth, increased thirst, decreased urine output (mild: one wet diaper or void in 6 hours; moderate to severe: fewer than one wet diaper or void in 6 hours), lack of tears when crying, and sunken eyes. It is important to also educate parents and caregivers of children younger than 18 years of age to avoid aspirin due to the potential risk of Reye's syndrome. Currently the Centers for Disease Control and Prevention is investigating increases in invasive group A strep infections, which include necrotizing fasciitis and streptococcal toxic shock syndrome, among children in the United States (CDC, 2024).

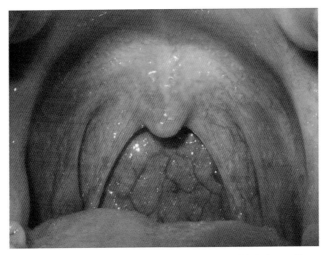

Fig. 24.1 Viral pharyngitis. Note the inflamed and erythematous pharynx. Viral pharyngitis may produce raised whitish to yellow lesions in the pharynx that are surrounded by erythema. (From Encyclopaedia Britannica. (2023). *Britannica.com encyclopedia.* https://www.britannica.com/science/pharyngitis.)

Rogers & Eastland, 2021). There is also opportunity for the microbiome normally found in the oropharynx to become pathogenic, causing disease when protective barriers or defensive mechanisms are weakened (Rogers, 2023; Rogers & Eastland, 2021). Once the first line of defense is breached, inflammation ensues.

The clinical manifestations associated with pharyngitis are linked to the pathophysiologic process of invading pathogens initiating an inflammatory response. The symptoms associated with infections, such as fever and malaise, are caused by this inflammatory response (Rogers, 2023; Rogers & Eastland, 2021). The erythema and warmth are a result of vasodilation and increased blood flow to the injured site. Edema (swelling) occurs in the nasal cavity and pharynx as exudate (fluid and cells) accumulates, which can lead to subsequent obstruction. Edema is usually accompanied by pain caused by pressure exerted by exudate accumulation, as well as the presence of soluble biochemical mediators such as prostaglandins and bradykinin. Certain infections, such as the rhinovirus, produce bradykinin and other inflammatory mediators that stimulate nerve endings within the pharynx, causing pain.

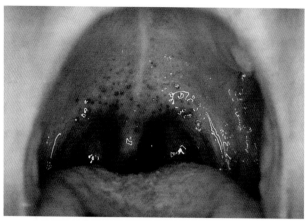

Fig. 24.2 Group A Streptococcus (GAS) Streptococcal pharyngitis. Note white exudates on erythematous swollen tonsils. (Courtesy CDC/Heinz F. Eichenwald, MD.)

BOX 24.2 ■ Diversity Considerations

Rheumatic heart disease (RHD) results from damage to heart valves caused by episodes of rheumatic fever, an autoimmune inflammatory reaction to group A streptococcus (GAS) pharyngitis, and claims over 288,000 lives each year. The vast majority of mortalities are in low- or middle-income countries, where poverty is widespread and individuals have limited access to health care. Many people do not have the means to cover the cost of care and may be unaware of the potential risk of RHD from untreated GAS. Another concern is overcrowding and poor living conditions. In high-income countries, the disease remains prevalent among immigrants, older adults, and indigenous peoples. RHD can be prevented by treating GAS with antibiotics (World Health Organization, 2020).

VIRAL PHARYNGITIS

The most common viral pathogens associated with acute pharyngitis are the rhinovirus and adenovirus. A rhinovirus enters through the nares and causes an inflammatory response. Adenoviruses differ from rhinoviruses in that there is direct invasion of the pharyngeal mucosa. However, an adenovirus can cause a similar inflammatory response, causing hyperemia of the pharynx (Fig. 24.1).

BACTERIAL PHARYNGITIS

Many bacteria have specialized surface structures that contribute to the structural integrity of biofilms and provide adherence to cells and tissue during invasion. The flagella, which allow the bacteria to move, express adhesins, allowing GAS bacterial adherence (Rogers, 2023; Rogers & Eastland, 2021). GAS is a highly adapted pathogen, with humans as its only known biological host (Bessen et al., 2018; Osowicki et al., 2019). It is the most common bacterial pathogen of pharyngitis and tends to colonize the oropharyngeal mucosal epithelium of the upper respiratory tract and the superficial layers of the epidermis (Bessen et al., 2018; Shulman et al., 2012). Once colonization is established, the organism can cause symptomatic pharyngitis (Fig. 24.2), with or without tonsillitis (Bessen et al., 2018). GAS can result in postinfection sequelae including acute poststreptococcal glomerulonephritis, acute rheumatic fever, and rheumatic heart disease (Box 24.2). The incubation period of GAS pharyngitis is approximately 2 to 5 days (CDC, 2024) (Box 24.3).

BOX 24.3 ■ Older Adult Considerations

A retrospective study found that less than 25% of the elderly adults presenting to the emergency department with sore throat had pharyngitis. However, it was found that only 46.7% had group A streptococcus (GAS) screening. In the patients who were tested for GAS, 42.9% were positive, which is more than twice the number found in the general or pediatric population. Elderly adults who have comorbid conditions, especially respiratory disease, and are highly suspect of GAS should be tested to initiate appropriate treatment with antibiotics. Residents at long-term care facilities often have underlying conditions and are vulnerable to invasive GAS infection. In fact, one study revealed that the incidence of invasive GAS among residents of long-term care facilities was almost six times higher than among community-based residents and that they were 1.5 times as likely to die from the infection as community-based patients. Providers have an opportunity to increase surveillance of this population to improve detection and secondary disease prevention. Residents should be provided the opportunity to receive an annual influenza immunization and pneumonia vaccine according to guidelines (Smith-Garcia et al., 2018; Thigpen et al., 2007).

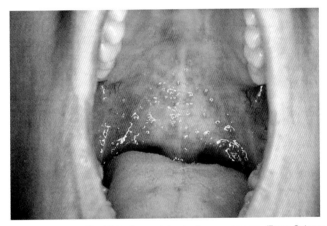

Fig. 24.3 Herpes simplex pharyngitis. Note the vesicles in the oropharynx. (From Science Photo Library. (2024). Sciencephoto.com. https://www.sciencephoto.com/keyword/herpetic-pharyngitis.)

SEXUALLY TRANSMITTED PHARYNGITIS

Two of the most common pathogens related to sexually transmitted pharyngitis are HSV and gonorrhea. HSV pharyngitis is caused by herpes simplex virus type 1 or 2. HSV-1 is typically spread via infected saliva and initially causes acute herpetic pharyngotonsillitis in adults (Fig. 24.3). Gonococcal pharyngitis is caused by the bacteria *Neisseria gonorrhoeae*, which is a gram-negative diplococcus (Lee & White, 2018). HSV-2 and gonococcal pharyngitis can occur after oral sexual contact with an infected partner (Lee & White, 2018; Rogers, 2023; Rogers & Eastland, 2021). The incubation period for HSV pharyngitis is 2 to 12 days (Workowski et al., 2021).

Physical Clinical Presentation

SUBJECTIVE

Most patients present with sudden onset of a sore throat that worsens when swallowing, fever, headache, and fatigue (CDC, 2024; Gottlieb et al., 2018). During the focused history, documentation should include the onset of symptoms; precipitating events; location, intensity, and quality of pain; progression of symptoms; alleviating and aggravating factors; previous episodes; and associated symptoms. Document allergies, ill contacts, autoimmune diseases, and medical, social, and family histories, including any accounts of rheumatic fever. The evaluation for acute pharyngitis should include the patient's sexual history with a record of high-risk behaviors, past and current histories of STIs, number of partners and their gender, and use of protection (Lee & White, 2018). GAS pharyngitis should be suspected in patients with an acute onset of sore throat predominately in winter or early spring with complaints of fever, odynophagia, absent cough, headache, nausea, vomiting, abdominal pain, and possible exposure to the illness (Gottlieb et al., 2018; Shulman et al., 2012). Viral pharyngitis should be suspected with symptoms of cough, rhinorrhea, hoarseness, oral ulcers, or conjunctivitis (CDC, 2024). Sexually transmitted pharyngitis should be suspected in patients with high-risk behaviors presenting with painful small oral vesicles.

OBJECTIVE*

Generalized: Fatigue; myalgia; **fever**
  Neurological: Headache
  HEENT: Conjunctivitis; coryza; **sore throat**; **odynophagia**; cough; hoarseness; mucosa erythema; pharyngeal erythema; tonsillar hypertrophy or inflammation with or without exudates (amount and color) and erythema; oral lesions; palatal petechia; neck stiffness; **trismus**; **uvular deviation**; **drooling**; **inability to swallow liquids**; **voice changes**
  Neck: Anterior cervical lymphadenopathy with tenderness; submental lymphadenopathy
  Cardiovascular: Tachycardia (with fever); **new murmur (with rheumatic fever)**
  Pulmonary: *Inspection:* Tachypnea
  Auscultation: **Stridor**; wheezing (with postnasal and oral drainage)
  Integumentary: Scarlatiniform rash

Evaluation and Differential Diagnoses
DIAGNOSTICS

- Rapid antigen detection test for group A beta-hemolytic streptococcus pharyngitis OR throat culture. Testing in adults is only recommended for patients whose clinical and epidemiologic features do not reliably discriminate between viral or bacterial infection and for patients suspected of STI etiology (Shulman et al., 2012).
- Centor score and modified Centor criteria or McIsaac score (Fine et al., 2012; Gottlieb et al., 2018; Shulman et al., 2012)
- Monospot test considered suspected infectious mononucleosis
- Viral culture or Tzanck smear for HSV pharyngitis (Johns Hopkins Medicine, n.d.; Moye, 2018)
- Culture, nucleic acid amplification test, and point-of-care nucleic acid amplification test cultures are available for detecting oropharyngeal gonococcal infection (Workowski et al., 2021).

DIFFERENTIAL DIAGNOSIS

- Peritonsillar abscess (Box 24.4)
- Epiglottitis
- Kawasaki disease
- Airway obstruction

---

*Hallmark signs are bolded and **Red flags are bolded and underlined**.

BOX 24.4 ■ Acute Care Considerations

Group A streptococcus pharyngitis may lead to peritonsillar abscess, a pus collection between the tonsillar capsule and the pharyngeal constrictor muscle. Peritonsillar abscess can become life threatening if it causes airway obstruction. If the oropharynx begins to lose its patency, it is imperative to maintain an airway, which may require immediate endotracheal intubation. Patients require intravenous antibiotics and intravenous steroids, and they are often dehydrated due to poor oral intake because of the swelling and pain and require fluid resuscitation (Klug et al., 2020; Wolford et al., 2023).

Plan
GUIDELINE RESOURCES

- Shulman, S. T., Bisno, A. L., Clegg, H. W., Gerber, M. A., Kaplan, E. L., Lee, G., Martin, J. M., & Van Beneden, C. (2012). Clinical practice guideline for the diagnosis and management of group A streptococcal pharyngitis: 2012 update by the Infectious Diseases Society of America. *Clinical Infectious Diseases*, *55*(10), e86–e102. https://doi.org/10.1093/cid/cis629.
- Centers for Disease Control and Prevention. (2021). *Summary of CDC STI treatment guidelines, 2021.* https://www.cdc.gov/std/treatment-guidelines/wall-chart.pdf.

Pharmacotherapy

- Medication
  - Antibiotic treatment is for bacterial pharyngitis or STI pharyngitis. Antibiotic treatment is not recommended for patients with negative rapid antigen detection test results. Viral pharyngitis should not be treated with antibiotics:
    - Penicillin V 250 mg four times daily or 500 mg twice daily for 10 days *OR*
    - Amoxicillin 50 mg/kg once daily (max = 1000 mg); alternate: 25 mg/kg (max = 500 mg) twice daily for 10 days (Algorithm 24.1)
  (Shulman et al., 2012; Workowski et al., 2021)
- If allergy to penicillin:
  - First-generation cephalosporins:
    - Cephalexin 20 mg/kg per dose twice daily (max = 500 mg/dose) for 10 days *OR*
    - Cefadroxil 30 mg/kg once daily (max = 1 g) for 10 days *OR*
    - Clindamycin 7 mg/kg per dose three times daily (max = 300 mg/dose) for 10 days *OR*
    - Clarithromycin 7.5 mg/kg per dose twice daily (max = 250 mg/dose) for 10 days *OR*
    - Azithromycin 12 mg/kg once (max = 500 mg), then 6 mg/kg (max = 250 mg) once daily for the next 4 days
- For HSV: Acyclovir, valacyclovir, or famciclovir (Workowski et al., 2021)
- For uncomplicated gonococcal pharyngitis: Ceftriaxone IM (St Cyr et al., 2020)
- Adjunctive therapy
  - Salt water oral rinse: 1/4 to 1/2 teaspoon of salt per cup (8 ounces [approximately 240 mL]) of warm water. The water should be gargled and then spit out (not swallowed).
  - Acetaminophen or nonsteroidal antiinflammatory drugs
  - Decongestant combined with antihistamine
- Smoking cessation aids if warranted

NONPHARMACOTHERAPY

- Educate
  - Good hand hygiene
  - Respiratory etiquette
  - Stay home from work or school until afebrile and for at least 12 to 24 hours after starting antibiotic therapy.
  - Monitor for complications: Peritonsillar abscess, retropharyngeal abscess, rheumatic fever, poststreptococcal glomerulonephritis
  - Complete the full course of antibiotic as prescribed.
- Lifestyle and behavioral modifications
  - Smoking cessation
- Complementary treatment
  - Complementary and alternative therapies with natural medicines and supplements may interact with prescription medications. Obtain a complete medication history.
- Referral
  - Consult otolaryngologist for recurrent infections or if no improvement after antibiotic treatment
  - Refer for counseling regarding behavioral, psychosocial, and medical implications of sexually transmitted pharyngeal infection
- Follow-up
  - Follow up within 48 to 72 hours if no improvement or worsening of symptoms

(CDC, 2021; CDC, 2024; Shulman et al., 2012)

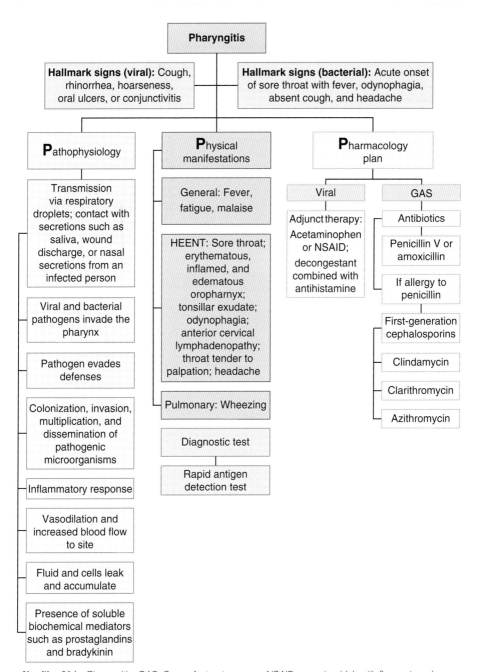

Algorithm 24.1 Pharyngitis. *GAS*, Group A streptococcus; *NSAIDs*, nonsteroidal antiinflammatory drugs.

References

Alzahrani, M. S., Maneno, M. K., Daftary, M. N., Wingate, L., & Ettienne, E. B. (2018). Factors associated with prescribing broad-spectrum antibiotics for children with upper respiratory tract infections in ambulatory care settings. *Clinical Medicine Insights: Pediatrics, 12,* 1179556518784300.

Bessen, D. E., Smeesters, P. R., & Beall, B. W. (2018). Molecular epidemiology, ecology, and evolution of group A streptococci. *Microbiology Spectrum, 6*(5) 10-1128.

Centers for Disease Control and Prevention. (2024, March 1). *Clinical Guidance for Group A Streptococcal Pharyngitis.* Retrieved September 9, 2024, https://www.cdc.gov/group-a-strep/hcp/clinical-guidance/strep-throat.html?CDC_AAref_Val–https://www.cdc.gov/groupastrep/diseases-hcp/strep-throat.html.

Cunha, B. A. (2017). A positive rapid strep test in a young adult with acute pharyngitis: Be careful what you wish for!. *IDCases, 10,* 58–59.

Fine, A. M., Nizet, V., & Mandl, K. D. (2012). Large-scale validation of the centor and McIsaac scores to predict group A streptococcal pharyngitis. *Archives of Internal Medicine, 172*(11), 847–852.

Gottlieb, M., Long, B., & Koyfman, A. (2018). Clinical mimics: An emergency medicine-focused review of streptococcal pharyngitis mimics. *Journal of Emergency Medicine, 54*(5), 619–629.

Johns Hopkins Medicine. (n.d.). Oral herpes. Retrieved September 7, 2024, https://www.hopkinsmedicine.org/health/conditions-and-diseases/herpes-hsv1-and-hsv2/oral-herpes#:~:text=Oral%20herpes%20can%20be%20difficult,herpes%20is%20antiviral%20oral%20medication.

Klug, T. E., Greve, T., & Hentze, M. (2020). Complications of peritonsillar abscess. *Annals of Clinical Microbiology and Antimicrobials, 19*(1), 32. https://doi.org/10.1186/s12941-020-00375-x.

Lee, M. J., & White, J. (2018). Sexually transmitted causes of urethritis, proctitis, pharyngitis, and cervicitis. *Medicine, 46*(6), 313–318.

Moye, M. (2018). *Herpes simplex virus.* In M. Rosenbach, K. Wanat, R. Micheletti, & L. Taylor (Eds.), *Inpatient dermatology (pp. 151–155).* Springer, https://doi.org/10.1007/978-3-319-18449-4_31.

Osowicki, J., Azzopardi, K. I., McIntyre, L., Rivera-Hernandez, T., Ong, C.-L. Y., Baker, C., Gillen, C. M., Walker, M. J., Smeesters, P. R., Davies, M. R., & Steer, A. C. (2019). A controlled human infection model of group A streptococcus pharyngitis: Which strain and why? *MSphere, 4*(1), e00647–e00718.

Ressner, R. A. (2020). Hidden harms in managing adult pharyngitis. *Military Medicine, 185*(9–10), e1385–e1386.

Rogers, J. L (2023). *Pathophysiology: The biologic basis for disease in adults and children* (9th ed.). Elsevier.

Rogers, J., & Eastland, T. (2021). Understanding the most commonly billed diagnoses in primary care: Acute pharyngitis. *Nurse Practitioner, 46*(5), 48–54. https://doi.org/10.1097/01.NPR.0000742908.69893.bb.

Shulman, S. T., Bisno, A. L., Clegg, H. W., Gerber, M. A., Kaplan, E. L., Lee, G., Martin, J. M., & Van Beneden, C. (2012). Clinical practice guideline for the diagnosis and management of group A streptococcal pharyngitis: 2012 update by the Infectious Diseases Society of America. *Clinical Infectious Diseases, 55*(10), e86–e102.

Smith-Garcia, J., Leggett, K., & Chan, S. B. (2018). Group A beta-hemolytic streptococcus pharyngitis in the elderly. *Annals of Emergency Medicine, 72*(4), S67–S68. https://doi.org/10.1016/j.annemergmed.2018.08.167.

St Cyr, S., Barbee, L., Workowski, K. A., Bachmann, L. H., Pham, C., Schlanger, K., Torrone, E., Weinstock, H., Kersh, E. N., & Thorpe, P. (2020). Update to CDC's treatment guidelines for gonococcal infection, 2020. *Morbidity and Mortality Weekly Report, 69*(50), 1911–1916.

Thigpen, M. C., Richards, C. L., Lynfield, R., Barrett, N. L., Harrison, L. H., Arnold, K. E., Reingold, A., Bennett, N. M., Craig, A. S., Gershman, K., Cieslak, P. R., Lewis, P., Greene, C. M., Beall, B., & Van Beneden, C. A. Active Bacterial Core Surveillance/Emerging Infections Program Network. (2007). Invasive group A streptococcal infection in older adults in long-term care facilities and the community, United States, 1998–2003. *Emerging Infectious Diseases, 13*(12), 1852–1859. http://doi.org/10.3201/eid1312.070303.

Wolford, R. W., Goyal, A., Syed, S. Y., & Schaefer, T. J. (2023), *Pharyngitis,* Retrieved September 7, 2024, https://www.ncbi.nlm.nih.gov/books/NBK519550.

Workowski, K. A., Bachmann, L. H., Chan, P. A., Johnston, C. M., Muzny, C. A., Park, I., Reno, H., Zenilman, J. M., & Bolan, G. A. (2021). Sexually transmitted infections treatment guidelines, 2021. *MMWR Recommendations and Reports, 70*(4), 1–187.

World Health Organization. (2020). *Rheumatic heart disease.* Retrieved September 7, 2024, https://www.who.int/news-room/fact-sheets/detail/rheumatic-heart-disease#:~:text=The%20disease%20results%20from%20damage,death%20or%20life%2Dlong%20disability.

Gastrointestinal System

SECTION OUTLINE

25 Abdominal Pain

26 Gastroesophageal Reflux Disease

27 Abdominal Hernia

28 Inflammatory Bowel Disease

29 Irritable Bowel Syndrome

30 Cholelithiasis

CHAPTER 25

Abdominal Pain

Julia L. Rogers

Differential Diagnoses for Abdomen Pain

Abdominal Pain

Abdominal pain is common and affects nearly everyone at some point in their life (Peery et al., 2019). In the United States there are approximately 6 million emergency department (ED) visits for abdominal pain annually (Peery et al., 2019). Abdominal pain can range from mild and self-limiting to severe and debilitating, even leading to mortality. The pain may be vague, specific, referred, acute, or chronic, making the diagnosis difficult. The abdomenal cavity houses vital organs of the digestive, urinary, endocrine, exocrine, circulatory, and parts of the reproductive systems. Hence many pathologies can cause abdominal pain, including neurologic, cardiopulmonary (Box 25.1), genitourinary, gastrointestinal (GI), musculoskeletal, and reproductive (Box 25.2). Abdominal pain etiology ranges from benign to life-threatening. While 90% of outpatient cases are manageable, 10% require immediate emergency care (Rogers & Schallmo, 2021). Key acute conditions necessitating ED referral include appendicitis, pancreatitis, bowel perforation (associated with acute diverticulitis), peritonitis, or bowel obstruction. In the adult population, common causes of abdominal pain in the outpatient setting include gastroenteritis, irritable bowel syndrome (IBS), gastritis, and urologic sources (Rogers & Schallmo, 2021) (see Chapters 26 and 29 for gastrointestinal conditions) (see Chapters 31 and 32 for genitourinary conditions). Chronic abdominal pain is defined as lasting 6 months or more, either intermittently or continuously, and can generally be managed in the outpatient setting (Charles et al., 2019).

Pathophysiology

Abdominal pain is initiated by the activation of abdominal nociceptive receptors (specialized sensory neurons) by mechanical and/or chemical stimuli. There are three afferent relays (first, second, and third order neurons) that respond to stimuli and send them to the brain to be processed. The brain then coordinates a response and sends it back to the source via efferent pathways (Algorithm 25.1). The type, quality, intensity, and location of pain are dependent on the relay response, which classifies pain as somatic, visceral, or referred (Banasik & Copstead, 2019; Penner & Fishman, 2023a; Spain, 2023). Because there are multiple relay pathways, it is possible to experience different types of pain in the same or separate areas of the body. Somatic pain arises from cutaneous or deep structures, occurring in bones, joints, connective tissue, and muscles (Banasik & Copstead, 2019; Spain, 2023). Somatic abdominal pain arises from the parietal peritoneum and tends to be asymmetric and well localized and described as sharp. Patients with somatic pain are often able to pinpoint the precise location of the pain because somatic innervation is unilateral and is intensified by sudden movement, deep inspiration, or application of pressure on the abdominal wall. An example of somatic pain is postoperative cholecystectomy pain. Visceral pain occurs in hollow and solid organs and is due to infiltration, compression, traction, stretch, or distension

> **BOX 25.1 ■ Older Adult Considerations**
>
> Recent research has explored the relationship between pain sensation and gut microbiota profiles in older adults with heart failure, a significant area of study given the high prevalence of pain in this population. The study investigated how gut microbiota composition might be associated with pain intensity and interference in heart failure patients. Findings suggest a potential link between specific gut bacterial taxa and pain experiences in these individuals. This research highlights the complex interplay between the gut microbiome and pain perception in heart failure, opening new avenues for understanding and potentially managing pain in this vulnerable population. The implications of this study could lead to novel approaches in pain management for heart failure patients, possibly involving interventions targeting the gut microbiome. (Chen et al., 2023).

> **BOX 25.2 ■ Diversity Considerations**
>
> Healthcare providers must consider unique physiological and pharmacological factors when evaluating abdominal pain in transgender and gender-diverse (TGD) populations. Gender-affirming hormone therapy can alter gastrointestinal physiology and liver function, potentially influencing pain perception and medication metabolism. Physical assessment should be conducted with sensitivity to gender identity, acknowledging that anatomical structures may not align with traditional expectations. Pharmacotherapy for abdominal pain in TGD individuals requires careful consideration of drug interactions with hormone therapies and potential impacts on gender-affirming treatments. Additionally, clinicians should be aware that stress related to gender identity and societal stigma may exacerbate gastrointestinal symptoms and pain experiences in TGD patients. Culturally competent care, including using appropriate language and respecting gender identity, is crucial for accurate diagnosis and effective treatment of abdominal pain in this diverse population.(Newman et al., 2023).

(Banasik & Copstead, 2019; Penner & Fishman, 2023a; Spain, 2023). The visceral afferents innervate abdominal visceral structures and bilaterally enter several spinal levels, causing diffuse pain (Banasik & Copstead, 2019; Rogers & Schallmo, 2021). For example, the small intestine visceral nerve enters the spinal cord at levels T8 to L1, aligning with the periumbilical area; therefore patients with an inflamed and distended appendix may locate the pain by moving their hand across the middle abdomen or periumbilical area (Penner & Fishman, 2023a). Visceral pain tends to be described as vague, cramping, dull, and aching. Referred pain is also visceral, but felt along the same skin dermatome or shared afferent neuropathway as the organ, and at a site distant to the original visceral pain site (Banasik & Copstead, 2019; Spain, 2023). Pain referred to multiple sites with different pain qualities is caused by simultaneous somatic and visceral innervation. One pain site may have an aching quality, but a distant site may be a well-localized pain. A patient who presents with acute cholecystitis reports dull, aching pain in the abdomen but also reports a distant well-localized pain in the right scapula; this is an example of referred pain.

Physical Clinical Presentation

SUBJECTIVE

Obtain a thorough history of present illness (HPI) and review of systems (ROS). For all pediatric patients, ask both the patient (if able to communicate) and the same questions to the parent or guardian accompanying the child (Box 25.3). Documentation should include the onset of symptoms; precipitating events; location, intensity, and quality of pain; progression of symptoms; alleviating and aggravating factors; previous episodes; and associated symptoms. The OPQRSTU assessment is just one mnemonic that can be used to conduct a complete history (Jarvis, 2020):

    O—Onset: "When did the pain start?" "What were you doing when the pain started?"

BOX 25.3 ■ Pediatric Considerations

Abdominal pain is a common complaint in pediatric patients, presenting diagnostic challenges due to the wide range of potential causes. While most cases of abdominal pain in children are due to benign conditions, a significant minority require surgical intervention. There are key symptoms associated with potentially serious conditions: vomiting, fever, and right lower quadrant pain, which are particularly indicative of possible surgical needs. These findings underscore the importance of thorough clinical assessment in pediatric abdominal pain cases. Providers should be alert to these specific symptoms, as they may signal the need for more intensive evaluation or surgical consultation. There is certainly an ongoing need to improve diagnostic accuracy and appropriate management of abdominal pain in pediatric populations. (Sforza et al., 2023).

P—Provoke or *palliative*; any aggravating and alleviating factors: "What makes the pain better or worse?"

Q—Quality or characteristics of pain (e.g., sharp, dull, tingling, burning) (Table 25.1): "What does your pain feel like?"

R—Region or *radiation*; the location of pain: "Point to the current location of your pain." "Where did the pain start?" "Does the pain radiate or move?"

S—Severity and *symptoms*, using a scale (e.g., numeric rating scale, visual analog scale, or Wong-Baker FACES Pain Rating Scale) to quantify pain level; it is important to use a pain intensity assessment tool appropriate for the patient's developmental level: "Rate your pain on a scale of 0 to 10 with 0 meaning no pain and 10 meaning the worst pain imaginable. How bad is the pain at its worst?" Ask about associated symptoms occurring with the pain (e.g., nausea, vomiting, fever): "What other symptoms are you experiencing?"

T—Time frame, duration, and frequency of pain: "Is this your first episode of pain?" "How long does the pain last?" "Does the intensity of pain change with time or position?"

U—You, the impact of pain on the patient's normal daily routine: "How is the pain affecting your life?" "Does it limit your function or activities?" "Are you able to work?" Are you able to perform activities of daily living such as bathing, dressing, toileting, walking, and eating?" (Jarvis, 2020; Rogers & Schallmo, 2021)

A comprehensive ROS aids in formulating precise differential diagnoses by elucidating associated symptoms (Table 25.2) (Goolsby & Grubbs, 2019; Penner & Fishman, 2023b). Document allergies as well as medical, social, family, and travel history. The intake of an accurate medical history is critical because patients with comorbid conditions such as type 2 diabetes mellitus may present with less pain due to neuropathic changes (see Chapter 14). The medical history should contain all previous diagnoses and a surgical history (specifically GI or abdominal surgeries). Inquire as to any recent sick contacts, travel domestically or internationally, emergency or urgent care visits, or hospitalizations. Review a current list of medications, any medications recently discontinued, and recent use of antibiotics, opioids, or complementary medications. Document any family history of GI disease or cancers (Rogers & Schallmo, 2021).

HPI or ROS:* Patient reports **hematemesis**; **hematochezia**; **severe vomiting**; **severe diarrhea**; **dysphagia**; **acute, accelerating chronic pain or acute pain, or new pain symptoms in chronic abdominal pain**; pain in relation to meals or bowel movement; odynophagia; rectal occult blood; nausea; vomiting; recent changes in stool color or consistency or in bowel habit; diarrhea; constipation; melena; bloating (Algorithm 25.1)

Genitourinary: Incontinence; dysuria; **hematuria**; frequency; urgency; hesitancy; polydipsia; polyuria; dark amber urine

---

*Hallmark signs are bolded but are dependent on etiology of abdominal pain and **Red flags are bolded and underlined**.

TABLE 25.1 ■ **Classification of Pain and Associated Disease**[a]

Classification of Pain	Visceral Pain	Somatoparietal Pain	Referred Pain
	Vague, poorly localized, crampy, burning, midline, restless, diaphoresis, pallor, nausea	Specific, localized, intense, guarding, worse with movement, respirations, cough	Abdomen to back or back to abdomen
Disease and/or organ association	Inflammation or injury to an organ	Inflammation within parietal perineum	Visceral pain referred away from the organ
	Appendix: Appendicitis	Infection	Appendicitis: Pain referred to the labia, testicle, or shaft of penis or lower quadrants of abdomen or lower back
	Gallbladder: Cholelithiasis or cholecystitis	Abscess	Gallbladder: Pain referred to right shoulder or back
	Stomach/gastrointestinal tract: Gastritis	Constipation	Stomach: Pain referred to mid-center upper back
	Kidney: Nephrolithiasis Bladder/ureter	Hematoma	Obturator hernia: Pain referred along medial aspect of thigh to knee (Howship–Romberg sign)
	Pancreas: Pancreatitis	Tumor: Iliopsoas, pelvic bone	Pancreas: Pain referred to left mid-back
	Liver: Cirrhosis	Injury to musculoskeletal system of abdomen	Liver: Pain referred to right shoulder
	Lung		Lung and diaphragm: Pain referred to left shoulder
	Malignancy or tumor Organ ischemia		

[a]This is not a comprehensive list.

Reproductive: Females should be screened for sexually transmitted diseases; pelvic inflammatory disease; premenopausal females should be asked about menstrual cycle history, contraceptive use, vaginal discharge and bleeding, dyspareunia, or dysmenorrhea; prostate hypertrophy

Psychiatric: Depression; anxious

OBJECTIVE*

Generalized: Weakness; fatigue; polyphagia; <u>fever</u>; <u>unintentional weight loss</u>; <u>loss of appetite</u>; <u>pain that awakens the patient from sleep</u>; <u>immediate severe pain</u>; chills

  Neurological: <u>Confusion</u>

  Cardiovascular: <u>Chest pain</u>; <u>tachycardia</u>; <u>hypotension</u>; <u>lower extremity edema</u>

  Pulmonary: *Inspection:* <u>Labored respirations</u>; <u>tachypnea</u>; <u>use of accessory muscles</u>; cough

TABLE 25.2 ■ Abdominal Pain Physical Assessment Clinical Manifestations

Inspection	Auscultation	Percussion	Palpation	Special Maneuvers
Jaundice association to **liver disease**	Decreased/absent bowel sounds association to **paralytic ileus or peritonitis**	Tympanic association to **gastric air**	Hepatomegaly association to **cirrhosis, hepatitis, right heart failure, cysts, malignancy**	Rebound tenderness association to **peritoneal inflammation**
Lack of bowel peristalsis association to **bowel obstruction**	Tinks or high-pitch bowel sounds association to **bowel obstruction**	Dull association to **liver or spleen**	Splenomegaly association to **infection, inflammation process**	Heel strike association to **peritoneal irritation or appendicitis**
Abdominal distention, change in contour or symmetry association to **fat, fluid, feces; fetus; flatus; fibroid; full bladder; fatal tumor; false pregnancy**	Borborygmi prolonged gurgles association to **gastroenteritis, hunger, early obstruction**	Flat association to **muscle or bone**	Aortic aneurysm association to **arteriosclerosis, hypertension, trauma**	Rovsing's sign association to **appendicitis**
Pulsations association to **aortic aneurysm**	Rushes association to **intestinal obstruction**	Resonant association to **lung involvement**	Growth or mass in abdominal organs association to **tumor benign or malignant**	Obturator sign association to **appendicitis**
	Rubs association to **inflammation, peritoneal surface of organ, tumor, infection, or splenic infarct**	Hyperresonant association to **emphysematous lung**		Psoas muscle sign association to **appendicitis**
	Splash association to **gas and fluid in a cavity OR free air in peritoneum or thorax**			Murphy's sign association to **cholecystitis**
	Bruits association to **aneurysm**			Shifting dullness association to **ascites**
				Scratch test association to **enlarged liver**
				Hepatojugular reflux association to **right sided heart failure**

From Goolsby, M. J., & Grubbs, L. (2023). Advanced assessment: Interpreting findings and formulating differential diagnoses (5th ed.). F.A. Davis Company. Used with permission.

Gastrointestinal: *Inspection:* **Abdominal distention/swelling**; rash; abdomen is asymmetrical; peristalsis; pulsations; discoloration

Auscultation: Hyper-/hypobowel sounds; bruits—aorta, iliac, or femoral arteries

Percussion: Dullness

Palpation: Tenderness; **rebound tenderness**; **abdominal rigidity**; **guarding**; **right upper or lower quadrant pain**; hepatomegaly (liver 0–1 cm below costal margin); mass; splenomegaly

Integumentary: Jaundice, pallor; rash

(See Fig. 25.1.)

(Ball, 2023; Dains et al., 2024; Goolsby & Grubbs, 2019; Penner & Fishman, 2023a, 2023b; Rogers & Schallmo, 2021; Spain, 2023)

Evaluation and Differential Diagnoses

DIAGNOSTICS

- Emergent abdominal pain with red flags*
  - Individuals presenting with red flag symptoms or who require emergency workup should be referred to the nearest ED.
- Nonemergent acute abdominal pain
  - Labs:
    - Complete blood count with differential
    - Complete metabolic panel
    - Amylase and lipase
    - Erythrocyte sedimentation rate
    - C-reactive protein
    - Urinalysis or urine dipstick
    - Pregnancy test (all females of child-bearing age)
  - Diagnostic imaging:
    - Abdominal ultrasound
- Chronic abdominal pain
  - Labs:
    - Complete blood count with differential
    - Complete metabolic panel
    - Amylase and lipase
    - Serum iron, total iron binding capacity, ferritin
    - Antitissue transglutaminase, IgA
    - Erythrocyte sedimentation rate
    - C-reactive protein
    - Hepatitis screening panel
    - Thyroid function panel if constipation or diarrhea
    - Pregnancy test for all females of child-bearing age
  - Diagnostic imaging:
    - Ultrasound
    - Computed tomography (CT) or magnetic resonance imaging (MRI) may be indicated, unless previously completed and normal

(Charles et al., 2019; Rogers & Schallmo, 2021; Spain 2023)

DIFFERENTIAL DIAGNOSIS

- See Tables 25.1 and 25.2 and Fig. 25.1 for possible differential diagnoses.

Sites and common causes of acute abdominal pain

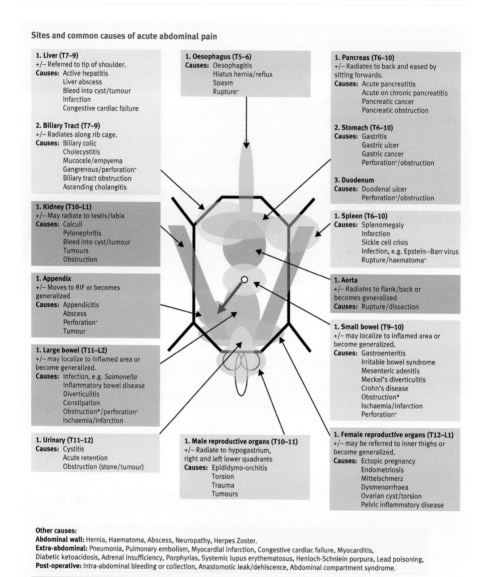

1. Liver (T7–9)
+/– Referred to tip of shoulder.
Causes: Active hepatitis
Liver abscess
Bleed into cyst/tumour
Infarction
Congestive cardiac failure

2. Biliary Tract (T7–9)
+/– Radiates along rib cage.
Causes: Biliary colic
Cholecystitis
Mucocele/empyema
Gangrenous/perforation*
Biliary tract obstruction
Ascending cholangitis

1. Kidney (T10–L1)
+/– May radiate to testis/labia
Causes: Calculi
Pylonephritis
Bleed into cyst/tumour
Tumours
Obstruction

1. Appendix
+/– Moves to RIF or becomes
generalized
Causes: Appendicitis
Abscess
Perforation*
Tumour

1. Large bowel (T11–L2)
+/– may localize to inflamed area or
become generalized.
Causes: Infection, e.g. *Salmonella*
Inflammatory bowel disease
Diverticulitis
Constipation
Obstruction*/perforation*
Ischaemia/infarction

1. Urinary (T11–12)
Causes: Cystitis
Acute retention
Obstruction (stone/tumour)

1. Oesophagus (T5–6)
Causes: Oesophagitis
Hiatus hernia/reflux
Spasm
Rupture*

1. Male reproductive organs (T10–11)
+/– Radiate to hypogastrium,
right and left lower quadrants
Causes: Epididymo-orchitis
Torsion
Trauma
Tumours

1. Pancreas (T6–10)
+/– Radiates to back and eased by
sitting forwards.
Causes: Acute pancreatitis
Acute on chronic pancreatitis
Pancreatic cancer
Pancreatic obstruction

2. Stomach (T6–10)
Causes: Gastritis
Gastric ulcer
Gastric cancer
Perforation*/obstruction

3. Duodenum
Causes: Duodenal ulcer
Perforation*/obstruction

1. Spleen (T6–10)
Causes: Splenomegaly
Infarction
Sickle cell crisis
Infection, e.g. Epstein–Barr virus
Rupture/haematoma*

1. Aorta
+/– Radiates to flank/back or
becomes generalized
Causes: Rupture/dissection

1. Small bowel (T9–10)
+/– may localize to inflamed area or
become generalized.
Causes: Gastroenteritis
Irritable bowel syndrome
Mesenteric adenitis
Meckel's diverticulitis
Crohn's disease
Obstruction*
Ischaemia/infarction
Perforation*

1. Female reproductive organs (T12–L1)
+/– may be referred to inner thighs or
become generalized.
Causes: Ectopic pregnancy
Endometriosis
Mittelschmerz
Dysmenorrhoea
Ovarian cyst/torsion
Pelvic inflammatory disease

Other causes:
Abdominal wall: Hernia, Haematoma, Abscess, Neuropathy, Herpes Zoster.
Extra-abdominal: Pneumonia, Pulmonary embolism, Myocardial infarction, Congestive cardiac failure, Myocarditis,
Diabetic ketoacidosis, Adrenal insufficiency, Porphyrias, Systemic lupus erythematosus, Henloch-Schnlein purpura, Lead poisoning,
Post-operative: Intra-abdominal bleeding or collection, Anastomotic leak/dehiscence, Abdominal compartment syndrome.

Key
(T) Segmental innervation of viscera.
* **Perforation** may be localized or generalized: NB Rebound pain, Guarding, Rigid abdomen +/– absent bowel sounds.
* **Causes of bowel obstruction:** (a) Luminal: Foreign body, Bezoars, Gallstone ileus (b) Mural: Tumours, Intussusception,
Benign strictures e.g. diverticula/Crohn's/ischaemic, (c) Extra-Mural: Adhesions, Hernia, Volvulus, Abdominal aortic aneurysm.

Fig. 25.1   Sites and causes of abdominal pain. (From Smith, J. K., & Lobo, D. N. (2012). Investigation of the acute abdomen. *Surgery, 30*(6), 296–305.)

Plan

GUIDELINE RESOURCES

- Mayumi, T., Yoshida, M., Tazuma, S., Furukawa, A., Nishii, O., Shigematsu, K., Azuhata, T., Itakura, A., Kamei, S., Kondo, H., Maeda, S., Mihara, H., Mizooka, M., Nishidate, T.,

Obara, H., Sato, N., Takayama, Y., Tsujikawa, T., Fujii, T., … Hirata, K. (2016). The practice guidelines for primary care of acute abdomen 2015. *Journal of General and Family Medicine*, *17*(1), 5–52. https://doi.org/10.14442/jgfm.17.1_5

- Refer to individual disease guidelines
  - Chapter 30: Cholelithiasis
  - Chapter 26: Gastroesophageal Reflux Disease
  - Chapter 28: Inflammatory Bowel Disease
  - Chapter 29: Irritable Bowel Syndrome
  - Chapter 31: Nephrolithiasis
  - Chapter 32: Urinary Tract Infection
  - Chapter 38: Benign Prostatic Hypertrophy
  - Chapter 39: Dysmenorrhea
  - Chapter 40: Sexually Transmitted Infections

Pharmacotherapy

- Acute abdominal pain with red flags*
  - ED (Box 25.4)
- Acute abdominal pain without red flags*
  - Medications per underlying etiology (Algorithm 25.1)
- Chronic abdominal pain
  - Medications per underlying etiology
- Smoking cessation aids should be offered to any person currently smoking tobacco.

(Charles et al., 2019; Rogers & Schallmo, 2021; Spain 2023)

NONPHARMACOTHERAPY

- Educate
  - Red flags:
    - Pain that
      - Awakens the individual from sleep
      - Persists longer than 6 hours and increases in intensity
      - Changes location
      - Causes nausea and vomiting or hematemesis
      - Worsens with walking or increased movement
      - Radiates to shoulder or back
    - Black tarry stools or hematochezia
    - Abdominal distention that is progressive

BOX 25.4 ■ Acute Care Considerations

Abdominal pain is a common presenting complaint in emergency departments (EDs), requiring careful evaluation and management. Recent research has focused on identifying predictors of unscheduled return visits with admission (URVAs) within 72 hours for patients initially presenting with abdominal pain. Understanding these risk factors is crucial for improving patient outcomes and optimizing resource allocation in acute care settings. Clinicians should be aware of potential indicators that may predispose patients to URVAs, as this knowledge can inform discharge planning and follow-up care. Implementing strategies based on these predictors could potentially reduce complications and enhance the overall quality of care for patients with acute abdominal pain. (Jiang et al., 2023).

- Decreased urine output or no urine output
- Fever
- Syncope or hypotension
- Weight loss
- Cause of abdomen pain if known
- Differential diagnoses
- Medication purpose and side effects
- Eliminate triggering foods, beverages, stressors
- Self-management
- Importance of vaccines
- Lifestyle and behavioral modifications
  - Diet: FODMAP (FODMAP stands for fermentable oligosaccharides, disaccharides, monosaccharides, and polyols. Types of carbohydrates that can be difficult for some people to digest, leading to gastrointestinal issues); heart healthy, low fat
  - Exercise
  - Smoking cessation
- Complementary treatment
  - Psychosocial rehabilitation
  - Cognitive behavioral therapy
  - Complementary and alternative therapies with natural medicines and supplements may interact with prescription medications. Obtain a complete medication history.
- Referral
  - Gastroenterologist
  - Identify and refer to specialty for treatment of comorbid conditions
- Follow-up
  - Office visit 1 to 2 weeks after hospital discharge
  - 1 month after starting any new medication or sooner if side effects
  - Every 3 to 6 months for chronic abdominal pain that has stabilized

(Charles et al., 2019; Rogers & Schallmo, 2021; Spain 2023)

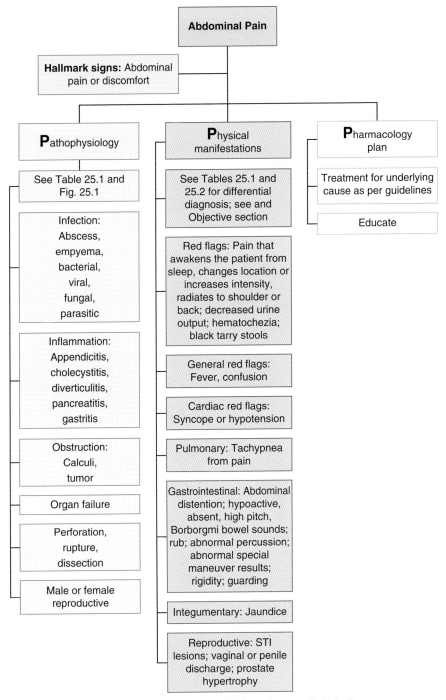

Algorithm 25.1 Abdominal Pain. *STI*, Sexually transmitted infection.

References

Ball, J. W., Dains, J. E., Flynn, J. A., Solomon, B. S., & Stewart, R. W. (2023). *Seidel's guide to physical examination: An interprofessional approach [E-book]* (9th ed.). Elsevier.

Banasik, J. L., & Copstead, L. C. (2019). *Pathophysiology* (6th ed.). Elsevier.

Charles, G., Chery, M., & Channell, M. K. (2019). Chronic abdominal pain: Tips for the primary care provider. *Osteopathic Family Physician, 11*(1), 20–26.

Chen, J., Wang, Z., Starkweather, A., Chen, M.-H., McCauley, P., Miao, H., Ahn, H., & Cong, X. (2023). Pain sensation and gut microbiota profiles in older adults with heart failure. *International Nursing Review.* https://doi.org/10.1097/NR9.0000000000000024.

Dains, J. E., Baumann, L. C., & Scheibel, P. (2024). *Advanced health assessment & clinical diagnosis in primary care* (7th ed.). Elsevier.

Goolsby, M. J., & Grubbs, L. (2019). *Abdomen.* In M. J. Goolsby, & L. Grubbs (Eds.), *Advanced health assessment: Interpreting findings and formulating differential diagnoses* (4th ed., pp. 275–325). F. A. Davis Company.

Jarvis, C. (2020). *Physical examination and health assessment* (7th ed.). Elsevier.

Jiang, Y., Jiang, Y., Xie, J., Zhao, X., Ye, L., & Zhu, Y. (2023). Predictors of 72-h unscheduled return visits with admission in patients presenting to the emergency department with abdominal pain. *European Journal of Medical Research, 28*(1), 336. https://doi.org/10.1186/s40001-023-01256-7.

Newman, K. L., Vélez, C., Paul, S., Radix, A. E., Streed, C. G., & Targownik, L. E. (2023). Research considerations in digestive and liver disease in transgender and gender-diverse populations. *Clinical Gastroenterology and Hepatology, 21*(10), 2443–2449. https://doi.org/10.1016/j.cgh.2023.03.017.

Peery, A. F., Crockett, S. D., Murphy, C. C., Lund, J. L., Dellon, E. S., Williams, J. L., Jensen, E. T., Shaheen, N. J., Barritt, A. S., Lieber, S. R., Kochar, B., Barnes, E. L., Fan, C., Pate, V., Galanko, J., Baron, T. H., & Sandler, R. S. (2019). Burden and cost of gastrointestinal, liver, and pancreatic diseases in the United States: Update 2018. *Gastroenterology, 156*(1), 254–272.e11.

Penner, R. M., & Fishman, M. B. (2024). In A. D. Auerbach, M. D. Aronson, & L. Kunins (Eds.), Retrieved September 12, 2024. *Causes of abdominal pain in adults.* http://www.uptodate.com/contents/causes-of-abdominal-pain-in-adults/print.

Penner, R. M., & Fishman, M. B. (2023). In A. D. Auerbach, M. D. Aronson, & L. Kunins (Eds.), Retrieved September 12, 2024. *Evaluation of the adult with abdominal pain.* http://www.uptodate.com.contents/evaluation-of-the-adult-with-abdominal-pain/print.

Rogers, J. L., & Schallmo, M. (2021). Understanding the most commonly billed diagnoses in primary care: Abdominal pain. *Nurse Practitioner, 46*(1), 13–20. http://doi.org/10.1097/01.NPR.0000724512.95721.68.

Sforza, M., Mancini, S., Biffanti, R., Gamba, P., & Zanatta, C. (2023). Abdominal pain in children: A retrospective study in a tertiary pediatric emergency department. *Frontiers in Pediatrics, 11.* Article 1118874. https://doi.org/10.3389/fped.2023.1118874.

Spain, S. (2023). Alterations in the digestive system. In J. L. Rogers (Ed.), *McCance & Huether's pathophysiology: The biologic basis for disease in adults and children* (9th ed.). Elsevier.

CHAPTER 26

Gastroesophageal Reflux Disease

Julia L. Rogers

Gastroesophageal Reflux Disease

Gastroesophageal reflux disease (GERD) is a chronic relapsing condition that affects all age groups, races, and genders. Risk factors include obesity, hiatal hernia, pregnancy, smoking, and alcohol use (Rogers & Eastland, 2021). Eating habits may also contribute to GERD, including consumption of acidic, high-fat foods as well as size and timing of meals, particularly with respect to sleep (Box 26.1).

Pathophysiology

The esophagus is a muscular tube that connects the pharynx to the stomach and is divided into three functional areas: the upper esophageal sphincter, the esophageal body, and the lower esophageal sphincter (LES). The muscular tone of the functional areas coordinates an organized pattern of contraction and relaxation to move contents in a forward direction (Rogers & Eastland, 2021). Transient LES relaxation is a normal physiologic response to gastric distention after eating food or drinking liquids that facilitates digestion. Frequent and prolonged relaxations, however, can contribute to GERD due to lowered LES pressure (Clarrett & Hachem, 2018) (Fig. 26.1). Other factors that can hinder the effectiveness of the antireflux barrier include abnormal crural diaphragm anatomy or function, hiatal hernia, impaired esophageal clearance, and delayed gastric emptying (Algorithm 26.1) (Clarrett & Hachem, 2018).

Parietal cells play a pivotal role in gastric homeostasis and are crucial in the pathophysiology of GERD because they secrete hydrochloric acid (HCl), which creates an acidic environment, acts as a bactericide against swallowed microorganisms, dissolves food fibers, and converts pepsinogen to pepsin (Rogers & Eastland, 2021; Spain, 2023). Pepsin breaks down the protein in food for digestion. HCl is harmful for the esophageal mucosa and can induce heartburn, chest pain, and mucosal lesions. Histamine stimulates HCl secretion by activating H2-type receptors of parietal cells and initiating a cascade of reactions that culminate in acid secretion (Rogers & Eastland, 2021; Spain, 2023). One reaction is the stimulation of gastric hydrogen potassium adenosine triphosphatase or proton pump, which responds by secreting gastric acid. The H2-type receptors and proton pump are important features related to pharmacologic treatments (Algorithm 26.1). GERD occurs when these gastric contents (acid, pepsin, or bile) flow backward into the esophagus. It is this process that causes the foul taste some may report in the mouth, along with throat irritation, inflammation, erosion, and cough.

Physical Clinical Presentation

SUBJECTIVE

The most common symptoms of GERD are substernal burning and discomfort, which patients often refer to as heartburn or indigestion, that occasionally radiates upward to the neck and throat. Another common complaint is a bitter taste in the mouth from gastric regurgitation.

BOX 26.1 ■ Diversity Considerations

Healthcare disparities affect the care of disease processes and are a growing concern internationally. Research guidelines, government institutions, and scientific journals continue to minimize disparities through policies regarding the collection and reporting of racial/ethnic data. One area where shortcomings remain is with gastroesophageal reflux disease (GERD), hence the importance of ensuring that diverse participants are included and accurately described within GERD research studies. This will advance evidence-based care, help prevent health care disparities, and ensure that care can be translated to all patients (Craven et al., 2018).

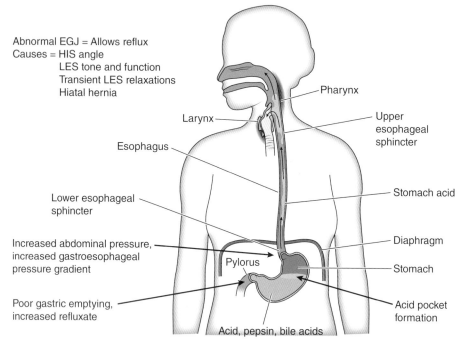

Abnormal EGJ = Allows reflux
Causes = HIS angle
       LES tone and function
       Transient LES relaxations
       Hiatal hernia

Pharynx

Larynx

Upper esophageal sphincter

Esophagus

Lower esophageal sphincter

Stomach acid

Increased abdominal pressure, increased gastroesophageal pressure gradient

Pylorus

Diaphragm

Stomach

Poor gastric emptying, increased refluxate

Acid pocket formation

Acid, pepsin, bile acids

Fig. 26.1   GI anatomy and pathophysiology of gastroesophageal reflux disease. *EGJ*, esophagogastric junction; *LES*, lower esophageal sphincter.

There are other manifestations patients may report that are considered extraesophageal or atypical symptoms. The most common are noncardiac chest pain followed by chronic cough with excessive mucus and throat clearing. The irritation of the throat from the cough and reflux can lead to sore throat, laryngitis, tonsilitis, odynophagia, and dental erosion.

During the focused history, documentation should include the onset of symptoms; precipitating events; location, intensity, and quality of pain; progression of symptoms; alleviating and aggravating factors; previous episodes; and associated symptoms. Document any allergies to medications as well as exposure to smoke and environmental or occupational irritants. Ask if the patient has been around any ill contacts and if they are a current or previous tobacco or marijuana user. Ask all pertinent questions in the past medical history to rule out myocardial infarction, aortic dissection, postnasal drip, rhinosinusitis, chronic obstructive pulmonary disease, sleep apnea, infection, and malignancy. A multitude of cardiac and pulmonary diseases can present with similar symptoms as GERD. Be sure to include family history of stomach, colon, or other

---

BOX 26.2 ■ Pediatric Considerations

A thorough history and physical examination in the evaluation of gastroesophageal reflux disease (GERD) is important to distinguish gastroesophageal reflux (GER) from GERD, identify possible complications of GERD, and exclude underlying, possibly serious or life-threatening disorders.

Several red flag clinical manifestations in children suggest a disorder other than GERD. For example, weight loss, lethargy, fever, excessive pain and irritability, and dysuria suggest systemic infection or urinary tract infection. While GER is common and often physiological in infants, GERD is the appropriate diagnosis when reflux symptoms are chronic (onset of regurgitation and/or any vomiting more than 6 months duration); there is increasing severity; or the symptoms are persistant beyond the typical age of resolution (between 12 months and 18 months of age). A bulging fontanel, macro/microcephaly, or seizures may represent intracranial pressure possibly from a brain tumor, meningitis, or hydrocephalus. Persistent forceful vomiting, nocturnal vomiting, or bilious vomiting can represent an intestinal obstruction, Hirschsprung's disease, intestinal atresia, or intussusception. Hematemesis may be cause for concern of an esophageal, stomach, or gastrointestinal bleed; acid-peptic disease; Mallory-Weiss tear; or reflux esophagitis. Chronic diarrhea may suggest food protein–induced gastroenteropathy. Rectal bleeding is concerning for bacterial gastroenteritis, inflammatory bowel disease, or acute surgical conditions. Abdominal distention is concerning for an obstruction, dysmotility, or an anatomic abnormality (Rosen et al., 2018). All pediatric symptoms should be reported to pediatric provider.

BOX 26.3 ■ Older Adult Considerations

Older adult patients represent a challenging population when diagnosing or treating gastroesophageal or laryngopharyngeal reflux because of their tendency to report atypical clinical manifestations. Working up the differential diagnoses can prolong the time to treatment. Another consideration is how aging leads to a defective, weakened, or incompetent antireflux barrier; abnormal esophageal clearance; reduced salivary production; altered esophageal mucosal resistance; and delayed gastric emptying, leading to complications of gastroesophageal reflux disease (GERD) such as esophagitis, esophageal stricture, Barrett's esophagus, and esophageal cancer. Older patients also have a higher proportion of hiatal hernias, found in 60% of those aged 60 years and older, which impairs the function of the lower esophageal sphincter (LES) and may impair the clearance of refluxed acid from the distal esophagus. In addition, older patients generally are prescribed multiple medications that decrease LES pressure, such as nitrates, calcium channel blockers, benzodiazepines, anticholinergics, and antidepressants. Due to the possibility of adverse events, consideration should be given to clearance outcomes of proton pump inhibitors and drug interactions in patients 65 years of age or older when determining therapeutic approaches (Authors original).

---

gastrointestinal cancers. Review current and past medications, specifically asking about medications that may cause cough such as angiotensin-converting enzyme (ACE) inhibitors (Durazzo et al., 2020; Maret-Ouda et al., 2020; Smith & Davila, 2023). Pediatric and geriatric patients may present differently (Boxes 26.2 and 26.3).

OBJECTIVE*

Generalized: <u>Weight loss unintentional</u>

HEENT: Sore throat; hoarse voice; laryngitis; tonsillitis; dental erosion; **<u>odynophagia</u>**; **<u>dysphagia</u>**; substernal chest burning and discomfort; epigastric pain

---

*Hallmark signs are bolded and <u>Red flags are bolded and underlined</u>.

BOX 26.4 ▪ Acute Care Considerations

Chronic gastroesophageal reflux disease (GERD) damages the normal esophageal squamous epithelium of the esophagus and replaces it with metaplastic columnar mucosa, causing Barrett's esophagus. Patients may be hospitalized with Barrett's esophagus for a few reasons. First, Barrett's esophagus is the only known precursor to the lethal esophageal adenocarcinoma; therefore patients may be hospitalized for treatment or complications from the cancer. Second, patients may be hospitalized for endoscopy procedures including biopsy, endoscopic resection, or endoscopic eradication therapy. It is vital to monitor any patient after endoscopic procedures for methemoglobinemia, a condition in which hemoglobin decreases its ability to carry oxygen. Methemoglobinemia is a complication that can happen after the use of topical anesthetic sprays (e.g., lidocaine or benzocaine), that are used for numbing the throat during the endoscopic procedures. The presentation is cyanosis with no significant alterations in diagnostics or labs except for the methemoglobin level. The treatment is methylene blue IV (Gao et al., 2022; Shaheen et al., 2022).

Cardiovascular: <u>Chest pain (noncardiac)</u>; regular rate rhythm; normal S1/S2; murmur; rub; gallop

Pulmonary: *Inspection:* **Cough; excessive phlegm/throat clearing.** *Auscultation:* Wheezing

Gastrointestinal: <u>Hematemesis</u>; **coffee ground emesis**; **black tarry stools**; <u>hematochezia</u>; nausea; <u>vomiting</u>

(Ball, 2023; Dains et al., 2024; Durazzo et al., 2020; Spain, 2023)

Evaluation and Differential Diagnoses

DIAGNOSTICS

- Presenting symptoms (typical, atypical, or alarm)
- Esophagogastroduodenoscopy (EGD) to evaluate esophageal mucosa
- Reflux monitoring by gastroenterologist to assess pH and esophageal acid
- Complete blood count (CBC); anemia concern for gastrointestinal bleed

(Katz et al., 2022; Smith & Davila, 2023)

DIFFERENTIAL DIAGNOSIS

- Cardiac disease (myocardial infarction; aortic dissection)
- Pulmonary disease (chronic obstructive pulmonary disease; asthma; postnasal drip; rhinosinusitis; effusion; sleep apnea; embolism; infection; or malignancy)
- Reaction or side effect from angiotensin-converting enzyme (ACE) inhibitors
- Peptic ulcer disease
- Barrett's esophagus and carcinoma (Box 26.4)

Plan

GUIDELINE RESOURCES

- Katz, P. O., Dunbar, K. B., Schnoll-Sussman, F. H., Greer, K. B., Yadlapati, R., & Spechler, S. J. (2022). ACG clinical guideline for the diagnosis and management of gastroesophageal reflux disease. *American Journal of Gastroenterology, 117*(1), 27–56. https://doi.org/10.14309/ajg.0000000000001538.

Pharmacotherapy

- Medications: Typical symptoms
  - Proton pump inhibitor (PPI) once daily 30 to 60 minutes before breakfast:
    - 8-week trial of empiric PPI treatment daily:
      - If symptoms improve or resolve, a presumptive diagnosis of GERD can be made.
      - If symptoms do not improve or resolve or if they return after PPI is stopped, EGD is recommended.
      - If EGD is not diagnostic for GERD, reflux monitoring should be done while patient is off pharmacotherapy to confirm GERD diagnosis.
- Medications: Atypical or extraesophageal symptoms
  - Once all other potential causes have been ruled out and the patient has typical and atypical symptoms, initiate PPI twice daily (bid): 30 to 60 minutes before breakfast and 30 to 60 minutes before dinner.
    - Complete 8-to-12-week trial of empiric treatment with PPI bid:
      - If symptoms improve or resolve, a presumptive diagnosis of GERD can be made.
      - Discontinue routine use of PPI if there is no evidence of esophagitis or Barrett's esophagus and symptoms are well controlled with trial, and use only as needed.
  - If symptoms do not improve or resolve, EGD is recommended.
  - If only atypical symptoms are present, reflux testing is recommended before PPI therapy.
- Medications: Alarm symptoms
  - Perform EGD as the first test for diagnosis
- Medications: Nonerosive reflux disease
  - Use PPI on demand or intermittently.
- Assess medications that can lower LES pressure during medication reconciliation. Reduce, change, or eliminate possible medications that lower LES pressure and lead to GERD symptoms.
  - Calcium channel blockers, nitrites, anticholinergics, tricyclic antidepressants, sildenafil, hormone replacement therapy, oral contraceptives, bisphosphonates, and beta-adrenergic agonists
- Surgical management: Performed by gastroenterologist
  - Antireflux surgery is recommended for patients with severe reflux esophagitis:
    - Fundoplication
    - Magnetic sphincter augmentation
    - Transoral incisionless fundoplication
    - Radiofrequency
- Smoking cessation aids should be offered to any person currently smoking tobacco.
(Mungan & Pinarbasi Simsek, 2017; Katz et al., 2022; Smith & Davila, 2023)

NONPHARMACOTHERAPY

- Educate
  - Trigger foods and beverages
  - Eating smaller meals
  - Eat dinner at least 2 to 3 hours prior to bedtime
  - Elevate the head of the bed
  - Left-side sleeping
  - Self-management
  - Disease progression

- Medications that may exacerbate symptoms
- Medication compliance
- Lifestyle and behavioral modifications
  - Weight reduction if overweight or obese to maintain normal body mass index
  - Diet: Eliminate trigger foods and beverages (e.g., citrus, high-fat foods, coffee, carbonated beverages, alcohol)
  - Exercise
  - Smoking cessation
- Complementary treatment
  - Complementary and alternative therapies with natural medicines and supplements may interact with prescription medications. Obtain a complete medication history.
- Referral
  - Gastroenterologist:
    - Alarm symptoms
    - EGD testing
    - Esophagitis or Barrett's esophagus
    - Surgical management
  - Identify and refer to specialist for treatment of comorbid conditions
- Follow-up
  - Office visit at the end of PPI trial
  - Office visit 2 weeks after PPI trial has ended
  - Routine follow-up every 3 to 6 months until controlled

(Mungan & Pinarbasi Simsek, 2017; Katz et al., 2022; Smith & Davila, 2023)

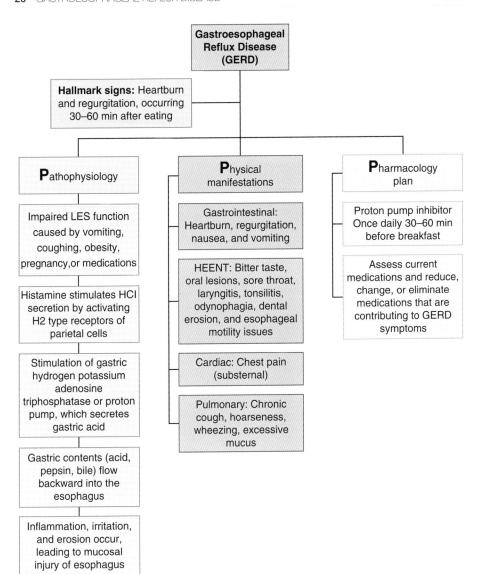

Algorithm 26.1 Gastroesophageal Reflux Disease. *GERD*, Gastroesophageal reflux disease; *HCl*, hydrochloric acid; *LES*, lower esophageal sphincter; *PPI*, proton pump inhibitor.

References

Ball, J. W., Dains, J. E., Flynn, J. A., Solomon, B. S., & Stewart, R. W. (2023). *Seidel's guide to physical examination: An interprofessional approach [E-book]* (9th ed.). Elsevier.

Clarrett, D. M., & Hachem, C. (2018). Gastroesophageal reflux disease (GERD). *Missouri Medicine, 115*(3), 214.

Craven, M. R., Kia, L., O'Dwyer, L. C., Stern, E., Taft, T. H., & Keefer, L. (2018). Systematic review: Methodological flaws in racial/ethnic reporting for gastroesophageal reflux disease. *Diseases of the Esophagus, 31*(3), dox154. https://doi.org/10.1093/dote/dox154.

Dains, J. E., Baumann, L. C., & Scheibel, P. (2024). *Advanced health assessment & clinical diagnosis in primary care* (7th ed.). Elsevier.

Durazzo, M., Lupi, G., Cicerchia, F., Ferro, A., Barutta, F., Beccuti, G., & Pellicano, R. (2020). Extra-esophageal presentation of gastroesophageal reflux disease: 2020 update. *Journal of Clinical Medicine, 9*(8), 2559. http://doi.org/10.3390/jcm9082559.

Gao, H., Basri, R., & Tran, M. H. (2022). Acquired methemoglobinemia: A systematic review of reported cases. *Transfusion and Apheresis Science, 61*(2), 103299.

Katz, P. O., Dunbar, K. B., Schnoll-Sussman, F. H., Greer, K. B., Yadlapati, R., & Spechler, S. J. (2022). ACG clinical guideline for the diagnosis and management of gastroesophageal reflux disease. *American Journal of Gastroenterology, 117*(1), 27–56.

Lechien, J. R. (2022). Treating and managing laryngopharyngeal reflux disease in the over 65s: Evidence to date. *Clinical Interventions in Aging, 17*, 1625–1633. https://doi.org/10.2147/CIA.S371992.

Maret-Ouda, J., Markar, S. R., & Lagergren, J. (2020). Gastroesophageal reflux disease: A review. *JAMA, 324*(24), 2536–2547.

Mungan, Z., & Pinarbasi Simsek, B. (2017). Which drugs are risk factors for the development of gastroesophageal reflux disease? *Turkish Journal of Gastroenterology, 28*(Suppl 1), S38–S43. http://doi.org/10.5152/tjg.2017.11.

Rogers, J., & Eastland, T. (2021). Understanding the most commonly billed diagnoses in primary care: Gastroesophageal reflux disease. *Nurse Practitioner, 46*(4), 50–55. http://doi.org/10.1097/01.NPR.0000737196.69218.b6.

Rosen, R., Vandenplas, Y., Singendonk, M., Cabana, M., DiLorenzo, C., Gottrand, F., Gupta, S., Langendam, M., Staiano, A., Thapar, N., Tipnis, N., & Tabbers, M. (2018). Pediatric gastroesophageal reflux clinical practice guidelines: Joint recommendations of the North American Society for Pediatric Gastroenterology, Hepatology, and Nutrition and the European Society for Pediatric Gastroenterology, Hepatology, and Nutrition. *Journal of Pediatric Gastroenterology and Nutrition, 66*(3), 516–554. https://doi.org/10.1097/MPG.0000000000001889.

Shaheen, N. J., Falk, G. W., Iyer, P. G., Souza, R. F., Yadlapati, R. H., Sauer, B. G., & Wani, S. (2022). Diagnosis and management of Barrett's esophagus: An updated ACG guideline. *American Journal of Gastroenterology, 117*(4), 559.

Smith, W., & Davila, N. (2023). Gastroesophageal reflux disease: 2021 guideline updates and clinical pearls. *Nurse Practitioner, 48*(7), 24–25.

Spain, S. R. (2023). Alterations of digestive function. In J. L. Rogers (Ed.), *McCance & Huether's pathophysiology: The biologic basis of disease in adults and children*, (9th ed., pp. 1318–1342). Elsevier.

CHAPTER 27

Abdominal Hernia

Julia L. Rogers

Ventral Hernia

Abdominal Hernia

An abdominal hernia is a protrusion of intestine through an area of weakness in abdominal muscles or through the inguinal ring (Spain, 2023) (Fig. 27.1). A hernia can be classified as inguinal, ventral (umbilical and incisional), or femoral. The most common hernia is inguinal, which accounts for about 75% of cases. The most common ventral hernia is incisional following laparotomy (Söderbäck et al., 2018; Tran et al., 2023). A hernia may lead to a more serious process including obstruction, strangulation, perforation, or incarceration of the bowel. Risk factors associated with hernia are comorbid systemic chronic diseases including diabetes mellitus (see Chapter 14), renal failure, obesity, smoking, and malnutrition. Medications such as steroids and immunosuppressants can also increase the risk of developing an incisional hernia postsurgery. An individual is at higher risk if the surgery is an acute abdominal surgery done emergently, it involves a midline incision, or there is an associated infection (Dai et al., 2019; Tubre et al., 2018).

Pathophysiology

A hernia can be congenital or acquired (Box 27.1). Acquired hernias most commonly occur anteriorly, through the inguinal and femoral canals or umbilicus, or at sites of surgical scars (Algorithm 27.1). Inguinal hernias tend to have narrow orifices and large sacs; therefore they are of concern because of the risk of visceral protrusion (external herniation). Small bowel loops herniate most often, but portions of omentum or large bowel may also herniate and become entrapped. Pressure at the neck of the outpouching bowel may impair venous drainage, leading to stasis and edema. These changes increase the bulk of the herniated loop, leading to permanent entrapment (incarceration) and, over time, arterial and venous compromise (strangulation), which may result to infarction (Spain, 2023).

Incisional hernias develop due to improper healing in more than one layer of the abdominal wall and failure of the abdominal wall to close properly after any surgical procedure where the abdominal wall is incised (Söderbäck et al., 2018; Tubre et al., 2018). Less obvious hernias or those that are not well defined may develop from a weakness in one or more layers of the three abdominal muscles (Söderbäck et al., 2018; Spain, 2023; Tubre et al., 2018). A ventral hernia can predispose the patient to the classic complications of incarceration, obstruction, or strangulation. An incarcerated hernia cannot be reduced and therefore the contents of the hernial sac cannot be returned to the peritoneal cavity (Box 27.2). A strangulated hernia occurs when the blood supply to the viscera lying in the hernial sac is cut off, leading to ischemia (Spain, 2023). A strangulated hernia is a medical emergency.

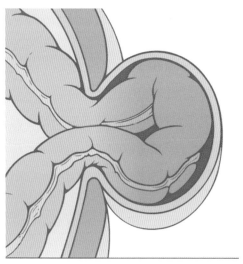

Fig. 27.1   Hernia. (From Kumar V., et al. (2018). Robbins basic pathology (10th ed.). Philadelphia: Elsevier).

BOX 27.1 ■ Pediatric Considerations

Hernias (i.e., congenital or acquired) occur in newborns and throughout childhood. The most common are inguinal hernias, which account for approximately 80% of all childhood hernias. Inguinal hernias occur more frequently in males than females. During the eighth month of gestation, an inguinal hernia may present from persistence of all or part of the processus vaginalis, the tube of peritoneum that precedes the testicle through the inguinal canal into the scrotum (in males) or the round ligament into the labia (in females). An inguinal hernia can be palpated as a thickening of the cord in the groin, and the silk glove sign can be elicited by rubbing together the sides of the empty hernial sac. Newborns may also have an umbilical hernia (Fig. 27.2). This occurs when fusion of the umbilical ring is incomplete at the point where the umbilical vessels exit the abdominal wall. Hernias may bulge or become more apparent when the infant cries or strains or when the older child strains, coughs, or stands for a long time (Triggs & Gilbert, 2023).

BOX 27.2 ■ Older Adult Considerations

Older adults are more susceptible to inguinal herniation due to weakening of abdominal musculature. This population is also at greater risk for mortality; therefore a prompt diagnosis is paramount to prevent mortality. Older adults may present with an incarcerated hernia and small bowel obstruction, which requires surgical intervention. However, there may be reluctance to perform diagnostics in the elderly, which leads to significant underdiagnosis, undertreatment, and increased mortality. The elderly present with clinical manifestations of constant severe pain in the right or left lower abdominal quadrant that worsens with coughing or straining. Physical examination reveals a hernia or mass that is nonreducible. Diagnosis should be confirmed by diagnostic imaging (computed tomography [CT] or magnetic resonance imaging [MRI]), in which case surgical intervention is indicated. Providers need to be diligent in early detection of surgical conditions to prevent fatal consequences of underdiagnosis or missed diagnosis (Brüggemann et al., 2021; Dains et al, 2024).

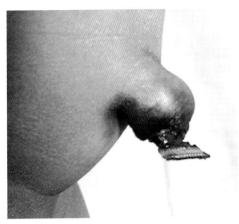

Fig. 27.2 Newborn with umbilical hernia. (From Zitelli, B. J., & Davis, H. W. (2007). *Atlas of pediatric physical diagnosis* (5th ed.). Mosby.)

BOX 27.3 ■ Diversity Considerations

Hernia repair exhibits global heterogeneity in surgical approaches with a spectrum of techniques ranging from tension-free mesh repairs to laparoscopic and robotic interventions, each associated with distinct morbidity profiles and recurrence rates. Lower socioeconomic status has been shown to be predictive of poorer surgical outcomes in hernia repair. However, more research is needed with regard to gender, race, and socioeconomic status on ventral hernia presentation, management, and outcomes. Culture and geography play a role in hernia-related healthcare with significant variation in care relative to gender, race, and socioeconomic status. Therefore providers must be diligent in providing consistent care for all patients with hernias (Cherla et al., 2018).

Physical Clinical Presentation

SUBJECTIVE

During the history, the healthcare provider should inquire about the circumstances and precipitating events leading up to the onset of hernia (e.g., heavy lifting, straining, surgery); symptoms; location, intensity, and quality of pain (e.g., intermittent, localized); progression of hernia and pain; and swelling. Also document whether the hernia is reducible; alleviating and aggravating factors (e.g., lifting, exertion, standing, straining, or coughing); previous hernia(s); and associated symptoms (Dains et al., 2024). Ask about red flags such as colicky abdominal pain, nausea, and vomiting that may suggest entrapment or strangulation. Individuals may report pain unilaterally in the right or left lower abdominal quadrant that may radiate to the groin or testicle. The pain is usually described as dull or aching. If the hernia is strangulated, the pain is severe. The pain tends to intensify with straining, lifting, bearing down, or movement of lower extremities (Dains et al., 2024; Spain, 2023; Tran et al., 2023). Document allergies, ill contacts, and medical, social, and family history (Box 27.3).

OBJECTIVE*

Examination should be performed with patient standing and supine (Algorithm 27.1).

Abdomen: *Inspection:* Perform with and without patient performing Valsalva's maneuver; suprapubic fullness; **asymmetrical distention or protrusion**

Palpation: Warmth, tenderness to **right or left lower quadrant; pain/tenderness with palpation; palpate for inguinal, incisional, femoral, and umbilical hernias**—uncomplicated hernia will reduce and **strangulated hernia will not reduce**; pain may radiate to groin or testicle; palpable mass inguinal ring of femoral area; bowel sounds present in uncomplicated hernias

Auscultate: Auscultate scrotum to distinguish loops of bowel from mass

Integumentary: Area around hernia may be discolored and warm

(Ball et al., 2023; Dains et al., 2024; Spain, 2023; Tran et al., 2023)

Evaluation and Differential Diagnoses

DIAGNOSTICS

- Ultrasound of abdomen (US)
- Computed tomography scan of abdomen (CT)

DIFFERENTIAL DIAGNOSIS

- Hydrocele, varicocele, spermatocele
- Testicular tumor or malignancy
- Enlarged lymph node
- Cyst
- Lipoma
- Psoas abscess

Plan

GUIDELINE RESOURCES

- Tran, H. M., MacQueen, I., Chen, D., & Simons, M. (2023). Systematic review and guidelines for management of scrotal inguinal hernias. *Journal of Abdominal Wall Surgery, 2,* 11195. https://doi.org/10.3389/jaws.2023.11195.
- Henriksen, N. A., Montgomery, A., Kaufmann, R., Berrevoet, F., East, B., Fischer, J., Hope, W., Klassen, D., Lorenz, R., Renard, Y., Garcia Urena, M. A., Simons, M. P., & European and Americas Hernia Societies. (2020). Guidelines for treatment of umbilical and epigastric hernias from the European Hernia Society and Americas Hernia Society. *British Journal of Surgery, 107*(3), 171–190. https://doi.org/10.1002/bjs.11489.
- Henriksen, N. A., Kaufmann, R., Simons, M. P., Berrevoet, F., East, B., Fischer, J., Hope, W., Klassen, D., Lorenz, R., Renard, Y., Garcia Urena, M. A., Montgomery, A., & on behalf of the European Hernia Society and the Americas Hernia Society. (2020). EHS and AHS guidelines for treatment of primary ventral hernias in rare locations or special circumstances. *BJS Open, 4*(2), 342–353. https://doi.org/10.1002/bjs5.50252.

---

*Hallmark signs are bolded and **Red flags are bolded and underlined**.

> **BOX 27.4 ■ Acute Care Considerations**
>
> Acute care is required for patients with nonreducible hernia or hernias that need surgical repair. The type of repair often determines the length of hospital stay and risk. There is a decreased risk of both incisional hernia and surgical-site occurrences in patients undergoing laparoscopic operations compared with open operations. Abdominal surgery can be performed by several minimally invasive approaches. It is suggested to avoid midline incisions for laparotomies and specimen extraction sites because that type of incision has the highest rate of hernia. The recommendation for suturing the closure of elective midline incisions is to use a continuous small-bites suturing technique with a slowly absorbable suture in order to avoid an incisional hernia (Deerenberg et al., 2022).

Pharmacotherapy

- Medications
  - Analgesic for pain (acetaminophen or ibuprofen) (Algorithm 27.1)
- Smoking cessation aids should be offered to any person currently smoking tobacco.

SURGICAL

- Hernia reducible
  - Referral for elective surgery
- Hernia not reducible
  - Emergent surgery
- Surgical repair
  - Open, laparoscopic, and robotic techniques
  - Mesh; provides strength for the repair and scaffold for the healing tissue (Box 27.4)

NONPHARMACOTHERAPY

- Educate
  - Prevention of hernia postsurgery
  - Conservative nonoperative treatment
  - Recurrence of hernia
  - Proper lifting techniques
- Lifestyle and behavioral modifications
  - Weight loss if obese to maintain a normal body mass index
  - Glucose control if diabetic
  - Smoking cessation if tobacco or vape user
- Complementary treatment
  - Complementary and alternative therapies with natural medicines and supplements may interact with prescription medications. Obtain a complete medication history.
- Referral
  - Surgery
  - Gastroenterologist
  - Identify and refer to specialist for treatment of comorbid conditions
- Follow-up
  - Emergency department for evaluation if pain suddenly worsens
  - Office visit every 3 to 6 months

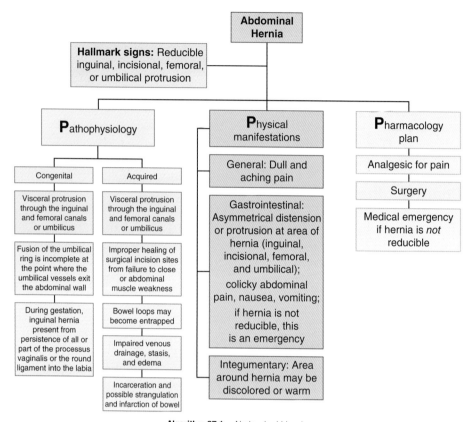

Algorithm 27.1   Abdominal Hernia

References

Ball, J. W., Dains, J. E., Flynn, J. A., Solomon, B. S., & Stewart, R. W. (2023). *Seidel's guide to physical examination* (10th ed.). Elsevier.

Brüggemann, R. A. G., Brouns, S. H. A., Mommers, E. H. H., & Spaetgens, B. (2021). The delicate balance between over- and underdiagnosis in older people: A simple inguinal hernia? *Age and Ageing, 50*(4), 1429. https://doi.org/10.1093/ageing/afab087.

Cherla, D. V., Poulose, B., & Prabhu, A. S. (2018). Epidemiology and disparities in care: The impact of socio-economic status, gender, and race on the presentation, management, and outcomes of patients undergoing ventral hernia repair. *Surgical Clinics of North America, 98*(3), 431–440. https://doi.org/10.1016/j.suc.2018.02.003.

Dai, W., Chen, Z., Zuo, J., Tan, J., Tan, M., & Yuan, Y. (2019). Risk factors of postoperative complications after emergency repair of incarcerated groin hernia for adult patients: A retrospective cohort study. *Hernia, 23*(2), 267–276.

Dains, J. E., Baumann, L. C., & Scheibel, P. (2024). *Advanced health assessment & clinical diagnosis in primary care* (7th ed.). Elsevier.

Deerenberg, E. B., Henriksen, N. A., Antoniou, G. A., Antoniou, S. A., Bramer, W. M., Fischer, J. P., Fortelny, R. H., Gök, H., Harris, H. W., Hope, W., Horne, C. M., Jensen, T. K., Köckerling, F., Kretschmer, A., López-Cano, M., Malcher, F., Shao, J. M., Slieker, J. C., de Smet, G. H. J., ... Muysoms, F. E. (2022). Updated guideline for closure of abdominal wall incisions from the European and American Hernia Societies. *British Journal of Surgery, 109*(12), 1239–1250. https://doi.org/10.1093/bjs/znac302.

Söderbäck, H., Gunnarsson, U., Hellman, P., & Sandblom, G. (2018). Incisional hernia after surgery for colorectal cancer: A population-based register study. *International Journal of Colorectal Disease, 33*(10), 1411–1417.

Spain, S. (2023). Alterations of digestive function. In J. L. Rogers (Ed.), *McCance & Huether's pathophysiology: The biologic basis for disease in adults and children*, (9th ed., pp. 1318–1374). Elsevier.

Tran, H. M., MacQueen, I., Chen, D., & Simons, M. (2023). Systematic review and guidelines for management of scrotal inguinal hernias. *Journal of Abdominal Wall Surgery, 2*, 11195.

Triggs, N. D., & Gilbert, C. (2023). The Child With Gastrointestinal Dysfunction. In M. J. Hockenberry, E. A. Duffy, & K. Gibbs (Eds.), Wong's nursing care of infants and children. (12th ed., pp. 860–866). Elsevier.

Tubre, D. J., Schroeder, A. D., Estes, J., Eisenga, J., & Fitzgibbons, R. J. (2018). Surgical site infection: The "Achilles heel" of all types of abdominal wall hernia reconstruction. *Hernia, 22*(6), 1003–1013.

CHAPTER 28

Inflammatory Bowel Disease

Julia L. Rogers

Crohn's Disease and Ulcerative Colitis

Inflammatory bowel disease (IBD) is characterized by remission and exacerbation of abdominal pain, diarrhea, hematochezia, fecal urgency, and weight loss (Spain, 2023). The most common chronic inflammatory intestinal disorders are Crohn's disease (CD) and ulcerative colitis (UC). Both disease processes are linked to chronic inflammation in the intestinal mucosa, cause ulcerations, and are autoimmune related (Goolsby & Grubbs, 2019; Spain, 2023). The prevalence of IBD is approximately 1.4 million people in the United States, with approximately 30,000 new cases annually (Spain, 2023). Risk factors include diet, psychological stress, viruses, and smoking.

CD presents in young individuals usually in their 20s or 30s as a progressive and debilitating disease. CD can affect any area of the gastrointestinal (GI) tract from the esophagus to the anus. CD has a cobblestone appearance and is characterized by inflammation and discontinuous transmural involvement of the GI tract known as skip lesions, most commonly in the proximal colon at the terminal ileum or cecum (Goolsby & Grubbs, 2019; Spain, 2023). The ulcerations of CD are deep fissures that commonly lead to fistulas.

UC also strikes individuals at a young age, with peak incidence between ages 15 and 25 years. UC has more of a continuous pattern in the colonic mucosa. The inflammation and ulcerations in UC are limited primarily to the mucosal layer within the sigmoid colon and rectum but can involve the entire colon (Goolsby & Grubbs, 2019; Spain, 2023). Superficial ulcerations are common due to the friable mucosa and may lead to crypt abscesses.

Pathophysiology

The pathogenesis of IBD involves a failure of the body's immune response to regulation, genetic predispositions, and environmental triggers that disrupt microbial flora (Algorithm 28.1 and Algorithm 28.2). The mucosal epithelium within the GI tract serves as a natural barrier to protect against invading pathogens. However, infective pathogens (e.g., bacteria and viruses), environmental factors (e.g., high-fat diet with increased intake of caffeine, gas-producing or spicy foods), stress (work or home), and smoking can alter or break down intestinal mucosa defense mechanisms, leading to the inflammation and ulcerations seen in IBD (Goolsby & Grubbs, 2019; Spain, 2023) (Fig. 28.1). The disrupted or damaged mucosa barrier allows pathogens and other antigens to pass more freely because of increased permeability. A natural defense mechanism that the body uses in a healthy state is the secretion of mucin, an antimicrobial that provides a layer of protection against pathogens. However, IBD decreases the secretion of mucin and leads to overstimulation of the gut immune system with an inflammatory response (Goolsby & Grubbs, 2019; Spain, 2023). Genetic susceptibility also plays an important role in the development of IBD due to the autoimmune process.

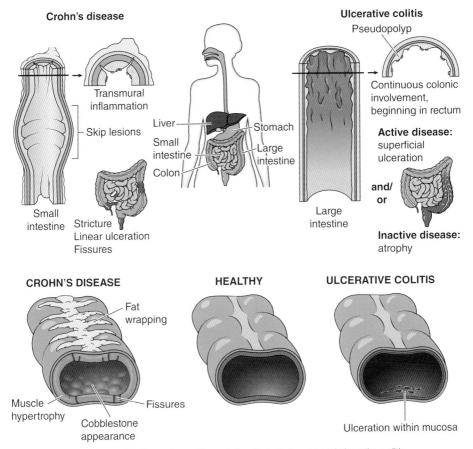

Fig. 28.1 Distribution patterns differentiating Crohn's disease and ulcerative colitis.

CROHN'S DISEASE

The inflammation and skip lesions associated with CD can be anywhere along the GI tract from the mouth to the rectum. Inflamed areas are mixed or alongside uninflamed areas, noncaseating granulomas, fistulas, fissures, and deep penetrating ulcers and are mostly seen in the distal small intestine and proximal large colon (Goolsby & Grubbs, 2019; Spain, 2023). The surface of the inflamed bowel usually has a characteristic cobblestone appearance resulting from the fissures and crevices that develop, surrounded by areas of submucosal edema (Algorithm 28.1). Smoking might contribute to the development of IBD by influencing the intestinal microbiome, as people with CD who smoke show a dysbiosis within their intestinal microbiota. There is a strong association between CD and nucleotide-binding oligomerization domain (CARD15/NOD2) gene mutations (Goolsby & Grubbs, 2019; Spain, 2023).

ULCERATIVE COLITIS

Inflammation at the base of the crypt of the Lieberkühn in the large intestine is the primary lesion of UC (Spain, 2023). UC generally initiates in the rectum and extends proximally through the entire colon (Algorithm 28.2). The inflammation causes continuous hyperemic, edematous, and dark red lesions limited to the mucosal epithelium (Goolsby & Grubbs, 2019; Spain, 2023). Severe inflammation leads to hemorrhage of the mucosa, causing small erosions to form and coalesce into ulcers in the mucosa, eventually forming abscesses and causing necrosis (Goolsby & Grubbs, 2019; Spain, 2023). The inflammation and destruction of the mucosa cause bleeding, cramping pain, and the urge to defecate. The loss of absorptive mucosal surface causes rapid colonic transit time, leading to frequent large volumes of watery diarrhea or diarrhea with passage of small amounts of blood and purulent mucus (Goolsby & Grubbs, 2019; Spain, 2023).

Physical Clinical Presentation

SUBJECTIVE

During the focused history, documentation should include the onset of symptoms; precipitating events; location, intensity, and quality of pain; progression of symptoms; alleviating and aggravating factors; previous episodes; and associated symptoms. The onset may be sudden and severe with complaints of diarrhea, fever, and abdominal tenderness, or it can be slow and gradual with mild cramps and an urge to defecate. Stool can be described as bloody with mucous or pus (Goolsby & Grubbs, 2019). Key questions can help differentiate the diagnosis. Table 28.1

TABLE 28.1 ■ Key Questions for History of Present Illness to Differentiate Crohn's Disease and Ulcerative Colitis

Feature	Crohn's Disease	Ulcerative Colitis
Pattern	Remission and exacerbations	Remission and exacerbations
Location of lesions	All of GI tract—mouth to anus; skip lesions common	Colon and rectum; no skip lesions
Area affected	Entire intestinal wall	Mucosal layer
Granuloma	Common cobblestone appearance	Rare
Abdominal pain	Common	Occasional; crampy
Pain with defecation	If anal fissures	Common
Urge to defecate, tenesmus, or urgency	Common	Common
Bloody stools	Less common	Common
Steatorrhea	Common	Rare
Stool characteristics	Diarrhea	Diarrhea: Frequent, large volumes of watery diarrhea, bloody or mucoid stools (10–20 stools/day)
		Constipation if rectum involved
Nocturnal diarrhea	Uncommon	When daytime symptoms are severe
Risks	Intestinal obstruction, weight loss, anal fissures, hemorrhoids, perirectal abscess, strictures, and fibrosis	Toxic megacolon, dehydration, weight loss, anemia, blood transfusions, anal fissures, hemorrhoids, perirectal abscess, strictures, fibrosis, obstruction, perforation, colonic dilation on abdominal radiographs
Extraintestinal manifestations	Arthritis, polyarthritis, fever, cutaneous lesions (erythema nodosum), episcleritis, uveitis, tachycardia, skin lesions, erythema nodosum, stomatitis, autoimmune anemia, hypercoagulability of blood, DVT, primary sclerosing cholangitis, ankylosing spondylitis, disorders of the liver, and sclerosing cholangitis	Arthritis, polyarthritis, fever, cutaneous lesions (erythema nodosum), episcleritis, uveitis, tachycardia, skin lesions, erythema nodosum, stomatitis, autoimmune anemia, hypercoagulability of blood, DVT, primary sclerosing cholangitis, ankylosing spondylitis, disorders of the liver, and sclerosing cholangitis

Adapted from Spain, S. (2023). Alterations of digestive function. In J. L. Rogers (Ed.), *McCance & Huether's pathophysiology: The biologic basis for disease in adults and children* (9th Ed. pp. 1318–1374), Mosby-Elsevier.

provides key features associated with each disease process, which can be used as a guide when asking an individual about the history of the present illness. Obtain a food diary of the last 24 hours to 7 days if possible. Document allergies, ill contacts, and medical, surgical, social, and family histories. Certain medications used to treat IBD are not given to individuals with previous cholecystectomy; therefore obtaining the surgical history is important. Individuals who report smoking currently have a twofold increase in risk of CD but only a moderate risk if they have quit smoking. Interestingly, there is a higher risk for UC in previous smokers who have quit within the last 12 months compared to those who currently smoke. Family history is an important component of the history because both CD and UC have a pattern of familial occurrence, are autoimmune disorders, and both can be accompanied by systemic manifestations. The incidence of IBD is 30 to 100 times greater if first-degree relatives have the diagnosis. IBD is autoimmune related; therefore ask if there is any family history of any autoimmune disease (Boxes 28.1, 28.2, and 28.3).

BOX 28.1 ■ Diversity Considerations

Patient diversity plays a major role in the pathogenesis and clinical manifestation of intestinal diseases and needs to be considered during diagnostic workup and plan of care. Factors such as gender, ethnicity, age, and socioeconomic status can affect the course of the patient's inflammatory bowel disease (IBD). For example, the medically underserved have poorer outcomes related to suboptimal health care, affecting more minorities and low-income groups. However, the initiation of biologics is helping to pave a pathway toward personalized individual care. Efforts on reducing health disparities will ensure that patients receive optimal preventative care to improve overall patient outcomes (Crohn's & Colitis Foundation, 2023; Hof et al., 2023).

BOX 28.2 ■ Pediatric Considerations

Pediatric inflammatory bowel disease may present differently than adult-onset disease. Children and adolescents with inflammatory bowel disease often have growth and developmental delays because of nutritional deficiencies and malnutrition associated with the disease. It can also influence mental health. In school-age children there is an increase in absenteeism in school, decreased extracurricular activity involvement, and overall decreased quality of life with underperformance in school. The health care provider needs to take a more holistic approach. Consideration should be given to promote weight-bearing exercise, improved nutrition, referral to psychology, and creation of a plan for school accommodations (Fuller, 2019).

BOX 28.3 ■ Older Adult Considerations

Clinical trials often do not include geriatric patients; therefore treatment guidelines are not always in the best interests of the elderly. Geriatric patients tend to have more comorbid conditions and polypharmacy and are increasingly frail. Elderly patients are often misdiagnosed because inflammatory bowel disease usually appears in the second or third decade of life; however, some individuals may present initially in the sixth or seventh decade of life. Symptoms may also vary in the older population, with hematochezia and extraintestinal manifestations being less common. There is an increase in hospitalizations, complications, and mortality in the elderly with inflammatory bowel disease as well. Health care providers must consider the potential complications in the geriatric population and be prepared to personalize treatment (Segal et al., 2020).

OBJECTIVE*

Generalized: Fever; malaise, **loss of appetite; weight loss; fatigue; night sweats**
HEENT: Dehydration, dry mucous membranes; episcleritis; uveitis; ocular lesions; oral lesions
Hematologic: Anemia, pale complexion
Cardiovascular: Tachycardia
Pulmonary: Labored respirations; tachypnea
Gastrointestinal: Abdominal pain; hematochezia; tenesmus;
Crohn's Disease: **abdominal tenderness over lesions;** nausea; vomiting; **diarrhea** with or without blood; pain with defecation; anorectal fissures; fistula; bowel strictures; **bowel obstruction; perforations; intraabdominal or perianal abscesses;**
Ulcerative Colitis: crampy abdominal pain; **diarrhea (frequent and large amounts if severe) with mucus or pus;** stool urgency; **toxic megacolon;** anal fissures, hemorrhoids, and **perirectal abscess; peritonitis** (Algorithms 28.1 and 28.2)
Musculoskeletal: Polyarthritis; arthropathies
Integumentary: Cutaneous lesions (erythema nodosum); ulcerations of perianal skin
Psychiatric: Depression; anxious
IBD is associated with extraintestinal (other than bowel) manifestations in up to 25% of patients and primarily affects the skin, joints, eyes, and liver.
(Ball et al., 2023; Dains et al., 2024; Goolsby & Grubbs, 2019; Spain, 2023)

Evaluation and Differential Diagnoses

DIAGNOSTICS

- Labs
  - Stool cultures for ova, parasites, and infection (e.g., *Clostridium difficile*)
  - Complete blood count; vitamin B12; folic acid due to anemia if ileum is involved, malabsorption of vitamin B12, folic acid, and vitamin D
  - Albumin to assess nutrition status
  - Electrolytes
- Diagnostic imaging
  - Computed tomography scan (CT) with contrast
  - Small bowel series or a capsule endoscopy (camera pill)
- Endoscopy
  - Sigmoidoscopy, colonoscopy, biopsy, histology

DIFFERENTIAL DIAGNOSIS

- Gastrointestinal infections: *C. difficile*
- Lactose intolerance
- Colon cancer (complication of UC)
- Intestinal adenocarcinoma (risk with CD)

Plan

GUIDELINE RESOURCES

- Feuerstein, J. D., Ho, E. Y., Shmidt, E., Singh, H., Falck-Ytter, Y., Sultan, S., Terdiman, J. P., Sultan, S., Cohen, B. L., Chachu, K., Day, L., Davitkov, P., Lebwohl, B., Levin, T. R.,

---

*Hallmark signs are bolded and <u>Red flags are bolded and underlined</u>.

Patel, A., Peery, A. F., Shah, R., Singh, S., Spechler, S. J. … Staller, K. (2021). AGA clinical practice guidelines on the medical management of moderate to severe luminal and perianal fistulizing Crohn's disease. *Gastroenterology*, *160*(7), 2496–2508. https://doi.org/10.1053/j.gastro.2021.04.022.

- Feuerstein, J. D., Isaacs, K. L., Schneider, Y., Siddique, S. M., Falck-Ytter, Y., Singh, S., Chachu, K., Day, L., Lebwohl, B., Muniraj, T., Patel, A., Peery, A. F., Shah, R., Sultan, S., Singh, H., Spechler, S., Su, G., Thrift, A. P., Weiss, J. M. … Weizman, A. V. (2020). AGA clinical practice guidelines on the management of moderate to severe ulcerative colitis. *Gastroenterology*, *158*(5), 1450–1461. https://doi.org/10.1053/j.gastro.2020.01.006.

Pharmacotherapy

- Medications: CD**
  - Moderate to severe disease for induction and maintenance of remission monotherapy (Algorithm 28.1):
    - anti-TNFα:
      - Infliximab
      - Adalimumab
      - Certolizumab pego
      - Ustekinumab
      - Vedolizumab
  - Naïve to biologic and immunomodulators:
    - Infliximab in combination with thiopurines for induction and remission
      - Adalimumab in combination with thiopurines for induction and remission
  - Corticosteroids for induction of remission but not for maintenance
  - CD and active perianal fistula without perianal abscess:
    - Infliximab *OR* adalimumab with ciprofloxacin for 12 weeks

(Feuerstein et al., 2021)

- Medications: UC**
  - Naïve to biologic agents:
    - Infliximab or vedolizumab rather than adalimumab, for induction of remission (Algorithm 28.2)
    - Tofacitinib only to be used in the setting of a clinical or registry study
  - Previously exposed to infliximab, nonresponsive:
    - Ustekinumab or tofacitinib rather than vedolizumab or adalimumab, for induction of remission
  - Induction of remission:
    - Biologic monotherapy (TNF-α antagonists, vedolizumab, ustekinumab) rather than thiopurine monotherapy
  - Combine TNF-α antagonists, vedolizumab, or ustekinumab with thiopurines or methotrexate, rather than biologic monotherapy or thiopurine monotherapy
  - Early use of biologic agents with or without immunomodulator therapy, rather than gradual step up after failure of 5-ASA
- See Box 28.4 for medications that are typically used in an acute care setting.
- Smoking cessation aids should be offered to any person currently smoking tobacco.

(Feuerstein et al., 2020)

**Refer to guidelines for specific medications to be used in specific circumstances and order.

BOX 28.4 ■ Acute Care Considerations

- Hospital medications
- In hospitalized adult patients with acute severe ulcerative colitis
  - Intravenous (IV) methylprednisolone dose equivalent of 40–60 mg daily rather than higher doses of IV corticosteroids to decrease risk of colectomy
  - Refractory to IV corticosteroids, use infliximab or cyclosporine

(Feuerstein et al., 2020)

NONPHARMACOTHERAPY

- Educate
  - Medications
  - Emergent red flags
  - Elimination of triggering foods
  - Self-management
  - Disease progression
- Lifestyle and behavioral modifications
  - Diet: CD—During an acute phase focus on an elemental diet that is low in residue and easy to digest. Consume a high-calorie, high-protein diet to support nutrient absorption and recovery. It is important to only intake necessary fats and minimize fiber, which can exacerbate symptoms.
  - Diet: UC—Avoid caffeine, lactose (milk), highly spiced foods, and gas-forming foods
  - Smoking cessation
- Complementary treatment
  - Psychosocial rehabilitation
  - Complementary and alternative therapies with natural medicines and supplements may interact with prescription medications. Obtain a complete medication history.
- Referral
  - Surgery:
    - CD: Surgical resection of damaged bowel, drainage of abscess, or repair of fistula tracts
    - UC: Surgical removal of the rectum and entire colon with the creation of an ileostomy or ileoanal anastomosis
  - Gastroenterologist
  - Identify and refer for treatment of comorbid conditions:
    - Complications of short bowel syndrome include malabsorption, diarrhea, and nutritional deficiencies
- Follow-up
  - Follow-up visit every 3 to 6 months
  - Colonoscopy per guidelines for cancer screening

(Feuerstein et al., 2020, 2021; Goolsby & Grubbs, 2019)

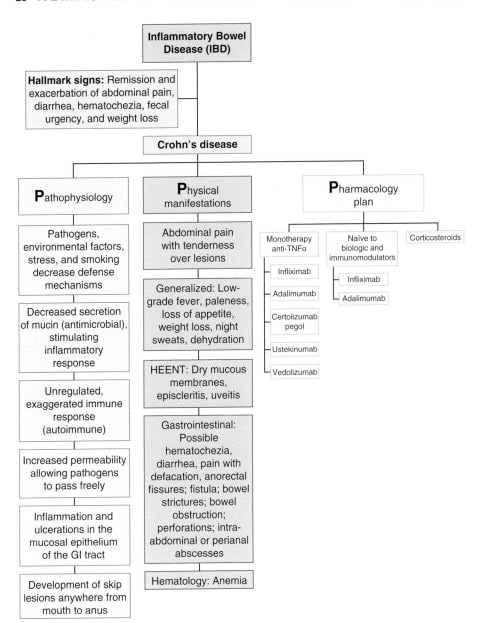

Algorithm 28.1   Inflammatory Bowel Disease: Crohn's Disease.

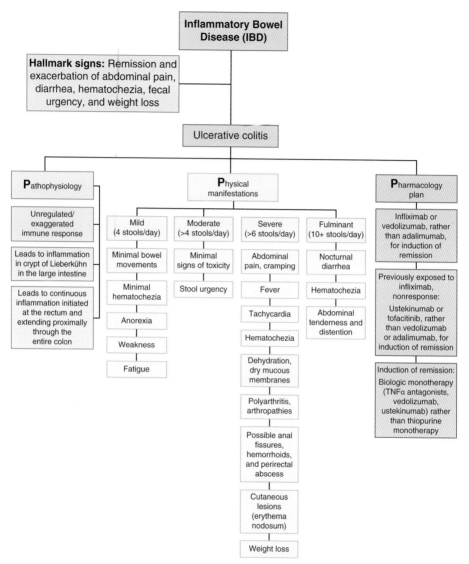

Algorithm 28.2   Inflammatory Bowel Disease: Ulcerative Colitis.

References

Ball, J. W., Dains, J. E., Flynn, J. A., Solomon, B. S., & Stewart, R. W. (2023). *Seidel's guide to physical examination* (10th ed.). Elsevier.

Crohn's & Colitis Foundation. (2024). Diversity, equity & inclusion. Retrieved September 12, 2024, https://www.crohnscolitisfoundation.org/about/diversity.

Dains, J. E., Baumann, L. C., & Scheibel, P. (2024). *Advanced health assessment & clinical diagnosis in primary care* (7th ed.). Elsevier.

Feuerstein, J. D., Ho, E. Y., Shmidt, E., Singh, H., Falck-Ytter, Y., Sultan, S., & Weiss, J. M. (2021). AGA clinical practice guidelines on the medical management of moderate to severe luminal and perianal fistulizing Crohn's disease. *Gastroenterology, 160*(7), 2496–2508.

Feuerstein, J. D., Isaacs, K. L., Schneider, Y., Siddique, S. M., Falck-Ytter, Y., Singh, S., & Terdiman, J. (2020). AGA clinical practice guidelines on the management of moderate to severe ulcerative colitis. *Gastroenterology, 158*(5), 1450–1461.

Fuller, M. K. (2019). Pediatric inflammatory bowel disease: Special considerations. *Surgical Clinics, 99*(6), 1177–1183.

Goolsby, M. J., & Grubbs, G. L. (2019). *Advanced assessment: Interpreting findings and formulating differential diagnoses* (4th ed.). F. A. Davis Company.

Hof, T., Thimme, R., & Hasselblatt, P. (2023). Diversity in gastroenterology: A focus on inflammatory bowel diseases. *Deutsche Medizinische Wochenschrift, 148*(9), 519–527. https://doi.org/10.1055/a-1892-4878.

Segal, J. P., Htet, H. M. T., Limdi, J., & Hayee, B. H. (2020). How to manage IBD in the 'elderly'. *Frontline Gastroenterology, 11*(6), 468–477.

Spain, S. (2023). Alterations of digestive function. In J. L. Rogers (Ed.), *McCance & Huether's pathophysiology: The biologic basis for disease in adults and children*, (9th ed., pp. 1318–1374). Mosby-Elsevier.

CHAPTER 29

Irritable Bowel Syndrome

Julia L. Rogers

Diarrhea, Constipation, and Mixed

Irritable bowel syndrome (IBS) is a gut–brain interaction disorder manifested by recurrent abdominal pain and alterations in stool form and/or frequency (Spain, 2023) (Algorithm 29.1). IBS is chronic, with a relapsing and remitting pattern. It is categorized into bowel habit subtypes including predominant diarrhea (IBS-D), predominant constipation (IBS-C), or a mix of both (IBS-M) (Chang et al., 2022; Lembo et al., 2022). IBS-D accounts for approximately 40% of cases, IBS-C accounts for 30%, and IBS-M accounts for 30% (Pimentel, 2016). IBS affects individuals of all ages, races, and genders, but females tend to be affected more than males. The onset of menarche in females often increases symptoms, indicating a connection to hormones. While IBS is not life threatening, the clinical manifestations associated with the syndrome lead to poor quality of life with psychological comorbidities and decreased socialization.

Pathophysiology

The pathophysiology of IBS involves abnormalities in gastrointestinal (GI) motility and secretion, visceral sensation and permeability, gut–brain interplay in both adults and pediatric populations (Box 29.2), gut microbiota and immune function, metabolite production, and psychosocial stress (Chang et al., 2022; Holtmann et al., 2016). The central nervous system (CNS), peripheral nervous system (PNS), and enteric nervous system (ENS) are all involved (Algorithm 29.1). The ENS controls the effector systems of the GI tract including musculature, secretory glands, and blood vessels. Nearly every neurotransmitter class found in the CNS is present in the ENS (Fig. 29.1).

Serotonin (5-HT) is an important neurotransmitter in the ENS and CNS and has a major role in the pathophysiology of IBS. The intestinal enterochromaffin cells store 90% of the body's total stores of serotonin and function as sensory transducers of intestinal stimuli. For example, when there is high intralumenal pressure, serotonin is released, activating the intrinsic and extrinsic primary afferent sensory neurons in the PNS that translate the stimulus information to the CNS, which responds to the PNS by causing a contraction of smooth muscle in the gut, promoting GI motility (Holtmann et al., 2016). The nausea that some individuals have with IBS is triggered when serotonin is released into the GI tract faster than it can be digested. Visceral hypersensitivity is common in IBS and originates in either the PNS or CNS, causing mild to severe abdominal pain and/or cramping. This is often treated with antispasmodics, which reduce smooth muscle contraction and possibly visceral hypersensitivity (Holtmann et al., 2016; Lembo et al., 2022).

IBS-D

IBS-D involves disordered bile salt metabolism, enhanced intestinal permeability, and sensitivity (Holtmann et al., 2016). Bile salt malabsorption and the increased intestinal absorption of water cause excess fluid in the GI tract, leading to increased colonic transit and expulsion of large amounts of watery diarrhea. Pharmacotherapy includes medication (loperamide) that inhibits

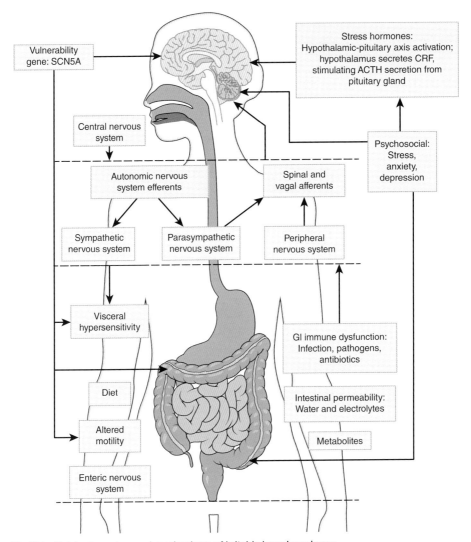

Fig. 29.1 Gut–brain system and mechanisms of irritable bowel syndrome.
ACTH, Adrenocorticotropic hormone; *CRF*, corticotropin-releasing factor; *GI*, gastrointestinal.

peristalsis, decreases secretary activity, and prolongs intestinal transit time (Lembo et al., 2022). Other medications such as the selective 5-HT$_3$ antagonists (alosetron) work to slow gastric motility and decrease visceral pain (Lembo et al., 2022).

IBS-C

The pathophysiology of IBS-C involves decreased intestinal permeability inhibiting the influx of fluid and electrolytes (chloride and bicarbonate). This decreases GI motility and delays colonic transit, causing the common symptoms of bloating and hard stool. There is a symbiotic relationship between constipation and increased visceral hypersensitivity causing hyperalgesia. The pressure that builds in the GI tract from bloating initiates the release of serotonin and subsequently the cascade of communications between the ENS, PNS, and CNS. The result is smooth muscle contractions in the GI tract to propel contents forward and improve motility.

Initial pharmacotherapy with an osmotic laxative increases absorption of water into the GI tract, making the stool softer and increasing peristalsis. Similarly, a partial agonist of the 5-HT$_4$ receptor (tegaserod) can be used to treat IBS-D by stimulating GI motility and increasing fluid absorption in the GI tract (Chang et al., 2022). Other pharmacotherapy agents (linaclotide and plecanatide) stimulate the guanylate cyclase C (GC-C) receptor, causing fluid and electrolyte (chloride and bicarbonate) secretion and reducing visceral hypersensitivity by inhibiting colonic nociceptors (Chang et al., 2022). Increasing water secretion into the intestinal lumen by inhibiting the GI sodium/hydrogen exchanger isoform and decreasing the absorption of sodium and phosphate is yet another method for treating IBS-D (tenapanor). Some of the pharmacotherapies not only relieve the constipation but have been found to have antinociceptive effects (Chang et al., 2022).

IBS may also be caused by a postinflammatory response due to an infectious or noninfectious process that disrupts the normal intestinal microbiota and activates the immune response (Holtmann et al., 2016). The manifestations that align with an intestinal infection (e.g., bacterial enteritis) include low-grade fever, fatigue, and increased leukocytes (Lembo et al., 2022). Treatment is a broad-spectrum antibiotic (rifaximin) to eradicate Gram-negative and Gram-positive anaerobic and aerobic bacteria until the causative agent is known through a culture (Lembo et al., 2022). Acute enteric infections commonly precipitate the onset of IBS (Holtmann et al., 2016).

Another pathophysiologic process that is linked to all IBS subtypes is psychosocial or epigenetic factors, which could be primary or secondary (Chang, 2022; Holtmann et al., 2016; Lembo et al., 2022). There is an interaction between the neuroendocrine system, neuroimmune system, autonomic nervous system, and pain modulatory responses that results in the physical manifestations of IBS (see Fig. 29.1). This is more common in individuals who have current psychosocial stressors and/or experienced early life trauma, abuse, or emotional stress. Chronic stress can influence sensory and motor function through the corticotropin-releasing hormone and catecholaminergic signaling (Holtmann et al., 2016). Environmental stress activates the secretion of the corticotropin-releasing factor from the hypothalamus and stimulates adrenocorticotropic hormone secretion from the pituitary gland, leading to the release of major hormone stress and cortisol. This cascade affects human organs, including the brain and gut. There is an anatomical connection between the GI tract and the CNS, but it extends to include endocrine, humoral, metabolic, and immune routes of communication as well (Ancona et al., 2021). Tricyclic antidepressants (TCAs) are prescribed for all IBS subtypes with a psychosocial component. TCAs are used to treat IBS symptoms due to their peripheral and central (i.e., supraspinal and spinal) actions, which can affect motility, secretion, and sensation (Chang, 2022; Lembo et al., 2022).

Physical Clinical Presentation

SUBJECTIVE

This diagnosis of IBS-D, IBS-C, and IBS-M is based on the medical history, physical examination, evaluation of GI symptoms, and Rome IV symptom-based criteria (Lembo et al., 2022). Therefore it is of upmost importance to take a detailed history when IBS is suspected or is part of the differential. The history of present illness documentation should include the onset of symptoms (abdominal pain, diarrhea, constipation); previous episodes; precipitating events; location, intensity, and quality of pain; frequency of bowel movements; progression of pain and bowel movements; changes in stool form or frequency; description of stool form (hard, loose, mushy, or watery); any straining, urgency, or feeling of incomplete evacuation with passage of stool; alleviating and aggravating factors such as relief with defecation; and associated symptoms such as passage of mucus or blood with bowel movements, bloating, or abdominal distention (Algorithm 29.1).

Document allergies, ill contacts, autoimmune diseases, and medical, social, and family histories. The patient should be asked directly about any alarm signs during the history of present illness, review of systems, and past medical history. **Alarm signs include an individual over the age of 50 years, unintentional weight loss, rectal bleeding, nocturnal diarrhea, iron deficiency anemia, hemorrhoids, or anal fissures**[*]. Document any family history of colon cancer, inflammatory bowel disease (ulcerative colitis or Crohn's disease), or celiac disease (Lembo et al., 2022).

OBJECTIVE*

Generalized: **Unintentional weight loss**
Hematologic: **Anemia**
Gastrointestinal: **Hematochezia**; **diarrhea**; **constipation**; **bloating**; **abdomen distention**; **rectal bleeding** not from hemorrhoids or anal fissures; hypo/hyperactive bowel sounds
Psychiatric: Depression; anxiety
(Ball et al., 2023; Chang, 2022; Dains et al., 2024; Goolsby & Grubbs, 2019; Lembo et al., 2022; Spain, 2023)

Evaluation and Differential Diagnoses

DIAGNOSTICS

- Rome IV criteria met for the past 3 months with onset of symptoms at least 6 months prior to diagnosis
  - Recurrent abdominal pain on average at least 1 day weekly in the past 3 months, associated with two or more of the following criteria:
    - Related to defecation
    - Change in frequency of stool
    - Change in form (appearance) of stool
  - Abdominal pain required to be present at least 1 day weekly on average during past 3 months
  - See Box 29.3 for older adult considerations
- Rome IV IBS subtype diagnostic criteria
  - IBS-D: <25% stools lumpy and hard and ≥25% stools loose or watery
  - IBS-C: ≥25% stools lumpy and hard and <25% stools loose or watery
  - IBS-M: ≥25% stools lumpy and hard and ≥25% stools loose or watery
- Rome IV IBS subtypes
  - Type 1: Separate hard pebbles and difficulty defecating
  - Type 2: Sausage shape and lumpy stool
  - Type 3: Sausage shape with cracks on surface of stool
  - Type 4: Sausage shape with smooth surface, soft stool
  - Type 5: Edges apparent on soft blobs of stool
  - Type 6: Edges ragged on mushy stool
  - Type 7: Liquid, no solid stool
- Labs (only if needed and diagnostic criteria above not met)
  - Complete blood count
  - C-reactive protein
  - Fecal calprotectin
  - Celiac serologies

---

[*]**Hallmark signs are bolded** and **Red flags are bolded and underlined**.

- Sigmoidoscopy or colonoscopy with biopsy (only if needed)
- Stool examinations for infection or other causes (only if needed)

(Chang, 2022; Drossman & Hasler, 2016; Lembo et al., 2022)

DIFFERENTIAL DIAGNOSIS

- Colon cancer
- Inflammatory bowel disease (Crohn's disease or ulcerative colitis)
- Ulcer

Plan

GUIDELINE RESOURCES

- Chang, L., Sultan, S., Lembo, A., Verne, G. N., Smalley, W., & Heidelbaugh, J. J. (2022). AGA clinical practice guideline on the pharmacological management of irritable bowel syndrome with constipation. *Gastroenterology*, *163*(1), 118–136. https://doi.org/10.1053/j.gastro.2022.04.016
- Lembo, A., Sultan, S., Chang, L., Heidelbaugh, J. J., Smalley, W., & Verne, G. N. (2022). AGA clinical practice guideline on the pharmacological management of irritable bowel syndrome with diarrhea. *Gastroenterology*, *163*(1), 137–151. https://doi.org/10.1053/j.gastro.2022.04.017

*Pharmacotherapy***

- Medications: IBS-D (Algorithm 29.1)
  - First line, mild:
    - Loperamide for diarrhea
    - Bile acid sequestrant (colestipol) for diarrhea
    - Antispasmodics:
      - Hyoscine
      - Dicyclomine
      - Peppermint oil
  - Second line, moderate:
    - Rifaximin 550 mg three times daily for 14 days
      - Recurrence of IBS-D: Re-treat with rifaximin up to two more times with same dose
    - TCA low dose if persistent abdominal pain and/or psychological symptoms
    - Eluxadoline 100 mg twice daily:
      - Contraindicated if history of cholecystectomy or more than 3 alcoholic beverages consumed daily
  - Third line, severe:
    - Alosetron: The US Food and Drug Administration (FDA) has restricted use to cases of severe IBS-D in females under a risk-management program.
- Medications: IBS-C (Algorithm 29.1)
  - First line, mild:
    - Polyethylene glycol laxatives (over the counter) for constipation
    - Antispasmodics for abdominal pain:
      - Hyoscine

**Selection of medication should be individualized based on clinical features and needs of the patient.

- Dicyclomine
- Peppermint oil
- Second line, moderate:
  - Linaclotide 290 mg once daily
  - Lubiprostone:
    - FDA approved for 8 mg twice daily for females with IBS-C
  - Plecanatide 3 mg once daily
  - Tenapanor 50 mg twice daily
- Third line, severe:
  - Tegaserod:
    - FDA limited approval for 6 mg twice daily for females with IBS-C who are younger than age 65 years and have no history of myocardial infarction, stroke, transient ischemic attack, or angina
  - TCA if persistent abdominal pain and/or psychological symptoms
- Smoking cessation aids should be offered to any person currently smoking tobacco.

NONPHARMACOTHERAPY

- Educate
  - Disease process and subtypes
  - Self-management
- Lifestyle and behavioral modifications
  - Diet low in fermentable oligosaccharides, disaccharides, monosaccharides, and polyols (FODMAP) (Black et al., 2022)
  - Avoid triggering foods and beverages:
    - Caffeine, lactose, spiced foods, and gas-forming foods
  - Consider social determinants of health (see Box 29.1)

BOX 29.1 ■ Diversity Considerations

Older patients are predisposed to malnutrition because of oral disease due to poor dentation, tooth loss, and chewing deficiencies related to cognitive decline, absence of prosthetic appliances, and hyposalivation. Older patients that are subject to poor social determinants of health and socioeconomic factors such as food insecurity also play a role in poor nutrition. Many individuals have limited control over food sources related to mobility and place of residence. It is important to be cognizant of these factors when considering a plan of care that includes dietary instruction (Luo et al., 2022).

BOX 29.2 ■ Pediatric Considerations

Dietary factors play an important role in the generation of symptoms in children with disorders of gut–brain interaction. The provider needs to consider the child as well as the parent or caregiver who will be purchasing and supplying the food if dietary modification is part of the treatment plan. Some dietary changes in the pediatric population that have been shown to be successful include:

- Colicky infants: Remove cow's milk from the infant's diet or from the maternal diet if breastfeeding.
- Regurgitation in children: Add thickeners to the formula or remove cow's milk from the infant's diet or from the maternal diet if breastfeeding.
- Children with pain-predominant gut–brain interaction: Use a soluble fiber supplement or a diet low in fermentable oligosaccharides, disaccharides, monosaccharides, and polyols.

(Nurko et al., 2022)

- Smoking cessation
- Complementary treatment
- See Box 29.4: Fecal microbiota transplantation as a possible treatment that requires acute care.
- Psychosocial rehabilitation
- Complementary and alternative therapies with natural medicines and supplements may interact with prescription medications. Obtain a complete medication history.
- Referral
- Psychologist or psychiatrist
- Gastroenterologist
- Identify and refer for treatment of comorbid conditions
- Follow-up
- Office visit 1 month after starting new medication
- Follow up every 3 to 6 months once stable

BOX 29.3 ■ Older Adult Considerations

The aging process brings on decreased pain sensitivity in most older adult patients. A population-based study revealed that abdominal pain with aging was virtually nonexistent. The decreased sensitivity to visceral pain may be the reason for lower prevalence rates of irritable bowel syndrome (IBS) in those aged 50 years and older. This could potentially be from a decrease in visceral pain–associated receptors and transient receptor expression. However, in a separate community-based survey, patients older than age 60 years were more likely to be diagnosed with IBS using Rome III criteria than those younger than age 60 years. Geriatric patients who are diagnosed with IBS are more likely to be prescribed tricyclic antidepressants (TCAs), selective serotonin reuptake inhibitors (SSRIs), and serotonin and norepinephrine reuptake inhibitors (SNRIs). This is concerning considering the documented anticholinergic effects, even at low doses. The Beers Criteria recommend avoiding antidepressants (i.e., TCAs, SSRIs, and SNRIs) in older adults due to the increased risk of falls. In comparing TCAs, SSRIs, and SNRIs, it is SSRIs that have the best safety profile in the elderly with the lowest potential for drug–drug interactions. However, the first line of treatment for IBS is to change the diet. Therefore a diet low in fermentable oligosaccharides, disaccharides, monosaccharides, and polyols (FODMAP), for example, should be considered before prescribing medication. However, the healthcare provider must consider the changes in older adults that may cause malnutrition if placed on such a strict diet (see Box 29.1). The 5Ms of Geriatrics framework can be utilized as a starting point when formulating a plan of care that is age friendly and includes pharmacologic modalities (neuromodulators, complementary and alternative medicines) and non-pharmacologic modalities (brain–gut behavioral therapies and diet-based therapies). The 5Ms of Geriatrics framework include *M*edications, *M*ind, *M*obility, *M*ulticomplexes, and what *M*atters most (Luo et al., 2022).

BOX 29.4 ■ Acute Care Considerations

Fecal microbiota transplantation (FMT) is becoming a more common treatment for irritable bowel syndrome (IBS). However, outcomes of randomized control trials have varied results. A published systematic review showed possible beneficial effects when FMT was delivered via endoscopy. While FMT appears to be safe compared to placebo in patients with IBS, there was not enough evidence to support the use of FMT for IBS (El-Salhy et al., 2023; Halkjær et al., 2023).

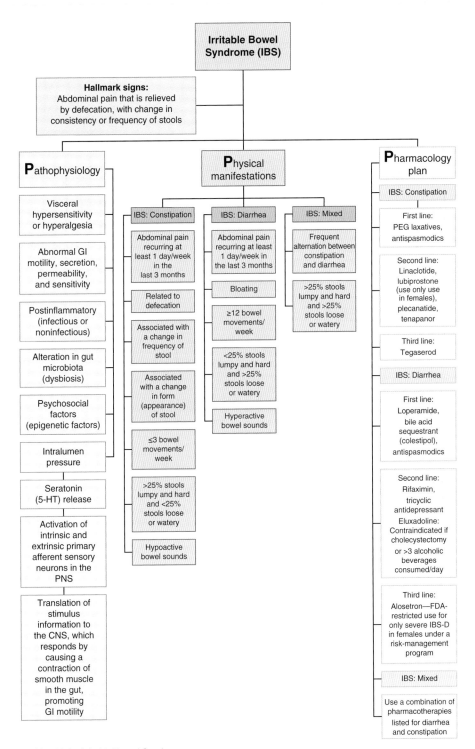

Algorithm 29.1 Irritable Bowel Syndrome.
CNS, Central nervous system; *FDA*, US Food and Drug Administration; *GI*, gastrointestinal; *PEG*, polyethylene glycol; *PNS*, peripheral nervous system.

References

Ancona, A., Petito, C., Iavarone, I., Petito, V., Galasso, L., Leonetti, A., Turchini, L., Belella, D., Ferrarrese, D., Addolorato, G., Armuzzi, A., Gasbarrini, A. & Scaldaferri, F. (2021). The gut-brain axis in irritable bowel syndrome and inflammatory bowel disease. *Digestive and Liver Disease, 53*(3), 298–305. doi: 10.1016/j.dld.2020.11.026.

Ball, J. W., Dains, J. E., Flynn, J. A., Solomon, B. S., & Stewart, R. W. (2023). *Seidel's guide to physical examination* (10th ed.). Elsevier.

Black, C. J., Staudacher, H. M., & Ford, A. C. (2022). Efficacy of a low FODMAP diet in irritable bowel syndrome: Systematic review and network meta-analysis. *Gut, 71*(6), 1117–1126.

Chang, L., Sultan, S., Lembo, A., Verne, G. N., Smalley, W., & Heidelbaugh, J. J. (2022). AGA clinical practice guideline on the pharmacological management of irritable bowel syndrome with constipation. *Gastroenterology, 163*(1), 118–136.

Drossman, D. A., & Hasler, W. L. (2016). Rome IV—Functional GI disorders: Disorders of gut-brain interaction. *Gastroenterology, 150*(6), 1257–1261.

Dains, J. E., Baumann, L. C., & Scheibel, P. (2024). *Advanced health assessment & clinical diagnosis in primary care* (7th ed.). Elsevier. https://pageburstls.elsevier.com/books/9780323832083.

El-Salhy, M., Gilja, O. H., & Hatlebakk, J. G. (2023). Factors affecting the outcome of fecal microbiota transplantation for patients with irritable bowel syndrome. *Neurogastroenterology & Motility, 36*(1), e14641.

Goolsby, M. J., & Grubbs, G. L. (2019). *Advanced assessment interpreting findings and formulating differential diagnoses* (4th ed.). F. A. Davis Company.

Halkjær, S. I., Lo, B., Cold, F., Christensen, A. H., Holster, S., König, J., & Petersen, A. M. (2023). Fecal microbiota transplantation for the treatment of irritable bowel syndrome: A systematic review and meta-analysis. *World Journal of Gastroenterology, 29*(20), 3185.

Holtmann, G. J., Ford, A. C., & Talley, N. J. (2016). Pathophysiology of irritable bowel syndrome. *Lancet Gastroenterology & Hepatology, 1*(2), 133–146.

Lembo, A., Sultan, S., Chang, L., Heidelbaugh, J. J., Smalley, W., & Verne, G. N. (2022). AGA clinical practice guideline on the pharmacological management of irritable bowel syndrome with diarrhea. *Gastroenterology, 163*(1), 137–151.

Luo, Y., Shah, B. J., & Keefer, L. A. (2022). Special considerations for the management of disorders of gut-brain interaction in older adults. *Current Treatment Options in Gastroenterology, 20*(4), 582–593.

Nurko, S., Benninga, M. A., Solari, T., & Chumpitazi, B. P. (2022). Pediatric aspects of nutrition interventions for disorders of gut-brain interaction. *American Journal of Gastroenterology, 117*(6), 995.

Pimentel, M. (2016). Update on irritable bowel syndrome diagnostics and therapeutics. *Gastroenterology & Hepatology, 12*(7), 442–445.

Spain, S. R. (2023). Alterations of digestive function. In J. L. Rogers (Ed.), *McCance & Huether's pathophysiology: The biologic basis for disease in adults and children*, (9th ed., pp. 1318–1374). Mosby-Elsevier.

CHAPTER 30

Cholelithiasis

Julia L. Rogers

Gallstones

Cholelithiasis

Cholelithiasis, commonly known as gallstones, are hard, stonelike pieces that develop within the gallbladder. Cholelithiasis is a widespread disorder, with an estimated worldwide prevalence of 10% to 15% and 20% to 40% of those individuals develop gallstone-related complications (Pisano et al., 2020). The risk factors for developing cholelithiasis are known as the six "f" risks (Algorithm 30.1). Individuals who are more prone to gallstones are *f*emale (gender at birth), are obese (*f*at), are aged 40 years and older (*f*orty), are White (*f*air skin tone) (Box 30.2), have a history of one or more pregnancies or use of oral contraception (*f*ertile), and have a familial history (*f*amily) (Goolsby & Grubbs, 2019; Spain, 2023). Gallstones can also occur at an earlier age (Box 30.1), usually after surgery, trauma, burns, sepsis, or critical illness (Goolsby & Grubbs, 2019). Obesity, diabetes mellitus (see Chapter 14), and insulin resistance predispose individuals to cholelithiasis and increase the risk of cholecystectomy. Other risk factors include rapid weight loss, Crohn's disease (see Chapter 28), cirrhosis, and diseases of the ileum (Spain, 2023).

Cholecystitis

Cholecystitis is an inflammation of the gallbladder that is generally caused by an obstruction of the gallbladder outlet from calculi, accounting for 80% to 90% of acute cholecystitis cases. The remaining cases (acalculous) are associated with sepsis, severe trauma, or infection of the gallbladder (Gallaher & Charles, 2022; Spain, 2023).

Pathophysiology

The pathophysiology of cholelithiasis is a complex interaction of genetic, environmental, local, systemic, and metabolic abnormalities. Cholelithiasis is initiated in the biliary tract as a result of either decreased metabolism of cholesterol and bilirubin or lack of motility of the gallbladder causing stasis of bile materials (Spain, 2023). The precursor to stone formation is biliary sludge within the gallbladder containing cholesterol, unconjugated bilirubin, bilirubin calcium salts, fatty acids, calcium carbonates, calcium phosphates, and mucin glycoproteins due to a decrease in the metabolism of these materials (see Algorithm 30.1). There are three main types of gallstones determined by their chemical composition. The most common type, cholesterol gallstones (containing 70% cholesterol), comprise up to 90% of gallstones. Cholesterol gallstones form in bile that is supersaturated with cholesterol produced by the liver. Supersaturation allows for formation of cholesterol crystals (microstones), which form into macrostones with the aggregation of crystals (Spain, 2023). The remaining black (hard) or brown (soft) pigment stones have less than 30% cholesterol and are composed of mucin glycoproteins and calcium salts. Stones can also be of a

---

BOX 30.1 ■ Pediatric Considerations

Jaundice in the pediatric population can be caused by several different processes. Hyperbilirubinemia, more commonly known as physiologic jaundice of the newborn, is frequently seen in newborns even before they leave the hospital. It can be related to the lack of maturity of bilirubin uptake and conjugation or poor caloric intake. It is easily treated with phototherapy and generally resolves within a few days. Biliary atresia is a rare congenital malformation that also causes jaundice in an infant. It is characterized by the absence or obstruction of extrahepatic bile ducts, resulting in neonatal cholestasis. Early diagnosis is essential because the obstruction of the bile canaliculi can lead to secondary biliary cirrhosis, portal hypertension, liver failure, and subsequent liver transplant, hence the importance of diagnosing and treating an infant with biliary atresia within the first 45 days of life (Spain, 2023).

BOX 30.2 ■ Diversity Considerations

Cholelithiasis is a common diagnosis in patients presenting to the emergency department (ED). Unless an emergent cholecystectomy is warranted, patients are treated for pain and discharged home to follow up with their primary care provider or surgeon to plan for a future laparoscopic cholecystectomy. However, for uninsured patients there is a lack of follow-up and subsequent return visits to the ED for care. Multiple studies have shown that uninsured patients and marginalized populations are at risk for greater ED utilization, highlighting the consequences of disparate access to care. Patients who are uninsured need to be provided with information on local resources and clinics for appropriate follow-up care for cholelithiasis. Furthermore, all patients should receive discharge instructions in their primary language about the diagnosis, symptoms, and plan of care for cholelithiasis, including dietary changes (Shenoy et al., 2022).

---

mixed composition. Decreased digestive movement, poor motility, incomplete postprandial emptying, and biliary stasis allow prolonged exposure to supersaturated bile, promoting gallbladder cholesterol stone formation. Stones are formed in three locations: the gallbladder or cystic duct (cholecystolithiasis), the extrahepatic bile duct (choledocholithiasis), and rarely the intrahepatic bile duct (hepatolithiasis). Cholesterol and black stones are more commonly formed within the gallbladder, whereas brown stones are formed in the bile ducts (Spain, 2023).

Bile stasis in the gallbladder causes inflammation and cholecystitis. Stones can accumulate and fill the entire gallbladder but lie dormant until the gallbladder becomes distended and inflamed, leading to cholecystitis. When the gallbladder contracts to release bile, stones may move into the cystic or common duct and become lodged. The obstruction causes the gallbladder to become more distended and inflamed, triggering the abrupt severe onset of pain. Pressure against the distended wall of the gallbladder decreases blood flow and may result in ischemia, necrosis, and perforation (Spain, 2023).

Physical Clinical Presentation

SUBJECTIVE

The presenting symptom of cholelithiasis and cholecystitis is epigastric or right upper abdominal pain (see Algorithm 30.1). The pain has a sudden onset and tends to increase steadily in intensity. The pain can persist from 30 minutes to up to 5 hours. The pain of biliary colic is usually located in the upper right quadrant or epigastric area and may be referred to the upper midback, right shoulder, or midscapular region and can be intermittent or steady (Goolsby & Grubbs, 2019). The patient may complain of associated symptoms such as fever, yellowing of eyes or skin, anorexia, fat intolerance, and/or abdominal pain 2 to 4 hours after eating. If Charcot's triad (fever/chills, jaundice, right upper quadrant pain) is present, it indicates that the stone is obstructing the common bile duct.

During the focused history, documentation should include the onset of symptoms; precipitating events; location, intensity, and quality of pain; progression of symptoms; alleviating and aggravating

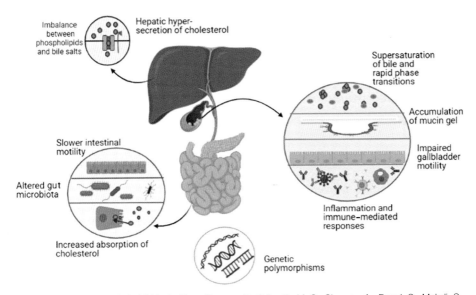

Fig. 30.1 Mechanisms of cholelithiasis. From Swarne, E., Srikanth, M. S., Shreyas, A., Desai, S., Mehdi, S., Gangadharappa, H. V., Suman, & Krishna, K. L. (2021). Recent advances, novel targets and treatments for cholelithiasis: A narrative review. *European Journal of Pharmacology, 908,* 174376. https://doi.org/10.1016/j.ejphar.2021.174376.

factors; previous episodes; and associated symptoms. Document allergies, ill contacts, and medical, social, and family histories. Surgical history should include any history of biliary surgery.

The common clinical manifestation associated with cholelithiasis, sudden onset of severe right upper quadrant abdominal or epigastric pain, occurs when gallstones block the bile duct, obstruct bile flow, and cause inflammation (Spain, 2023). There is the potential for symptoms to be acute or chronic based on the number of stones and whether the blockage is relieved by stone movement. Biliary colic is intermittent pain associated with transient calculi ductal obstruction. Acute cholecystitis from calculi usually subsides in 2 to 3 days, but in some cases it requires emergency cholecystectomy. In individuals with chronic recurrences, resolution usually results within 1 week (Goolsby & Grubbs, 2019). Acalculous cholecystitis tends to have an insidious onset because the clinical manifestations are disguised by the underlying condition(s) initiating the attack (Goolsby & Grubbs, 2019).

OBJECTIVE*

Generalized: Low-grade fever; chills; weakness; fatigue
    Neurological: Confusion
    Cardiovascular: Hypotension; tachycardia
    Pulmonary: <u>Labored respirations</u>; tachypnea (from pain)
    Gastrointestinal: Complaints of anorexia; postprandial pain; vomiting
    Inspection: **Nausea;** tea-colored urine
    Palpation: **Right upper quadrant pain; radiating pain to left scapula/shoulder; epigastric pain; abdominal guarding; rebound tenderness; enlarged gallbladder;** rigidity (see Algorithm 30.1)
    Percussion: Indirect fist percussion of the liver
    Auscultation: Bowel sounds decreased
    Special: Positive Murphy's sign

Hallmark signs are bolded and **<u>Red flags are bolded and underlined</u>. Italics represent special assessment techniques.*

Genitourinary: Hematuria
Integumentary: Jaundice; xanthomas; diaphoresis (see Box 30.1 for pediatric considerations with jaundice)
(Ball, 2023; Dains et al., 2024; Goolsby & Grubbs, 2019)

Evaluation and Differential Diagnoses

DIAGNOSTICS

- Labs
  - White blood cell count (WBC) elevated, leukocytes, neutrophils
  - C-reactive protein (CRP) elevated
  - Liver function tests (LFT) (elevated aspartate aminotransferase, alanine aminotransferase, alkaline phosphatase, bilirubin)
  - Amylase elevated with common bile duct obstruction
  - Lipase
- Diagnostic imaging
  - Abdominal ultrasound (gallbladder and biliary structures)
  - Abdominal computed tomography scan (CT)
  - Hepatobiliary iminodiacetic acid scan (HIDA)
  - Magnetic resonance imaging (MRI)
  - Magnetic resonance cholangiopancreatography (MRCP)
  - Endoscopic retrograde cholangiopancreatography
  - Percutaneous transhepatic cholangiography
  - Cholecystography (nuclear scan)

(Bonomo, 2024; European Association for the Study of the Liver [EASL], 2016; Goolsby & Grubbs, 2019; Gomi et al., 2018; Pisano et al., 2020; Spain, 2023)

DIFFERENTIAL DIAGNOSIS

- Acute abdomen
- Nephrolithiasis
- Peptic ulcer disease
- Pancreatitis

Plan

GUIDELINE RESOURCES

- IDSA 2024 Guideline Update on the Risk Assessment, Diagnostic Imaging, and Microbiological Evaluation of Complicated Intraabdominal Infections in Adults
- Bonomo, R. A., Tamma, P. D., Abrahamian, F. M., Bessesen, M., Chow, A. W., Dellinger, E. P., ... & Loveless, J. (2024). 2024 Clinical Practice Guideline update by the Infectious Diseases Society of America on complicated intra-abdominal infections: diagnostic imaging of suspected acute appendicitis in adults, children, and pregnant people. *Clinical Infectious Diseases*, ciae348. https://doi.org/10.1093/cid/ciae346.
- European Association for the Study of the Liver. (2016). EASL clinical practice guidelines on the prevention, diagnosis and treatment of gallstones. *Journal of Hepatology*, 65(1), 146–181. https://doi.org/10.1016/j.jhep.2016.03.005.
- Gomi, H., Solomkin, J. S., Schlossberg, D., Okamoto, K., Takada, T., Strasberg, S. M., Ukai, T., Endo, I., Iwashita, Y., Hibi, T., Pitt, H. A., Matsunaga, N., Takamori, Y., Umezawa, A., Asai, K., Suzuki, K., Han, H.-S., Hwang, T.-L., Mori, Y., ... Yamamoto, M. (2018). Tokyo

guidelines 2018: Antimicrobial therapy for acute cholangitis and cholecystitis. *Journal of Hepato-Biliary-Pancreatic Sciences, 25*(1), 3–16. https://doi.org/10.1002/jhbp.518.
- Pisano, M., Allievi, N., Gurusamy, K., Borzellino, G., Cimbanassi, S., Boerna, D., Coccolini, F., Tufo, A., Di Martino, M., Leung, J., Sartelli, M., Ceresoli, M., Maier, R. V., Poiasina, E., De Angelis, N., Magnone, S., Fugazzola, P., Paolillo, C., Coimbra, R., … Ansaloni, L. (2020). 2020 World Society of Emergency Surgery updated guidelines for the diagnosis and treatment of acute calculus cholecystitis. *World Journal of Emergency Surgery, 15*(1), 61. https://doi.org/10.1186/s13017-020-00336-x.

Pharmacotherapy

- Medications (Algorithm 30.1)
  - Nonsteroidal antiinflammatory drugs for pain control in biliary colic (Box 30.3):
    - Diclofenac, indomethacin, Mobic, ibuprofen
  - Antibiotics for complicated cholecystitis (Box 30.4)
  - Antispasmodics
  - Ezetimibe (selective cholesterol absorption inhibitor)
- Smoking cessation aids should be offered to any person currently smoking tobacco.
(EASL, 2016; Goolsby & Grubbs, 2019; Gomi et al., 2018; Pisano et al., 2020; Spain, 2023)

NONPHARMACOTHERAPY

- Educate
  - Eliminate triggering foods
  - Self-management
  - Disease prevention, diagnosis, treatment, and progression
- Lifestyle and behavioral modifications

BOX 30.3 ■ Older Adult Considerations

In the geriatric population it is important to review a current list of medications and past medical history when prescribing analgesics. The primary treatment for cholelithiasis and cholecystitis is pain control; however, there is increased risk of acute renal failure, gastrointestinal bleeding, and interactions with other medications in this population. Nonsteroidal antiinflammatory drugs should be avoided or used with extreme caution and frequent monitoring in geriatric patients. Because of the side effects associated with nonsteroidal antiinflammatory drugs, it is appropriate to use low-dose opioid medications. Initiate an opioid at 30% to 50% lower than the normal dose and titrate up for a short-term duration in patients older than age 65 years (Cash, 2024).

BOX 30.4 ■ Acute Care Considerations

In acute cholecystitis, the initial treatment for patients presenting to the emergency department or hospitalized with severe cholecystitis includes bowel rest, intravenous (IV) fluids for hydration, correction of electrolyte abnormalities, analgesics, and IV antibiotics. There are multiple factors to consider in selecting an empiric antimicrobial agent including local antibiogram, pharmacokinetics and pharmacodynamics, renal function, allergies, and previous use of antibiotics. A single broad-spectrum antibiotic is generally adequate. Piperacillin/tazobactam (3.375 g IV every 6 hours or 4.5 g IV every 8 hours), or ampicillin/sulbactam (3 g IV every 6 hours only if resistance is <20%), or cephalosporin or meropenem (1 g every 8 hours), or a fluoroquinolone are recommended as treatment regimens. Antiemetics can be used intravenously to help with nausea and vomiting (Gomi et al., 2018).

- Diet: Prevention—increase intake of polyunsaturated fat, monounsaturated fat (reduce cholesterol saturation in bile), caffeine, vitamin C (breaks down cholesterol in bile), and fiber. Reduce saturated fats and cholesterol intake. Stay hydrated with water intake (64 ounces per day)
- Exercise and maintenance of normal body weight and bidy mass index with gradual weight loss
- Smoking cessation
- Complementary treatment
  - Psychosocial rehabilitation
  - Vitamin C 2 g daily
  - Complementary and alternative therapies with natural medicines and supplements may interact with prescription medications. Obtain a complete medication history.
- Referral
  - Surgery for laparoscopic cholecystectomy
  - Gastroenterologist
  - Identify and refer to specialist for treatment of comorbid conditions
- Follow-up
  - 2 weeks after hospital discharge if hospitalized
  - Office visit every 3 to 6 months

(EASL, 2016; Goolsby & Grubbs, 2019; Gomi et al., 2018; Pisano et al., 2020; Spain, 2023)

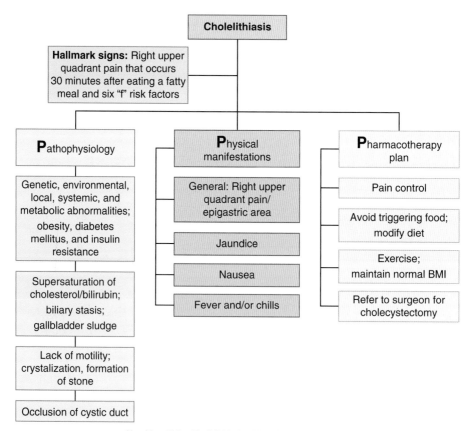

Algorithm 30.1 Cholelithiasis. *BMI,* Body mass index.

References

Ball, J. W., Flynn, J. E., Solomon, B. S., & Stewart, R. W. (2023). *Seidel's guide to physical examination: An interprofessional approach* (9th ed). St. Louis: Elsevier.

Bonomo, R. A., Tamma, P. D., Abrahamian, F. M., Bessesen, M., Chow, A. W., Dellinger, E. P., ... & Loveless, J. (2024). 2024 Clinical Practice Guideline update by the Infectious Diseases Society of America on complicated intra-abdominal infections: diagnostic imaging of suspected acute appendicitis in adults, children, and pregnant people. *Clinical Infectious Diseases*, ciae348. https://doi.org/10.1093/cid/ciae346.

Cash, J. (2024). *Adult gerontology practice guidelines* (3rd ed.). Springer.

Dains, J. E., Baumann, L. C., & Scheibel, P. (2024). *Advanced health assessment & clinical diagnosis in primary care* (7th ed). St. Louis: Elsevier.

European Association for the Study of the Liver. (2016). EASL clinical practice guidelines on the prevention, diagnosis and treatment of gallstones. *Journal of Hepatology, 65*(1), 146–181.

Gallaher, J. R., & Charles, A. (2022). Acute Cholecystitis. JAMA, *327*(10), 965–975.

Gomi, H., Solomkin, J. S., Schlossberg, D., Okamoto, K., Takada, T., Strasberg, S. M., & Yamamoto, M. (2018). Tokyo guidelines 2018: Antimicrobial therapy for acute cholangitis and cholecystitis. *Journal of Hepato-Biliary-Pancreatic Sciences, 25*(1), 3–16.

Goolsby, M. J., & Grubbs, G. L. (2019). *Advanced assessment: Interpreting findings and formulating differential diagnoses* (4th ed.). F. A. Davis Company.

Pisano, M., Allievi, N., Gurusamy, K., Borzellino, G., Cimbanassi, S., Boerna, D., & Ansaloni, L. (2020). 2020 World Society of Emergency Surgery updated guidelines for the diagnosis and treatment of acute calculus cholecystitis. *World Journal of Emergency Surgery, 15*(1), 1–26.

Shenoy, R., Kirkland, P., Jackson, N., DeVirgilio, M., Zingmond, D., Russell, M. M., & Maggard-Gibbons, M. (2022). Identifying vulnerable populations with symptomatic cholelithiasis at risk for increased health care utilization. *Journal of Trauma and Acute Care Surgery, 93*(6), 863–871.

Spain, S. R. (2023). Alterations of digestive function. In J. L. Rogers (Ed), *McCance & Huether's pathophysiology: The biologic basis for disease in adults and children* (9th ed., pp. 1318-1374). Elsevier.

Genitourinary System

SECTION OUTLINE

31 Nephrolithiasis
32 Urinary Tract Infection

CHAPTER 31

Nephrolithiasis

Julia L. Rogers

Kidney stones, Renal calculi and Urolithiasis

Nephrolithiasis

Nephrolithiasis, commonly known as renal calculi, kidney stones, or urolithiasis, are hard masses formed inside the kidneys from minerals and salts found within the body. Stones can be located anywhere along the urinary tract including in the kidneys, ureters, and urinary bladder. Stones present unilaterally in about 80% of individuals. The prevalence of kidney stones in the United States is approximately 11% in males and 7% in females. The risk of recurrence at 5 years is approximately 50% overall (Rogers, 2023; Khan et al., 2016). Stone formation is influenced by a number of factors, including age (before age 50 years), gender (male), race, geographic location (warm climate with high humidity), season (summer), fluid intake, diet, occupation, and genetic predisposition. Warmer climates with high humidity and rainfall influence a person's fluid intake and dietary patterns. Diseases that predispose individuals for stone formation are urinary tract infection (UTI) (see Chapter 32), hypertension (see Chapter 20), atherosclerosis (see Chapter 19), metabolic syndrome, obesity, and type 2 diabetes (see Chapter 14) (Goolsby & Grubbs, 2019; Rogers, 2023) (Fig. 31.1).

Pathophysiology

Human urine contains many ions capable of precipitating from solution and forming a variety of salts. The process of stone formation begins with supersaturation of one or more salts in the urine (Khan et al., 2016). Supersaturation, an essential component for free stone formation, is the presence of a higher concentration of a solute (salt) within a solvent (urine) than can be dissolved (Algorithm 31.1). This process allows the salts to change from a liquid to a solid state, forming crystals that grow from a small nucleus into larger stones through the crystallization or aggregation process. The normal flow of urine flushes most crystals out from the urinary tract. However, urinary stasis, anatomic abnormalities, or inflamed epithelium within the urinary tract may prevent elimination of crystals from the system, thus increasing the risk of stone formation. The urine does not need to remain continuously supersaturated for a stone to grow once its nucleus has precipitated from solution. The presence or absence of stone inhibitors (e.g., uromodulin [Tamm-Horsfall protein], potassium citrate, pyrophosphate, and magnesium), intermittent periods of supersaturation after the ingestion of a meal, dehydration from limited oral intake, or continued use of diuretics all play a role in stone formation and growth (Rogers, 2023).

Stones are classified according to the primary minerals (salts) that make up the stones. The most common stone types include calcium oxalate or calcium phosphate (70% to 80%), struvite (magnesium–ammonium–phosphate) (5% to 10%), and uric acid (5% to 10%) (Rogers, 2023). Cystine stones are rare (≤2%), as are stones that are formed from the metabolic effects of some

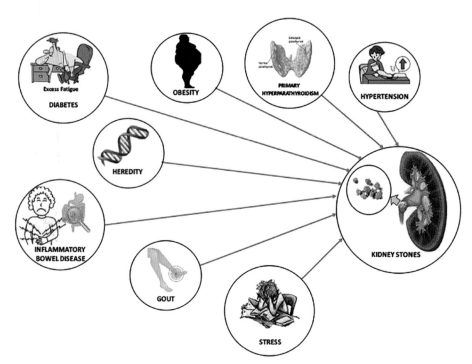

Fig. 31.1 Factors influencing nephrolithiasis. (From Devi, A. T., Nagaraj, R., Prasad, A., Lakkappa, D. B., Zameer, F., & Nagalingaswamy, N. P. M. (2022). Nephrolithiasis: Insights into biomimics, pathogenesis, and pharmacology. *Clinical Complementary Medicine and Pharmacology*, 3(11), 100077.)

medications (e.g., atazanavir, ceftriaxone, and N-acetyl-sulfadiazine). The pH of the urine influences the risk of precipitation and calculus formation. An alkaline urinary pH (pH >7.0) significantly increases the risk of calcium phosphate stone and struvite stone formation, whereas acidic urine (pH <5.0) increases the risk of uric acid stone formation. Cystine and xanthine also precipitate more readily in acidic urine (Rogers, 2023). Stones are also classified according to location and size. Staghorn calculi are large and fill the minor and major calyces. Nonstaghorn calculi are of variable size but tend to be smaller and are located in the renal calyces, in the renal pelvis, or at various sites along the ureter (Rogers, 2023).

Nephrolithiasis is a common cause of urinary tract obstruction. Urinary tract obstruction is a structural or functional abnormality that causes interference with the flow of urine at any site along the urinary tract. A kidney stone can be small enough to pass through the urinary tract or large enough to become lodged and completely obstruct the normal flow through the urinary tract. When the obstruction impedes urine flow it increases the risk of infection, increases hydrostatic pressure, dilates structures proximal to the blockage, and compromises renal function (Rogers, 2023). The size of a stone determines the likelihood that it will pass through the urinary tract and be excreted through micturition. Stones smaller than 4 mm have about a 50% chance of spontaneous (painful) passage, whereas stones that are larger than 6 mm have almost no chance of spontaneous passage (Rogers, 2023).

Hypercalciuria, hyperoxaluria, hyperuricosuria, hypocitraturia, mild renal tubular acidosis, crystal growth inhibitor deficiencies, and alkaline urine are associated with calcium stone formation. Hypercalciuria and hyperoxaluria are usually attributable to intestinal hyperabsorption and less commonly to a defect in renal calcium reabsorption. Hyperparathyroidism and bone demineralization associated with prolonged immobilization are also known to cause hypercalciuria (Rogers, 2023). Struvite stones may grow quite large and branch into a staghorn configuration and primarily contain magnesium, ammonium, and phosphate. Excessive uric acid secretion in the urine (e.g., gouty arthritis) causes uric acid stone formation. Uric acid is affected by consumption of purines (e.g., meat and beer) in the diet. Cystine and xanthine stone formation is from a genetic disorder of amino acid metabolism. The excess of cystinuria and xanthinuria in urine that is also acidic can cause cystine or xanthine stone formation (Rogers, 2023).

Physical Clinical Presentation

SUBJECTIVE

Hematuria and flank pain, referred to as renal colic, are the most common clinical manifestations of nephrolithiasis. Nausea, vomiting, and lower urinary tract symptoms such as dysuria, urinary urgency, frequency, or hesitancy are also often present. A fever is not usually present unless there is an infective process, an obstructed kidney, or another inflammatory process coexisting. A comprehensive history of present illness and physical examination of all abdominopelvic organ systems is essential to rule out other important or life-threatening conditions (Thia & Chau, 2022).

During the focused history, documentation should include the onset and duration of symptoms; precipitating events; location, intensity, and characteristics of pain; progression of symptoms; alleviating and aggravating factors; previous episodes; and associated symptoms. The location and characteristics of pain provide clues as to where the stone may be located along the urinary tract. Pain can be incapacitating or mild and may be accompanied by nausea and vomiting. Renal colic is pain directly related to dilation and spasm of smooth muscles related to ureteral obstruction. Moderate to severe pain that originates in the flank and radiates to the groin usually indicates obstruction of the renal pelvis or proximal ureter. Colic that radiates to the lateral flank or lower abdomen typically indicates obstruction in the midureter (Rogers, 2023). Symptoms of urinary urgency, frequency, or incontinence generally indicate obstruction of the lower ureter or ureterovesical junction. Gross or microscopic hematuria may be present depending on the size and shape of the stone as well as damage caused to the walls of ureters from stone movement.

Document allergies, ill contacts, and medical, social, and family histories. Include any medical conditions, dietary habits, or medications that predispose to stone development. The most common conditions associated with stone disease include dehydration, hyperparathyroidism, gout, hyperthyroidism, renal tubular acidosis type 1, obesity, type 2 diabetes mellitus (see Chapter 14), and malabsorptive gastrointestinal states due to bowel resection, bariatric surgery, or bowel disease (Pearle et al., 2014) (Box 31.1). Nutritional factors are associated with stone disease and linked to stone type. Document the amount and type of fluid intake per day, protein consumption including the type and amount, and foods containing high oxalate, calcium, or sodium, as well as intake of fruits and vegetables. The healthcare provider should always include all over-the-counter supplements within the dietary history (Pearle et al., 2014). The

---

BOX 31.1 ■ Older Adult Considerations

There is a rise in prevalence of nephrolithiasis in the geriatric population that is linked to other co-morbidities, such as metabolic syndrome, and polypharmacy. Another concern with aging adults is the change in urine habits such as increased frequency, urinary incontinence, and incomplete bladder emptying. All of which contribute to increased risk of urinary tract infection and therefore increased risk of stone formation. Older patients often have a higher risk of requiring surgery for stone removal because of the complexity and size of stones (Schulz et al., 2023).

provider should assess the patient's use of any stone-provoking medications or supplements (probenecid, protease or lipase inhibitors, triamterene, chemotherapy, vitamin C, vitamin D, calcium, and carbonic anhydrase inhibitors such as topiramate, acetazolamide, or zonisamide) (Pearle et al., 2014).

OBJECTIVE*

Generalized: Fatigue; <u>**fever; chills**</u>
Neurological: <u>**Confusion**</u>
Cardiovascular: Tachycardia (from pain/renal colic)
Pulmonary: *Inspection:* Tachypnea (from pain/renal colic)
Gastrointestinal: Moderate to severe costovertebral angle tenderness; soft, tender, mild distention (if obstructed); hypoactive bowel sounds; vomiting
Genitourinary: Hematuria; renal colic (squirming in pain, pacing, unable to lie still); incontinence; dysuria; frequency; urgency; hesitancy; <u>**pyuria**</u>
Reproductive: Suprapubic tenderness; testis tender
Psychiatric: May appear anxious from renal colic pain (Algorithm 31.1)
(Ball et al., 2023; Dains et al., 2024; Goolsby & Grubbs, 2019; Rogers, 2023)

Evaluation and Differential Diagnoses

DIAGNOSTICS

- Labs: Electrolytes, creatinine, uric acid, vitamin D, and parathyroid hormone to identify any underlying medical conditions associated with stone disease (e.g., primary or secondary hyperparathyroidism or gout)
- Urinalysis dipstick to obtain urine pH and microscopic evaluation to assess for infection and identify crystals pathognomonic of stone type. The presence of high urine pH (>7.0) or urea-splitting organisms such as Proteus species raises the possibility of struvite stones.
- Urine electrolytes
- Urine cystine if known family history
- Urine culture only if urinalysis suggestive of UTI or in patients with recurrent UTIs
- 24-hour urine analysis (performed twice) to determine urinary saturation of stone-forming salts. Consider metabolic testing for individuals with family history of stone disease, recurrent UTIs, malabsorptive intestinal disease or resection, obesity, or medical conditions predisposing individual to stones.
- Stone composition analysis may help determine plan of care as certain medical conditions and medications are associated with specific stone compositions (e.g., calcium phosphate stone composition likely associated with primary hyperparathyroidism or distal renal tubular acidosis and use of carbonic anhydrase inhibitors).
- Kidney, ureter, and bladder radiograph or digital tomogram
- Renal ultrasound (preferred initial imaging modality for children and pregnant females)
- Noncontrast computed tomography (CT) scan (initial imaging for initial presentation)
(Fulgham et al., 2013; Pearle et al., 2014; Rogers, 2023)

---

*Hallmark signs are bolded and <u>**Red flags are bolded and underlined**</u>.

> **BOX 31.2 ■ Acute Care Considerations**
>
> Obstructing ureteral stones can lead to urinary tract infections (UTIs), acute kidney injury (AKI), and urosepsis. It is important to obtain a urinalysis, renal function tests, and complete blood count to determine if any of these are present. The patient should be on broad spectrum antibiotics until the urine culture returns and the specific organism is identified and then the antibiotic can be adjusted appropriately. Continue to monitor renal function throughout the hospital stay. Interestingly, AKI is associated with a greater risk of kidney stones in the future, which increases with higher stages of AKI (Cheikh Hassan et al., 2023; Lim et al., 2022).

DIFFERENTIAL DIAGNOSIS

- Hyperparathyroidism: Primary hyperthyroidism is suspected with high serum calcium (S. Ca), elevated urine calcium (Ca), and parathyroid hormone in midrange, whereas low vitamin D levels may mask primary hyperparathyroidism or contribute to secondary hyperparathyroidism.
- Complicated upper UTI (i.e., pyelonephritis) (see Chapter 32)
- Cholelithiasis or cholecystitis
- Acute pancreatitis

Plan

GUIDELINE RESOURCES

- Pearle, M. S., Goldfarb, D. S., Assimos, D. G., Curhan, G., Denu-Ciocca, C. J., Matlaga, B. R., Monga, M., Penniston, K. L., Preminger, G. M., Turk, T. M. T., & White, J. R. (2014). Medical management of kidney stones: AUA guideline. *Journal of Urology, 192*(2), 316-324. http://dx.doi.org/10.1016/j.juro.2014.05.006.

Pharmacotherapy

- Medications (Algorithm 31.1)
  - Calcium oxalate *OR* calcium phosphate stone formers:
    - Thiazide diuretics**:
      - Hydrochlorothiazide 25 mg orally twice daily or 50 mg orally daily *OR*
      - Chlorthalidone 25 mg orally daily *OR*
      - Indapamide 2.5 mg orally daily:
        Potassium supplement if needed for hypokalemia from diuretics
  - Calcium oxalate, calcium phosphate, or uric acid stone formers:
    - Potassium citrate
    - Allopurinol: Recurrent calcium oxalate stones with hyperuricosuria and normal urine calcium. Do not routinely offer as first-line therapy for uric acid stone formers.
  - Cystine stone formers:
    - Increase fluid, restrict sodium and protein, and improve urine alkalinization:
      - Potassium citrate

---

*Appropriate for both calcium oxalate and calcium phosphate stone formers and high-risk first-time stone formers (e.g., solitary kidney, hypertension, large stone burden, or refractory to other risk-mitigating maneuvers).

- Cysteine-binding drugs as second-line therapy:
  - Tiopronin
- Struvite stone formers:
  - Urease inhibitor, acetohydroxamic acid (AHA) (closely monitor for phlebitis and hypercoagulable phenomena); use only after surgical options have been exhausted
- Antibiotics for complication of infection: UTI; urosepsis (see Chapter 32)
  - See Box 31.2.
- Smoking cessation aids should be offered to any person currently smoking tobacco.
- Vaccines: Influenza annually, pneumococcal, COVID-19, and zoster according to Centers for Disease Control and Prevention guidelines and recommendations

(Pearle et al., 2014; Rogers, 2023)

NONPHARMACOTHERAPY

- Educate
  - Clinical manifestations of infection
  - Disease progression
  - Medications prescribed, purpose, and appropriate use
  - Self-management
  - See Box 31.3.
- Lifestyle and behavioral modifications
  - Dietary changes can be made based on identification of metabolic, environmental, and dietary consumption risk factors (Pearle et al., 2014).

BOX 31.3 ■ Pediatric Considerations

Healthcare provider goals in urinary tract obstruction are to identify signs and symptoms associated with an obstruction, assist or perform diagnostic procedures, and provide education about the disease and plan of care to the patient and to their caregiver(s). When preparing parents and children for procedures, the provider should explain the procedure and potential complications in terms the patient and/or caregiver(s) can understand before they sign consent. Parents and children need emotional support and counseling during the potentially lengthy management of urinary disorders. Since parents are the primary caregivers during infancy and childhood, they need assistance in learning to manage the care of the child and in detecting subtle signs of urinary tract infection or complications of procedures (Kelly, 2024).

BOX 31.4 ■ Diversity Considerations

Healthcare providers need to self-reflect on potential implicit bias when caring for individuals who present with pain. Nephrolithiasis is a condition that can cause mild to severe pain depending on stone movement and placement. However, there are multiple studies that report racial and ethnic disparities in analgesia for patients presenting to the hospital with renal colic. More initiatives need to be enacted toward improving treatment and access to care for vulnerable populations with stone disease. Implementing community- and population-based interventions to decrease the risks of kidney stones needs to be a priority. Interventions could focus on ways to improve food security, which may lead to dietary changes and thus decrease obesity and diabetes. Improving access to outpatient services could prevent unnecessary hospital emergency room visits. The disparities documented in imaging, analgesia, availability of stone removing procedures, and metabolic evaluation could be improved with more accessibility (Crivelli et al., 2021).

- Diet: Dietary Approaches to Stop Hypertension diet:
  - Increase fruits and vegetables in calcium stone and uric acid stone formers with relatively low urinary citrate.
  - Limit nondairy animal protein in calcium stone and uric acid stone formers.
  - Recommend calcium intake of 1000–1200 mg daily in calcium stone formers.
  - Limit oxalate-rich foods in calcium oxalate stone formers with high urinary oxalate.
  - Restrict oxalate-rich foods in calcium oxalate stone formers.
  - Low salt (≤2300 mg daily)
  - High fluid intake: Preferably water (amount based on 24-hour urine collection with a goal of 2.5 L of urine output daily) (Pearle et al., 2014)
  - See Box 31.4.
- Complementary treatment
  - Avoid vitamin C, turmeric, cranberry tablets, and other over-the-counter supplements unless recommended by a specialist.
  - Complementary and alternative therapies with natural medicines and supplements may interact with prescription medications. Obtain a complete medication history.

(Pearle et al., 2014)
- Referral (identify and refer for treatment of comorbid conditions)
  - Nephrologist
  - Urologist
  - Dietitian
- Follow-up
  - Obtain a single 24-hour urine for stone risk factors within 6 months of initial treatment to assess response to pharmacotherapy and patient adherence. Urinary testing should be tailored to individual patient and stone type. Then, obtain 24-hour urine annually unless increased frequency is necessitated by stone activity.
  - If patient remains stone free on treatment regimen for an extended period of time, discontinuation of follow-up testing may be considered.
  - Repeat stone analysis for patients not responding to treatment.
  - Labs to monitor for potential side effects of pharmacotherapy (e.g., electrolytes, glucose, liver function tests, complete blood count)
  - Monitor for persistent or recurrent UTI in struvite stone formers.
  - One-year imaging interval is recommended for stable patients.

(Pearle et al., 2014; Rogers, 2023)

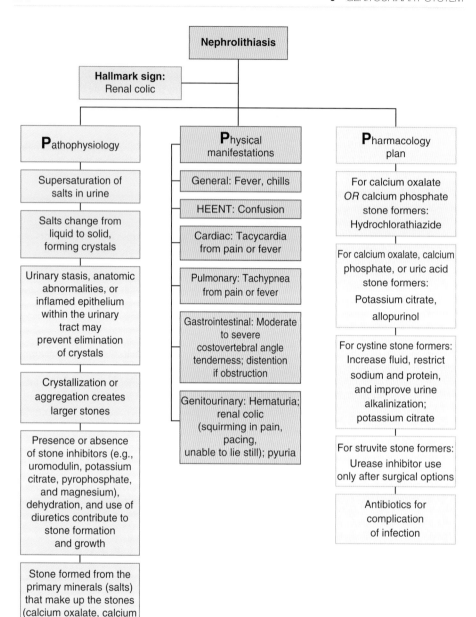

Algorithm 31.1 Nephrolithiasis

References

Ball, J. W., Dains, J. E., Flynn, J. A., Solomon, B. S., & Stewart, R. W. (2023). *Seidel's guide to physical examination: An interprofessional approach* (9th ed.). Elsevier.

Cheikh Hassan, H. I., Murali, K., Lambert, K., Lonergan, M., McAlister, B., Suesse, T., & Mullan, J. (2023). Acute kidney injury increases risk of kidney stones—a retrospective propensity score matched cohort study. *Nephrology, 38*(1), 138–147. https://doi.org/10.1093/ndt/gfac023.

Crivelli, J. J., Maalouf, N. M., Paiste, H. J., Wood, K. D., Hughes, A. E., Oates, G. R., & Assimos, D. G. (2021). Disparities in kidney stone disease: A scoping review. *Journal of Urology, 206*(3), 517–525. https://doi.org/10.1097/JU.0000000000001846.

Dains, J. E., Baumann, L. C., & Scheibel, P. (2024). *Advanced health assessment & clinical diagnosis in primary care* (7th ed.). Elsevier.

Fulgham, P. F., Assimos, D. G., Pearle, M. S., & Preminger, G. M. (2013). Clinical effectiveness protocols for imaging in the management of ureteral calculous disease: AUA technology assessment. *Journal of Urology, 189*(4), 1203–1213.

Goolsby, M. J., & Grubbs, G. L. (2019). *Advanced health assessment: Interpreting findings and formulating differential diagnoses* (4th ed.). F. A. Davis Company.

Kelly, M. S. (2024). The child with genitourinary dysfunction. In M. J. Hockenberry, E. A. Duffy, & K. D. Gibbs (Eds.), *Wong's nursing care of infants and children*. (12th ed., pp. 762–811). Elsevier.

Khan, S. R., Pearle, M. S., Robertson, W. G., Gambaro, G., Canales, B. K., Doizi, S., Traxer, O., & Tiselius, H. G. (2016). Kidney stones. *Nature Reviews Disease Primers, 2*, 16008. https://doi.org/10.1038/nrdp.2016.8.

Lim, W., Suhail, M., & Diaz, K. (2022). A case of bilateral infected kidney stones presenting with septic shock and acute kidney injury. *Cureus, 14*(2), e22506. https://doi.org/10.7759/cureus.22506.

Pearle, M. S., Goldfarb, D. S., Assimos, D. G., Curhan, G., Denu-Ciocca, C. J., Matlaga, B. R., & White, J. R. (2014). Medical management of kidney stones: AUA guideline. *Journal of Urology, 192*(2), 316–324.

Rogers, J. (2023). Alterations of the renal and urinary tract. In J. L. Rogers (Ed.), *McCance & Huether's pathophysiology: The biologic basis for disease in adults and children* (9th ed.). Elsevier.

Schulz, A. E., Green, B. W., Gupta, K., Patel, R. D., Loloi, J., Raskolnikov, D., & Small, A. C. (2023). Management of large kidney stones in the geriatric population. *World Journal of Urology, 41*(4), 981–992.

Thia, I., & Chau, M. (2022). *Renal tract stones—diagnosis and management*. IntechOpen.

CHAPTER 32

Urinary Tract Infection

Julia L. Rogers

Cystitis and Pyelonephritis

Urinary tract infections (UTIs) are the second most common infection in the United States and account for more than 10 million outpatient office visits annually (Burchum & Rosenthal, 2021). UTIs are classified as lower (cystitis) or upper (pyelonephritis) and further categorized as uncomplicated, complicated, recurrent, relapsing, or catheter associated. Uncomplicated UTIs can be acute, sporadic, or recurrent. Uncomplicated UTIs are limited to nonpregnant females with no relevant anatomical or functional abnormalities within the urinary tract and no comorbidities (Kang et al., 2018; Lajiness & Lajiness, 2019; Rogers, 2020). A complicated UTI often presents with systemic signs and symptoms and incorporates all UTIs not defined as uncomplicated. UTIs in immunocompromised patients, in males, and associated with fevers, stones, urinary obstruction, catheters, or sepsis or involving the kidneys are considered complicated. Recurrent UTI is considered when there are two independent culture-proven episodes of acute bacterial cystitis and associated symptoms within 6 months or three episodes within 1 year.

Pathophysiology

Urinary tract infections (UTIs) are characterized by inflammation of the urinary epithelium, typically caused by bacteria originating from the gastrointestinal tract (Rogers, 2023; Walsh & Collys, 2017). The infection process can be categorized into lower UTIs, confined to the bladder, and upper UTIs, involving the kidneys. In lower UTIs, bacteria ascend from the urethra to the bladder, while in upper UTIs (acute pyelonephritis), bacteria replicate in the bladder, ascend to the kidneys via the ureters, or spread through the bloodstream (Kang et al., 2018; Walsh & Collys, 2017). Several natural protective factors within the genitourinary system avert UTIs. Micturition, or urination, flushes most bacteria out of the urethra; body's maintenance of low pH and high urea osmolality; presence of uromodulin and uroepithelium secretions; and periurethral mucus-secreting glands that trap bacteria before they can ascend from the proximal urethra to the bladder (Rogers, 2023). Males have additional barriers, including longer urethra and secretions from the prostate (Rogers, 2023). The closure of the ureterovesical junction during bladder contraction prevents urine reflux, thereby preventing ascension of bacteria from the distal urethra to the ureters and kidneys, deterring an upper UTI. The presence of UTI occurs when bacteria are able to circumvent or overwhelm the body's defense mechanisms (Algorithm 32.1). There are pathogens that have the virulence to rapidly reproduce, resist bactericidal effects of complement, and express toxins. One such pathogen is *Escherichia coli* (*E. coli*), which is responsible for more than 80% of uncomplicated UTIs (Burchum & Rosenthal, 2021). Gram-positive cocci, especially *Staphylococcus saprophyticus*, account for 10% to 15% of community-associated urinary infections (Burchum & Rosenthal, 2021). Hospital-associated UTIs are frequently caused by Gram-negative bacilli such as *Klebsiella*, *Proteus*, *Enterobacter*, *Providencia*, and *Pseudomonas* species; *staphylococci*; and *enterococci* (Burchum & Rosenthal, 2021). The mechanisms of bacterial colonization are complex. Uropathogenic strains

Bacterial factors   **Host factors**   **Pathogenesis**

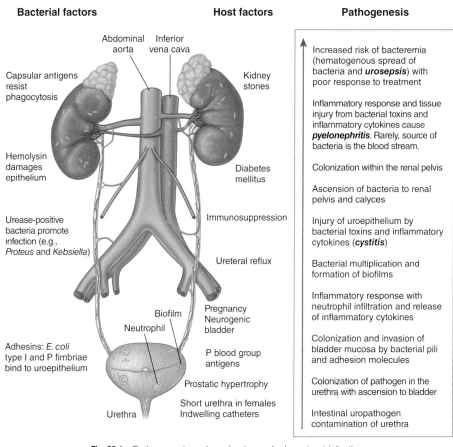

Capsular antigens resist phagocytosis

Hemolysin damages epithelium

Urease-positive bacteria promote infection (e.g., *Proteus* and *Kebsiella*)

Adhesins: *E. coli* type I and P fimbriae bind to uroepithelium

Abdominal aorta
Inferior vena cava

Kidney stones

Diabetes mellitus

Immunosuppression

Ureteral reflux

Biofilm
Neutrophil
Pregnancy
Neurogenic bladder

P blood group antigens

Prostatic hypertrophy

Short urethra in females
Indwelling catheters

Urethra

Increased risk of bacteremia (hematogenous spread of bacteria and **urosepsis**) with poor response to treatment

Inflammatory response and tissue injury from bacterial toxins and inflammatory cytokines cause **pyelonephritis**. Rarely, source of bacteria is the blood stream.

Colonization within the renal pelvis

Ascension of bacteria to renal pelvis and calyces

Injury of uroepithelium by bacterial toxins and inflammatory cytokines (**cystitis**)

Bacterial multiplication and formation of biofilms

Inflammatory response with neutrophil infiltration and release of inflammatory cytokines

Colonization and invasion of bladder mucosa by bacterial pili and adhesion molecules

Colonization of pathogen in the urethra with ascension to bladder

Intestinal uropathogen contamination of urethra

Fig. 32.1 Pathogenesis and mechanisms of urinary tract infection.

of *E. coli* have fingerlike projections that bind to receptors on the uroepithelium. Consequently, the uropathic strains resist flushing during normal micturition and have flagella that propel them upstream. Certain bacterial species can enhance their virulence by acting together to form a biofilm that enhances colonization and resists innate host defense mechanisms and antimicrobial therapy (Fig. 32.1). Several risk factors increase the risk of UTIs. Females are at higher risk of UTI than males due to an anatomically shorter urethra with relative proximity to the anus, increasing possibility of bacterial contamination. Females who are sexually active, pregnant, or postmenopausal; use spermicides; or are being treated with antibiotics are at even greater risk (Kang et al., 2018; McLellan & Hunstad, 2016; Walsh & Collys, 2017). Other individuals at higher risk for UTIs include older adults, individuals with indwelling catheters, and patients with comorbid conditions (e.g., type 2 diabetes mellitus, neurogenic bladder, or urinary tract obstruction) (Rogers, 2023). Not all bacteria in the urine provoke an inflammatory response or an infection. When this occurs, it is a condition called asymptomatic bacteriuria, which does not harm urinary function (Rogers, 2023). The clinical manifestations connected with UTIs directly relate to the inflammatory process within the genitourinary system (Box 32.1). The inflammation in the bladder wall stimulates stretch receptors, initiating symptoms of bladder fullness with small volumes of urine and producing the urgency and frequency of urination associated with cystitis (Rogers, 2023). Stimulation of sensory nerves, located just beneath the urothelium, can invoke suprapubic, flank, or low back pain,

---

BOX 32.1 ■ Diversity Considerations

There is limited literature on the relationship between socioeconomic factors and urinary tract infections. One of the issues is the lack of nationwide population-based data from primary health care settings. However, the available studies show that unmet social needs are associated with an increased incidence of genitourinary conditions as well as worse symptom severity. Healthcare providers can help mitigate the negative effects of social determinants of health by screening for, addressing, and documenting any barriers or areas of concern for the patient (Jansaker & Sundquist, 2021; Stewart & Dedmon, 2022; Zwaschka et al., 2022).

BOX 32.2 ■ Older Adult Considerations

Urinary tract infection (UTI) is common in older adults, but the clinical manifestations are atypical. Common subjective and objective findings are urinary incontinence, poor appetite, drowsiness, frequent falls, hypotension, tachycardia, and delirium. UTI manifests mainly as delirium or confusion in the absence of fever. The usual diagnostic approach for delirium is to determine if there is a neurologic etiology. However, the majority of elderly patients presenting with delirium are the result of an infection, and the diagnostic approach should include a urine dipstick or urinalysis. Teaching older adults about managing bladder problems and drinking enough fluids can help prevent UTIs. Early treatment can keep UTIs from becoming serious enough that they require hospitalization (Dutta et al., 2022; Healthy People 2030, n.d.).

BOX 32.3 ■ Acute Care Considerations

Acute pyelonephritis is a common medical complication of pregnancy and is responsible for 12% of antepartum admissions to the intensive care unit. Pregnant females are at a greater risk of sepsis and septic shock from pyelonephritis, which makes the diagnosis of sepsis critical because a delay in treatment with antibiotics is associated with increased mortality. The findings in current studies propose soluble suppressor of tumorigenicity 2 (sST2) as a biomarker to identify patients at risk for bacteremia. Pregnant patients with acute pyelonephritis and bacteremia have a higher plasma sST2 concentration than those with a negative blood culture. In nonpregnant adults and in children, sST2 has been proposed as a biomarker for sepsis because elevated concentrations correlate with worse outcomes and increased mortality (Chatterton et al., 2023).

---

as well as dysuria. The timing of pain during urination can indicate the location of pathology. Pain occurring at the start of urination may indicate urethral pathology whereas pain occurring at the end of urination typically indicates bladder origin (Michels & Sands, 2015).

Physical Assessment

SUBJECTIVE

The most important subjective criteria for initially diagnosing a simple UTI are presenting symptoms of dysuria, increased urinary frequency, urgency, hematuria, and incontinence. Other complaints include malodorous urine, nocturia, and new onset of suprapubic pain (Ball et al., 2023; Kang et al., 2018). Complicated UTI symptoms include all of those listed above, along with systemic findings such as fever, chills, flank pain, or acute mental status changes, especially in the older adult population (Box 32.2). Individuals may report a history of cystitis symptoms lasting more than 7 days, known antibiotic resistance, recurrent UTI, permanent Foley or suprapubic catheter. The provider should be aware of high-risk patient populations, such as pregnant women

---

BOX 32.4 ■ Pediatric Considerations

Urinary tract infection (UTI) is one of the most common bacterial infections in childhood. There is a growing concern of antibiotic resistance in the pediatric population with the increasing prevalence of pediatric community–acquired UTI by extended spectrum beta-lactamase-producing *Escherichia coli*. UTIs affect approximately 11% of females and 4% of males by age 16 years, but infection varies by age, gender, and circumcision status. Continuous antibiotic prophylaxis has been used in the past for recurrent UTI; however, it is no longer recommended in children with previous UTI, recurrent UTI, vesicular reflux, hydronephrosis, or neurogenic bladder (Autore et al., 2023; Collingwood et al., 2023a, 2023b; Leung et al., 2019).

(Box 32.3), persons that are immunocompromised, have a history of renal failure, renal transplant, neurogenic or dysfunctional bladder, or are immediate posturologic surgery. Some pediatric patients are also at a higher risk (Box 32.4). A medical history of vaginitis, prostatitis, sexually transmitted infections (see Chapter 40), bladder stones (see Chapter 31), reactive arthritis (see Chapter 8), and genitourinary dermatitis may align with a complicated UTI or provide clues of potential differential diagnoses (Ball et al., 2023; Kang et al., 2018; Rogers, 2020).

OBJECTIVE*

The physical exam is typically normal for uncomplicated UTIs.

Generalized: *Fever, chills*

Neurological: *Confusion or mental status changes* (more common in geriatric population)

Cardiovascular: *Tachycardia; hypotension*

Gastrointestinal: Nausea; vomiting

Genitourinary: Urinary frequency; urinary urgency; incontinence; hematuria; dysuria; suprapubic tenderness; hesitancy

Integumentary: Inspection for dermatologic conditions related to fungal infection or irritation and breakdown from incontinence (Algorithm 32.1)

(Ball et al., 2023; Kang et al., 2018; Michels & Sands, 2015)

Evaluation and Differential Diagnoses

DIAGNOSTICS

- Urinalysis with urine culture and sensitivity
- Urine dipstick: Positive nitrates and leukocyte esterase on the dipstick analysis are accurate indicators of a UTI.
- Ultrasound (kidney and/or bladder)
- Computed tomography (CT) scan: Reserve use for complicated UTI (febrile), atypical symptoms, inadequate response to antibiotic treatment, or obstruction suspected
- Cystoscopy and upper tract imaging should not be routinely obtained in the patient presenting with a recurring UTI.
- Screening for asymptomatic bacteriuria is only recommended for pregnant females and individuals who will be undergoing invasive urologic procedures.

(Nicolle et al., 2019)

---

*Hallmark signs are bolded and **Red flags are bolded and underlined**. A patient with a complicated UTI may present with systemic symptoms. *Systemic symptoms are italicized.*

DIFFERENTIAL DIAGNOSES

- Overactive bladder
- Interstitial cystitis/bladder pain syndrome
- Urolithiasis
- Sexually transmitted infection

Plan

GUIDELINE RESOURCES

- American Urological Association. (2022). Recurrent uncomplicated urinary tract infections in women: AUA/CUA/SUFU guideline (2022). https://www.auanet.org/guidelines-and-quality/guidelines/recurrent-uti.
- Gupta, K., Hooton, T. M., Naber, K. G., Colgan, R., Miller, L. G., Moran, G. J., Nicolle, L. E., Raz, R., Schaeffer, A. J., Soper, D. E., & Florida, M. (2011). International clinical practice guidelines for the treatment of acute uncomplicated cystitis and pyelonephritis in women: A 2010 update by the Infectious Diseases Society of America and the European Society for Microbiology and Infectious Diseases. *Clinical Infectious Diseases, 52*(5), e103–e120. https://doi.org/10.1093/cid/ciq257.
- National Institute for Health and Care Excellence. (2018). Urinary tract infection (lower): Antimicrobial prescribing. https://www.nice.org.uk/guidance/ng109.
- Nicolle, L. E., Gupta, K., Bradley, S. F., Colgan, R., DeMuri, G. P., Drekonja, D., Eckert, L. O., Geerlings, S. E., Köves, B., Hooton, T. M., Juthani-Mehta, M., Knight, S. L., Saint, S., Schaeffer, A. J., Trautner, B., Wullt, B., & Siemieniuk, R. (2019). Clinical practice guideline for the management of asymptomatic bacteriuria: 2019 update by the Infectious Diseases Society of America. *Clinical Infectious Diseases, 68*(10), e83–e110. https://doi.org/10.1093/cid/ciy1121.

Pharmacotherapy

- Initial pharmacotherapy should be tailored based on the infecting uropathogen if known from culture.
- Empiric pharmacotherapy for unknown pathogens is dependent on severity, local resistance patterns, and local antibiogram for the treatment of symptomatic UTIs.
- Do not treat asymptomatic bacteriuria with antibiotics.

ACUTE UNCOMPLICATED CYSTITIS

Current treatment guidelines recommend three options for first-line treatment of acute uncomplicated cystitis (Algorithm 32.1):
- Nitrofurantoin 100 mg twice daily for 5 days *OR*
- Trimethoprim/sulfamethoxazole 160/800 mg [1 double-strength tablet] twice daily for 3 days *OR*
- Fosfomycin 3 g in a single dose

**Use fluoroquinolone where prevalence of resistance of community uropathogen(s) is not known to exceed 10%.

***If prevalence of fluoroquinolone resistance exceeds 10%, an initial intravenous dose of a long-acting parenteral antimicrobial (e.g., ceftriaxone) or a consolidated 24-hour dose of an aminoglycoside is recommended.

Second-line treatment options for acute uncomplicated cystitis include fluoroquinolones or beta-lactam. Because of antimicrobial resistance, these are not considered first-line therapy (Gupta et al., 2011; Kang et al., 2018):

- Fluoroquinolone** Refer to "Guidline Resources" section above for dosages
- Beta-lactam*** Refer to "Guidline Resources" section above for dosages

No posttreatment test of cure urinalysis or urine culture in asymptomatic patients is needed (Anger et al., 2019; Nicolle et al., 2019).

PYELONEPHRITIS, COMPLICATED UTI

Current pharmacotherapy guidelines for pyelonephritis (not requiring hospitalization) recommend empiric therapy with a broader-spectrum antibiotic while awaiting culture and sensitivity results (Gupta et al., 2011; Kang et al., 2018). Once the uropathogen is known, continue the current antibiotic regimen if the pathogen is susceptible, or change to a microorganism-specific antibiotic based on susceptibility (Gupta et al., 2011; Kang et al., 2018) (Algorithm 32.1).

- Fluoroquinolones**
  - Ciprofloxacin 1000 mg extended release for 7 days OR
  - Levofloxacin 750 mg for 5 days
- Beta-lactam***
  - Ceftriaxone 1 g initial IV dose***

The US Food and Drug Administration recommends both clinical response (symptom resolution with no new UTI symptoms) *and* microbiological response (urine culture) <1000 CFU/mL to determine the eradication of complicated UTIs (Wagenlehner et al., 2020).

NONPHARMACOTHERAPY

- Educate
  - Correct use of antibiotics regarding dosing, completing full treatment even if feeling better, and avoiding inappropriate antimicrobial drug use
  - Self-care practices: Urinate regularly and postcoital voiding; wipe genitalia from the front toward the back after micturition; avoid douching; avoid scrubbing and use of harsh cleansing products on the genitalia.
- Lifestyle and behavioral modifications
  - Adequate oral hydration
  - Avoid common irritants: Coffee, citrus, and spermicides
  - Engage in safe-sex practices.
- Complementary treatment
  - Complementary and alternative therapies with natural medicines and supplements may interact with prescription medications. Obtain a complete medication history.
- Referral
  - Consider a referral to a specialist in urology for gross hematuria, incontinence, relapsing infections, and complicated infections.
  - Obstruction, urosepsis, and septic shock are medical emergencies that require referral to the emergency department.
- Follow-up
  - No follow-up is required for UTI unless symptoms remain or worsen.

(Clemens et al., 2022; Kang et al., 2018; McLellan & Hunstad, 2016; Mohiuddin, 2019)

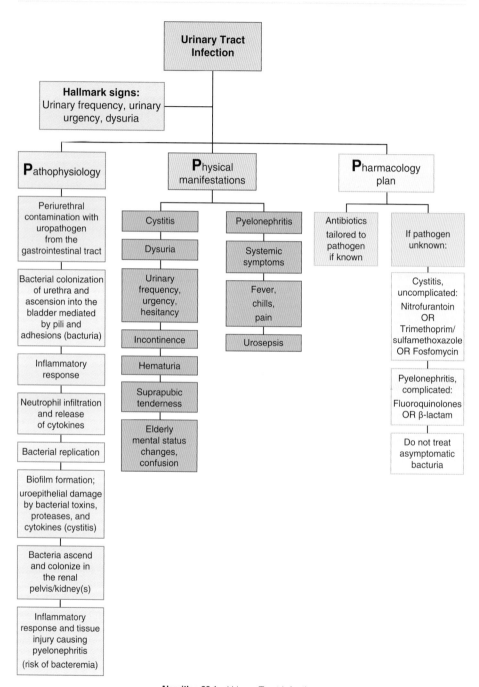

Algorithm 32.1   Urinary Tract Infection

References

Anger, J., Lee, U., Ackerman, A. L., Chou, R., Chughtai, B., Clemens, J. Q., Hickling, D., Kapoor, A., Kenton, K. S., Kaufman, M. R., Rondanina, M. A., Stapleton, A., Stothers, L., & Chai, T. C. (2019). Recurrent uncomplicated urinary tract infections in women: AUA/CUA/SUFU guideline. *Journal of Urology, 202*(2), 282–289.

Autore, G., Bernardi, L., Ghidini, F., La Scola, C., Berardi, A., Biasucci, G., Marchetti, F., Pasini, A., Capra, M. E., Castellini, C., Cioni, V., Cantatore, S., Cella, A., Cusenza, F., De Fanti, A., Della Casa Muttini, E., Di Costanzo, M., Dozza, A., & Gatti, C., … The Uti-Ped-Er Study Group. (2023). Antibiotic prophylaxis for the prevention of urinary tract infections in children: Guideline and recommendations from the Emilia-Romagna pediatric urinary tract infections (UTI-Ped-ER) Study Group. *Antibiotics, 12*(6), 1040. https://doi.org/10.3390/antibiotics12061040.

Ball, J. W., Dains, J. E., Flynn, J. A., Solomon, B. S., & Stewart, R. W. (2023). *Seidel's guide to physical examination* (10th ed.). Elsevier Health Sciences.

Burchum, J., & Rosenthal, L. D. (2021). *Lehne's pharmacotherapeutics for advanced practice nurses and physician assistants* (2nd ed.). Elsevier Health Sciences.

Chatterton, C., Romero, R., Jung, E., Gallo, D. M., Suksai, M., Diaz-Primera, R., Erez, O., Chaemsaithong, P., Tarca, A. L., Gotsch, F., Bosco, M., & Chaiworapongsa, T. (2023). A biomarker for bacteremia in pregnant women with acute pyelonephritis: Soluble suppressor of tumorigenicity 2 or sST2. *Journal of Maternal-Fetal & Neonatal Medicine, 36*(1), 2183470. https://doi.org/10.1080/14767058.2023.2183470.

Collingwood, J. D., Yarbrough, A. H., Boppana, S. B., & Dangle, P. P. (2023a). Increasing prevalence of pediatric community-acquired UTI by extended spectrum β-lactamase-producing E. coli: Cause for concern. *Pediatric Infectious Disease Journal, 42*(2), 106–109. https://doi.org/10.1097/INF.0000000000003777.

Collingwood, J. D., Wang, L., Aban, I. B., Yarbrough, A. H., Boppana, S. B., & Dangle, P. P. (2023b). Risk factors for community acquired pediatric urinary tract infection with extended-spectrum-β-lactamase Escherichia coli: A case-control study. *Journal of Pediatric Urology, 19*(1), 129.e1–129.e7. https://doi.org/10.1016/j.jpurol.2022.10.020.

Clemens, J. Q., Erickson, D. R., Varela, N. P., & Lai, H. H. (2022). Diagnosis and treatment of interstitial cystitis/bladder pain syndrome. *Journal of Urology, 208*(1), 34–42.

Dutta, C., Pasha, K., Paul, S., Abbas, M. S., Nassar, S. T., Tasha, T., Desai, A., Bajgain, A., Ali, A., & Mohammed, L. (2022). Urinary tract infection induced delirium in elderly patients: A systematic review. *Cureus, 14*(12), e32321. https://doi.org/10.7759/cureus.32321.

Gupta, K., Hooton, T. M., Naber, K. G., Wullt, B., Colgan, R., Miller, L. G., Moran, G. J., Nicolle, L. E., Raz, R., Schaeffer, A. J., & Soper, D. E. (2011). International clinical practice guidelines for the treatment of acute uncomplicated cystitis and pyelonephritis in women: A 2010 update by the Infectious Diseases Society of America and the European Society for Microbiology and Infectious Diseases. *Clinical Infectious Diseases, 52*(5), e103–e120.

Jansåker, F., Li, X., & Sundquist, K. (2021). Sociodemographic factors and uncomplicated cystitis in women aged 15–50 years: a nationwide Swedish cohort registry study (1997–2018). *The Lancet Regional Health - Europe 4*(78) 100108. https://doi.org/10.1016/j.lanepe.2021.100108.

Kang, C. I., Kim, J., Park, D. W., Kim, B. N., Ha, U. S., Lee, S. J., Yeo, J. K., Min, S. K., Lee, H., & Wie, S. H. (2018). Clinical practice guidelines for the antibiotic treatment of community acquired urinary tract infections. *Infection and Chemotherapy, 50*(1), 67–100.

Lajiness, B., & Lajiness, M. J. (2019). 50 years of urinary tract infections and treatments: Has much changed? *Urologic Nursing, 39*(5), 235–239.

Leung, A. K. C., Wong, A. H. C., Leung, A. A. M., & Hon, K. L. (2019). Urinary tract infection in children. *Recent Patents on Inflammation & Allergy Drug Discovery, 13*(1), 2–18. https://doi.org/10.2174/18722 13X13666181228154940.

McLellan, L. K., & Hunstad, D. A. (2016). Urinary tract infection: Pathogenesis and outlook. *Trends in Molecular Medicine, 22*(11), 946–957.

Michels, T. C., & Sands, J. E. (2015). Dysuria: Evaluation and differential diagnosis in adults. *American Family Physician, 92*(9), 778–786.

Mohiuddin, A. K. (2019). Alternative management of uncomplicated cystitis in women. *Journal of Urology and Nephrology, 2*(2), 147–151.

Nicolle, L. E., Gupta, K., Bradley, S. F., Colgan, R., DeMuri, G. P., Drekonja, D., Eckert, L. O., Geerlings, S. E., Köves, B., Hooton, T. M., Juthani-Mehta, M., Knight, S. H., Saint, S., Schaeffer, A. J., Trautner, B., Wullt, B., & Siemieniuk, R. (2019). Clinical practice guideline for the management of asymptomatic bacteriuria: 2019 update by the Infectious Diseases Society of America. *Clinical Infectious Disease, 68*(10), 1611–1615.

Rogers, J. (2023). Alterations of renal and urinary tract function. In J. L. Rogers (Ed.), *McCance and Huether's pathophysiology: The biologic basis for disease in adults and children* (9th ed., pp. 1232–1269). Mosby-Elsevier.

Rogers, J. (2020). Understanding the most commonly billed diagnoses in primary care: Urinary tract infections. *Nurse Practitioner, 45*(11), 35–40. http://doi.org/10.1097/01.NPR.0000718516.64801.27.

Stewart, C. W., & Dedmon, D. (2022). Impact of social determinants of health on adherence to urinary tract infection treatment recommendations: A scoping review. *[Doctoral project, University of Tennessee Health Science Center]. UTHSC Digital Commons.* http://doi.org/10.21007/con.dnp.2022.0022; https://dc.uthsc.edu/dnp/22.

U.S. Department of Health and Human Services. (n.d.). Reduce the rate of hospital admissions for urinary tract infections among older adults – OA-07. Healthy People 2030. https://health.gov/healthypeople/objectives-and-data/browse-objectives/infectious-disease/reduce-rate-hospital-admissions-urinary-tract-infections-among-older-adults-oa-07.

Wagenlehner, F. M. E., Bjerklund Johansen, T. E., Cai, T., Koves, B., Kranz, J., Pilatz, A., & Tandogdu, Z. (2020). Epidemiology, definition and treatment of complicated urinary tract infections. *Nature Reviews Urology, 17*(10), 586–600.

Walsh, C., & Collys, T. (2017). The pathophysiology of urinary tract infections. *Surgery, 35*(6), 293–298.

Zwaschka, T. A., Sebesta, E. M., Gleicher, S., Kaufman, M. R., Dmochowski, R. R., & Reynolds, W. S. (2022). The cumulative effect of unmet social needs on noncancerous genitourinary conditions and severity of lower urinary tract symptoms. *Neurourology and Urodynamics, 41*(8), 1862–1871. https://doi.org/10.1002/nau.25038.

Integumentary System

SECTION OUTLINE

33 Acne Vulgaris

34 Contact Dermatitis

35 Psoriasis

36 Malignant Skin Lesions

37 Integumentary Infections

CHAPTER 33

Acne Vulgaris

Jodi Allen ▪ Corrine M. Djuric

Acne Vulgaris

Acne vulgaris is one of the most common cutaneous conditions in the United States and one of the most common skin complaints seen in primary care. Approximately 85% of teenagers are affected by acne vulgaris, with the highest prevalence occurring between ages 12 and 25 years (Patel & Cohen, 2021). In recent years, diagnosis is on the rise in females aged 25 to 35 years (Shah et al., 2021). Although 80% of acne vulgaris cases occur in females, it is often more severe in males, with typical improvement as the person ages (Box 33.1) (Nicol & O'Haver, 2023). Acne vulgaris is present across all ethnic groups; however, ethnic differences in presentation have been identified (Box 33.2) (Shah et al., 2021). Risk for and severity of acne vulgaris increases in persons who have a family history of the diagnosis (Heng & Chew, 2020). A person's diet can increase their risk for acne vulgaris, especially if it is composed of high-fat and sugary foods. Prevalence of acne vulgaris in overweight and obese persons has been found to be higher than in normal and underweight persons (Heng & Chew, 2020). Acne presentation can range from mild to disfiguring and can cause significant psychological distress, low self-esteem, anxiety, and depression (Box 33.3) (Patel & Cohen, 2021).

Pathophysiology

Acne vulgaris development begins in the sebaceous gland and hair follicle, called the pilosebaceous unit, which are located primarily on the face, upper chest, upper arms, and back. Obstruction in the follicular canal by debris can cause noninflammatory and inflammatory changes. In noninflammatory acne vulgaris, the comedones are open or closed, with accumulated debris that causes obstruction, distention, and thinning of the follicular canal wall. Open comedones present as "blackheads" and closed comedones present as "whiteheads." Comedones reflect a defect in the desquamation at the opening of the pilosebaceous follicle. Shedding does not occur or is reduced, causing the epithelial cells along with keratin and sebum debris to become sticky and form blockages (see Algorithm 33.1). Inflammatory acne, or nodulocystic acne, develops when the closed comedone follicular wall erupts. This event causes sebum to be expelled into the surrounding dermis, forming inflammatory pustules and nodules that can be quite painful. Noninflammatory, open and closed, and inflammatory lesions can occur in the same person. The main hormones responsible for the development of acne vulgaris are androgens (dehydroepiandrosterone sulfate and testosterone) that are manufactured in large amounts during puberty (Nicol & O'Haver, 2023).

Physical Clinical Presentation

SUBJECTIVE

During the focused history, documentation should include the onset of symptoms; precipitating events; location, intensity, and quality of pain (if any); progression of symptoms; alleviating and aggravating factors; previous episodes; and associated symptoms. Persons with acne vulgaris will

BOX 33.1 ■ Older Adult Considerations

While rare, older adults can develop acne vulgaris. Older adults who experience depression, anxiety, and high levels of stress, often related to loss of a loved one or inability to live independently, can suddenly see acne vulgaris appear. Despite aging, the body continues to produce hormones such as testosterone in response to stress, which can cause sebaceous glands to increase oil production. Reducing stress levels and proper skin hygiene are the best treatment for older adults with acne vulgaris, as pharmacologic treatment side effects can be exacerbated with age and comorbid conditions (Home Care Assistance, 2020).

BOX 33.2 ■ Diversity Considerations

Ethnic differences in presentation of acne vulgaris have been identified, specifically in darker skin types. Papular lesions are the most common type of acne lesion identified in persons across all skin types; however, postinflammatory hyperpigmentation and hyperpigmented macules more commonly affect those with darker skin types. Black persons tend to have more comedonal acne while White and Asian persons tend to have more inflammatory acne. Hispanic persons tend to have more pustular lesions with subsequent scarring versus Asian and Black persons. Keloidal scarring, which is not a common complication of acne, tends to be identified in darker skin types as well. Understanding the variety of presentations across different skin types in acne vulgaris can provide insight to person-centered treatment (Powers et al., 2022).

BOX 33.3 ■ Pediatric Considerations

The overwhelming majority of persons cared for with acne vulgaris will be those within the pediatric population. Acne typically starts at the onset of puberty (in females, age 12 to 13 years; in males, age 14 to 15 years) and can ebb and flow in comedone and/or lesion development. While not a serious physical disorder, acne vulgaris has been associated with psychological distress and decreased emotional well-being. Depression screening tools such as the modified PHQ-9 for adolescents/teens should be used to aid in identification of depression and suicidal ideation (Bland, 2020).

typically present with comedones and/or nodulocystic lesions to the face, upper chest, upper arms, and/or back and admit to self-treatment with over-the-counter products that do not often alleviate the acne, leaving skin dry and irritated. Ascertain which over-the-counter products were tried and failed. Menses, sports participation, and stress can exacerbate acne in females and stress and sports participation can exacerbate acne in males. Persons will not report pain unless nodulocystic acne is present. Asking about family history of acne vulgaris can further guide diagnosis as can a social history that identifies a high-fat/high-sugar diet consumed by the person. A medication review can identify a secondary cause of acne vulgaris, specifically corticosteroids, thyroid hormones, certain antibiotics, and antiepileptic drugs. Some cosmetic products and generally poor skin hygiene can cause acne vulgaris to proliferate (Patel & Cohen, 2021).

OBJECTIVE*

Musculoskeletal: **Pain in bones or joints** with inflammatory acne (Box 33.4)

Integumentary: **<5-mm dome-shaped, smooth skin-colored white or gray papules or <5-mm papules with a central orifice containing brown or black material** (noninflammatory

---

*Hallmark signs are bolded and Red flags are bolded and underlined.

BOX 33.4 ■ Acute Care Considerations

Acne fulminans is a rare acute eruption of large inflammatory nodules in addition to ulcers and hemorrhagic crusts that is often mistaken for other dermatologic infections. This condition most frequently affects male adolescents with preexisting acne. It is most often triggered by isotretinoin therapy but can occur spontaneously. Systemic symptoms such as fever, malaise, and pain in bones and joints often manifest. Laboratory abnormalities such as leukocytosis, anemia, and elevated erythrocyte sedimentation rate (ESR) or C-reactive protein levels can aid in identification. Osteolytic lesions of the bone, most commonly at the sternum, clavicles, sacroiliac joints, or hips, can be identified on X-ray. Swift treatment is needed to decrease the risk of severe scarring of the affected tissue(s) (McKegney & Schneider, 2022).

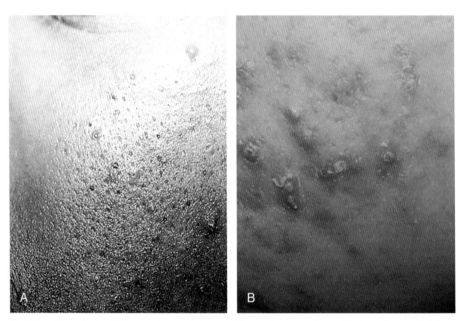

Fig. 33.1   Acne vulgaris. (A) Acne vulgaris with few noninflammatory comedones. (B) Comedones with inflammatory pustules. (From Zitelli, B. J., McIntire, S. C., & Nowalk, A. J. (2012). *Zitelli and Davis' atlas of pediatric physical diagnosis* (6th ed.). St. Louis, MO: Saunders.)

acne); **superficial (<5 mm) papules and pustules or deep, inflamed, tender papules (>5 mm)** (inflammatory acne) (Figs. 33.1 and 33.2) (see Algorithm 33.1)

Psychiatric: Feelings of sadness related to lack of self-esteem secondary to acne (Zaenglein et al., 2016)

Evaluation and Differential Diagnoses

DIAGNOSTICS

- No laboratory or imaging studies are required for the diagnosis of acne vulgaris. Patients with signs of hyperandrogenism or early onset puberty should be evaluated for this separately (Patel & Cohen, 2021).

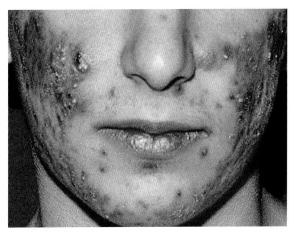

Fig. 33.2 Nodulocystic acne vulgaris. (From Paller, A. S., & Mancini, A. J. (2016). *Hurwitz clinical pediatric dermatology, a textbook of skin disorders of childhood and adolescence* (5th ed.). Philadelphia, Elsevier.)

DIFFERENTIAL DIAGNOSES

- Rosacea: Will present with erythema, telangiectasias, and papules or pustules on the central face but will not have comedones; is more common in adults and older adults
- Molluscum contagiosum: Caused by a virus and not specific to pilosebaceous units. The lesion appears as a firm, localized, dome-shaped papule (2–5 mm) with a shiny surface and central indentation but lacking the presence of open or closed comedones.
- Folliculitis: Lacks the presence of comedones and will be pruritic

(Nicol & O'Haver, 2023)

Plan

GUIDELINE RESOURCES

- Zaenglein, A. L., Pathy, A. L., Schlosser, B. J., Alikhan, A., Baldwin, H. E., Berson, D. S., Bowe, W. P., Graber, E. M., Harper, J. C., Kang, S., Keri, J. E., Leyden, J. L., Reynolds, R. V., Silverberg, N. B., Stein, L. F., Tollefson, M. M., Weiss, J. A., Dolan, N. C., Sagan, A. A., … Bhushan, R. (2016). Guidelines of care for the management of acne vulgaris. *Journal of the American Academy of Dermatology*, *74*(5), 945–973.e33. https://doi.org/10.1016/j.jaad.2015.12.037

Pharmacotherapy

The treatment of acne vulgaris is determined by severity (mild, moderate, or severe) (see Algorithm 33.1).

- Mild (primarily noninflammatory comedones with occasional small papules)
  - Benzoyl peroxide (BP) *OR* topical retinoid** *OR* topical combination therapy (BP + antibiotic, retinoid[2] + antibiotic, or retinoid[2] + BP + antibiotic):

**Avoid use of retinoid or isotretinoin in pregnant females. Any female who is of childbearing age planning to start isotretinoin (pregnancy category X) must have two negative pregnancy tests within 1 week of prescribing and two reliable forms of contraception (unless abstinence is their chosen method). Monthly pregnancy tests must be done thereafter. The female must maintain effective contraception 1 month before, during, and after therapy due to isotretinoin being a potent teratogen (Skidmore-Roth, 2022).

- Benzoyl peroxide:
  - 2.5% to 20% gel; 5% to 10% cream; 5% to 20% lotion or wash
- Topical retinoids:
  - Tretinoin: 0.025% to 0.1% cream or gel
  - Tazarotene: 0.05% to 0.1% cream, gel, or foam
  - Adapalene: 0.1% to 0.3% cream; 0.1% lotion
- Topical antibiotic:
  - Clindamycin: 1% solution, lotion or gel
  - Erythromycin: 2% solution, cream, gel, or lotion
- Moderate (mainly inflammatory lesions such as papules and pustules)
  - Topical combination therapy:
    - BP + antibiotic *OR* retinoid[2] + BP *OR* retinoid[2] + BP + antibiotic *OR* oral antibiotic + topical retinoid[2] + BP *OR* oral antibiotic + topical retinoid[2] + BP + topical antibiotic:
      - Oral antibiotics (doxycycline and minocycline are more effective than tetracycline; use for limited to shortest duration possible; reserve erythromycin use for those who cannot use tetracyclines, such as pregnant females or children <8 years of age):
        - Minocycline: 50–100 mg orally twice daily
        - Doxycycline: 50–100 mg orally twice daily
        - Tetracycline: 250–500 mg orally twice daily initially then 125–500 mg daily when improvement noted
        - Erythromycin: 250–500 mg orally twice daily
- Severe (lesions are mostly nodules and cysts)
  - Oral antibiotics + topical combination therapy (BP + antibiotic *OR* retinoid[2] + BP *OR* retinoid[2] + BP + antibiotic *OR* oral isotretinoin[2])

(Zaenglein et al., 2016)

NONPHARMACOTHERAPY

- Educate
  - Person and family about acne vulgaris, treatments (including length of treatment), likely side effects of treatment, and avoidance of exacerbation triggers (e.g., high-fat/high-sugar diet, infrequently washed sports paraphernalia, cosmetic products, and stress), and provide support related to psychological stressors
  - Proper skin hygiene, including washing the face twice daily with mild soap such as Dove, Neutrogena, or Aveeno cleansing bar. Avoid scrubbing, rubbing, picking, and squeezing acne. Comedone extractors can cause scarring and should not be used.
  - All products used on the face should be labeled as "noncomedogenic."
  - Use of sunscreen with all acne medication
- Lifestyle
  - Diets with a low glycemic load have been found to reduce acne lesions; diets with increased omega-3 and omega-6 fatty acid intake have been shown to improve acne vulgaris as well (Baldwin & Tan, 2021).
  - Stress reduction activities
- Referral
  - Dermatology if there is poor response to standard treatment or at any point when the treatment modality exceeds the experience of the clinician. If the person has severe acne vulgaris and/or desires to use isotretinoin, they should be evaluated and monitored by Dermatology.

- Follow-up
  - Every 4 to 6 weeks to monitor response to treatment and until lesions resolve or only a few new lesions appear every 2 weeks
  - Evaluate oral antibiotic use at least every 3 to 4 months.

(Eichenfield et al., 2021; Zaenglein et al., 2016)

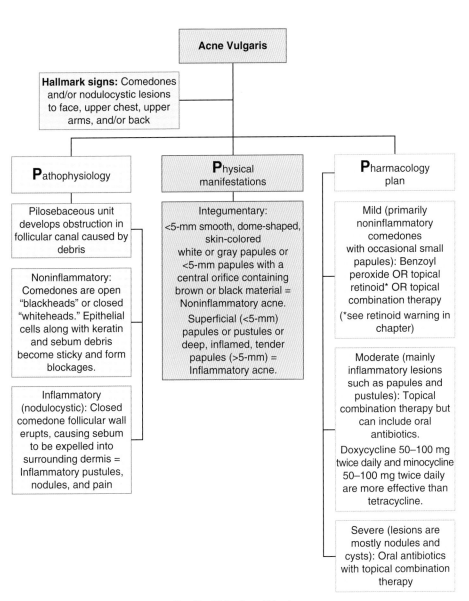

Algorithm 33.1   Acne Vulgaris

References

Baldwin, H., & Tan, J. (2021). Effects of diet on acne and its response to treatment. *American Journal of Clinical Dermatology, 22*(1), 55–65. https://doi.org/10.1007/s40257-020-00542-y.

Bland, T. B (2020). Dermatologic disorders. In D. L. Maaks, N. Starr, M. A. Brady, N. M. Gaylord, M. Driessnack, & K. G. Duderrstadt (Eds.), *Burns' pediatric primary care* (7th ed., pp. 593–596). Elsevier.

Eichenfield, D. Z., Sprague, J., & Eichenfield, L. F. (2021). Management of acne vulgaris, a review. *Journal of the American Medical Association, 326*(20), 2055–2067. https://doi.org/10.1001/jama.2021.17633.

Heng, A. H. S., & Chew, F. T. (2020). Systematic review of the epidemiology of acne vulgaris. *Scientific Reports, 10*, 5754. https://doi.org/10.1038/s41598-020-62715-3.

Home Care Assistance (2020). *Why do some seniors get acne?* https://www.homecareassistanceanchorage.com/what-causes-acne-in-older-adults/#:~:text=Seniors%20who%20experience%20depression%2C%20anxiety,aging%20adults%20may%20become%20stressed.

McKegney, C. C., & Schneider, D. (2022). A case of acne fulminans. *Journal of Pediatric Health Care, 36*(6), 603–606. https://doi.org/10.1016/j.pedhc.2022.06.005.

Nicol, N. H., & O'Haver, J (2023). Alterations of the integument in children. In R. L. Rogers (Ed.), *McCance and Huether's pathophysiology: The biologic basis for disease in adults and children* (9th ed., pp. 1541–1546). Mosby-Elsevier.

Patel, K., & Cohen, B. A. (2021). Acne vulgaris in teenagers. *Contemporary Pediatrics, 38*(8), 32. https://www.contemporarypediatrics.com/view/acne-vulgaris-in-teenagers.

Powers, C., Huynh, T., & Badon, H. (2022). Dermatologic differences in a diverse population. *Contemporary Pediatrics, 40*(5), 14–17. https://www.contemporarypediatrics.com/view/dermatologic-differences-diverse-population.

Shah, N., Shukla, R., Chaudhari, P., Patil, S., Patil, A., Nadkarni, N., & Goldust, M. (2021). Prevalence of acne vulgaris and its clinic-epidemiological pattern in adult patients: Results of a prospective, observational study. *Journal of Cosmetic Dermatology, 20*(11), 3672–3678. https://doi.org/10.1111/jocd.14040.

Skidmore-Roth, L. (2022). *Mosby's nursing drug reference* (35th ed.). Elsevier.

Zaenglein, A. L., Pathy, A. L., Scholsser, B. J., Alikhan, A., Baldwin, H. E., Berson, D. S., Bowe, W. P., Graber, E. M., Harper, J. C., Kang, S., Keri, J. E., Leyden, J. L., Reynolds, R. V., Silverberg, N. B., Stein, L. F., Tollefson, M. M., Weiss, J. A., Dolan, N. C., Sagan, A. A., … Bhushan, R. (2016). Guidelines of care for the management of acne vulgaris. *Journal of the American Academy of Dermatology, 74*(5), 945–973. https://doi.org/10.1016/j.jaad.2015.12.037.

Contact Dermatitis

Jodi Allen ▓ Corrine M. Djuric

Allergic and Irritant Contact Dermatitis

Contact dermatitis (CD) is an overarching term describing an eczematous eruption caused by either a delayed hypersensitive reaction to an allergen (allergic contact dermatitis or ACD) or a direct irritation to the skin from a substance (irritant contact dermatitis or ICD) (Box 34.1). The process is marked by a nonspecific inflammatory response and intracellular edema (Nicol & O'Haver, 2023). A prior exposure is not a factor in either reaction. An estimated 5.7 million health care visits per year are related to CD (Fonacier & Feldman, 2020). All age groups are affected, though females slightly more so than males, with an increased prevalence in infants (Box 34.2) and older adults (Box 34.3). Of all cases of occupational skin disease in industrialized countries, 85% to 95% are directly related to CD, with the hands being the most common site for manifestation (Fonacier & Feldman, 2020). All persons are at risk for developing CD, though age, occupation, and history of atopic dermatitis increase risk (Nicol & O'Haver, 2023). The most common allergens to cause AD are nickel, neomycin, fragrance mix, cobalt, and poison ivy, the latter which is thought to be the most common cause in the United States (Fig. 34.1). The most common irritants to cause ICD are detergents, cleansers, moisturizers, and shampoos (Fig. 34.2) (Nicol & O'Haver, 2023).

Pathophysiology

ALLERGIC CONTACT DERMATITIS

ACD begins with the contact of an offending agent with the skin. A T cell–mediated allergic response follows. The first phase, the sensitivity phase, occurs when the allergen penetrates the stratum corneum of the epidermis and is taken up by Langerhans cells. The antigens get identified on the surface of the cells and contact T lymphocytes. Clonal expansion and cytokines create a proliferation of the antigen-specific T lymphocytes and migrate back to the epidermis. This phase can take days or months. The second phase, the elicitation phase, occurs when antigen-specific T lymphocytes present in the skin combine with the subsequent exposures to the allergen to produce a localized inflammatory response (see Algorithm 34.1). The intensity of the response is dependent on the sensitizing ability of the allergen and the concentration of the allergen present (Nicol & O'Haver, 2023).

IRRITANT CONTACT DERMATITIS

ICD begins with a disruption of the outermost layer of the epidermis, the stratum corneum, after a single or repetitive exposure to an irritant. This disruption is typically caused by chemical or physical irritation, which increases transepidermal water loss (Nicol & O'Haver, 2023). The mechanisms of damage to the skin barrier are dependent on the intrinsic nature of the irritant

---

BOX 34.1 ■ **Acute Care Considerations**

Contact dermatitis does not often require acute care; however, the hypersensitivity reactions that can precipitate allergic contact dermatitis can also increase the risk for anaphylactic reactions. Irritant exposure that can precipitate irritant contact dermatitis can also increase the need for acute care, particularly if the exposure is prolonged, which can lead to a secondary chemical burn of the skin. Persons with allergic contact dermatitis and irritant contact dermatitis should be educated on signs of anaphylaxis and when to seek emergency care if this occurs. An allergist can assist in determining the severity of the allergen's effects and whether an EpiPen needs to be carried at all times (Fonacier et al., 2015).

BOX 34.2 ■ **Pediatric Considerations**

Diaper dermatitis (Fig. 34.2), a common form of irritant contact dermatitis, has decreased in prevalence since the development of disposable diapers. Chemical irritation occurs due to prolonged contact with urine and/or feces and mechanical irritation occurs from diapers rubbing on skinfolds. If a rash or irritation is noted around the child's anus, diarrhea is typically the cause; if a rash or irritation is noted on the skin but not on the skinfolds, urine is often responsible. Keeping the diaper area clean and dry is paramount to prevention, which usually requires frequent diaper changes. Protective barrier ointments such as Desitin or A&D at the first sign of irritation can limit severity. Leaving the usual diapered area open to air 3 to 4 times daily often alleviates this form of irritant contact dermatitis (Bland, 2020).

BOX 34.3 ■ **Older Adult Considerations**

Allergic contact dermatitis (ACD) is common in older adults. Those who have stasis dermatitis, chronic wounds, and chronic venous insufficiency have an increased prevalence of sensitization due to frequent exposure to topical treatments. This can cause challenges in prescribing topical treatments for ACD, which limits improvement of symptoms. Pruritis related to ACD that is left untreated can increase the risk for older adults to scratch and instigate secondary infections due in part to diminished immune function. A cascade of negative effects can ensue, highlighting the importance of allergen removal, allergen avoidance, and proper skin hygiene in the care of ACD in older adults (Lima et al., 2019).

---

itself. Damage to the skin barrier activates innate immune responses and ignites the inflammatory cascade (see Algorithm 34.2). Chronic ICD is less understood; however, it is postulated that chronic downregulation of the inflammatory response is responsible (Nicol & O'Haver, 2023).

Physical Clinical Presentation

SUBJECTIVE

Clinical presentation between ACD and ICD can be similar, making diagnosis challenging. During the focused history, documentation should include the onset of symptoms; precipitating events; location, intensity, and quality of pain (if any); progression of symptoms; alleviating and aggravating factors; previous episodes; and associated symptoms. Determining whether new or prolonged exposure to new or unusual substances has occurred is imperative to identify the potential trigger of ACD or ICD. Persons will typically report rash, pain, burning, and/or pruritis at the site(s) affected, though ACD typically produces more pruritis while ICD produces more burning. The most commonly affected sites are the hands, face, and neck, though any area of the skin can be affected. Asking about a previous history of atopic dermatitis as well as family history of atopic dermatitis and ACD is helpful to differentiate between ACD and ICD. Social history including occupational exposures can be beneficial in determining the underlying cause of either ACD or ICD (Bland, 2020; Nicol & O'Haver, 2023).

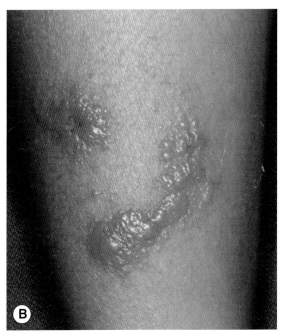

Fig. 34.1 Contact dermatitis, allergic. Characteristic linear vesicular eruption of the forearms related to exposure to poison ivy. (From Mancini, A. J., & Paller, A. S. (2020). *Paller and Mancini—Hurwitz clinical pediatric dermatology: A textbook of skin disorders of childhood and adolescence* (6th ed.). Elsevier.)

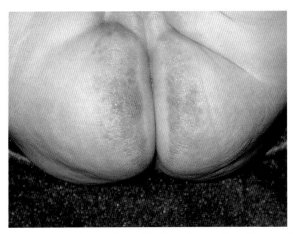

Fig. 34.2 Contact dermatitis, irritant. Diaper dermatitis. (From Sawyer, T., & Gleason, C. A. (2024). *Avery's diseases of the newborn* (11th ed.). Elsevier.)

OBJECTIVE*

A complete skin examination is needed, and the diagnosis of CD is typically based on clinical findings and history of exposure to an allergen or irritant. The area of involvement can provide clues as to the offending agent.

---

*Hallmark signs are bolded and <u>**Red flags are bolded and underlined**</u>.

> ### BOX 34.4 ■ Diversity Considerations
>
> Contact dermatitis (CD), including allergic contact dermatitis and irritant contact dermatitis, was once theorized to be less identified in persons of color due to their skin being less prone to contact sensitization. More recent published studies specific to patch testing demonstrate similar incidences of CD in both Black and White persons. Patch testing has identified nickel sulfate, bacitracin, and cobalt as the most prominent allergens causing allergic contact dermatitis in Black persons and nickel sulfate, neomycin, and formaldehyde as the most common causative agents in White persons. While nothing can be generalized with these findings, they identify the dissimilarities that can exist between ethnicities and the cause of CD as well as the importance of ensuring patch testing in all persons to alleviate the disorder (Okeke et al., 2022).

Cardiovascular/peripheral vascular: Tachycardia, elevated blood pressure (if significant pain response)

Integumentary: ACD—**vesicles, edema on an erythematous base**, ruptured vesicles with crusting; acute ICD—**sharply bordered areas of erythema, xerosis, and scaling**; chronic ICD—**hyperkeratosis, fissuring, hyperpigmentation, lichenification** (see Algorithms 34.1 and 34.2) (Bland, 2020; Nicol & O'Haver, 2023)

Evaluation and Differential Diagnoses

DIAGNOSTICS

No laboratory testing or diagnostics are required for the diagnosis of ICD; however, patch testing (Box 34.4) is the gold standard to diagnose and determine causative allergen(s) in ACD (Fonacier et al., 2015; Nicol & O'Haver, 2023).

DIFFERENTIAL DIAGNOSES

■ Atopic dermatitis: More chronic in nature and onset is typically in childhood. Presentation of lesions typically involves the flexure surfaces, and while there is an allergic component, there will be no preceding exposure to an irritant.
■ Psoriasis: More chronic in nature. Presentation of lesions typically involves the extensor surfaces, and there will be no preceding exposure to an allergen or irritant (see Chapter 35).
■ Scabies: Similar fissuring in the interdigit spaces can mimic CD. In scabies, burrows will be present over multiple warm locations of the body (waist, wrists, finger webs) without preceding exposure to an irritant or allergen. Pruritis will be more intense than ICD but may mimic ACD.
(Bland, 2020; Nicol & O'Haver, 2023)

Plan

GUIDELINE RESOURCES

■ Fonacier, L., Bernstein, D. I., Pacheco, K., Holness, D. L., Blessing-Moore, J., Khan, D., Lang, D., Nicklas, R., Oppenheimer, J., Portnoy, J., Randolph, C., Schuller, D., Spector, S., Tilles, S., & Wallace, D. (2015). Contact dermatitis: A practice parameter—Update 2015. *Journal of Allergy and Clinical Immunology: In Practice*, 3(3), S1–S39. https://doi.org/10.1016/j.jaip.2015.02.009

Pharmacotherapy

Once a diagnosis of CD is made, the offending agent should be identified and eliminated. For ACD, topical corticosteroids are recommended for acute, localized reactions and systemic corticosteroids are recommended for extensive, severe cases. For ICD, treatment with emollients and topical corticosteroids is recommended versus either therapy alone (see Algorithms 34.1 and 34.2).

- Topical corticosteroids: Use 2 to 3 times daily; will provide relief in 2 to 3 days, though it can take 2 to 3 weeks for complete healing. Ointment-based topical corticosteroids are preferred, and dose depends on severity and location.
- Systemic (oral) corticosteroids: 0.5 to 1 mg/kg daily (max 60 mg daily) for 7 days; reduce dose by 50% for 5 to 7 days, then taper to discontinue over 2 weeks if the area of allergic involvement is greater than 10% of the skin surface
- Emollients: Apply multiple times daily.

(Fonacier et al., 2015)

NONPHARMACOTHERAPY

- Educate
  - Person and family about the skin disorder, how to recognize triggers and prevent future contact, appropriate use of medication(s), and signs of exacerbation prompting further care
  - Importance of avoiding scratching and proper handwashing
- Lifestyle
  - Use of protective clothing, including gloves, particularly with occupational allergic/irritant exposure
- Referral
  - Severe cases of ACD or ICD and those persons who do not respond to typical treatment should warrant a referral to Dermatology; otherwise, this skin disorder can be effectively managed in primary care.
  - Allergist referral with ACD
- Follow-up
  - 1 week after treatment initiation to assess therapeutic response

(Bland, 2020; Fonacier et al., 2015)

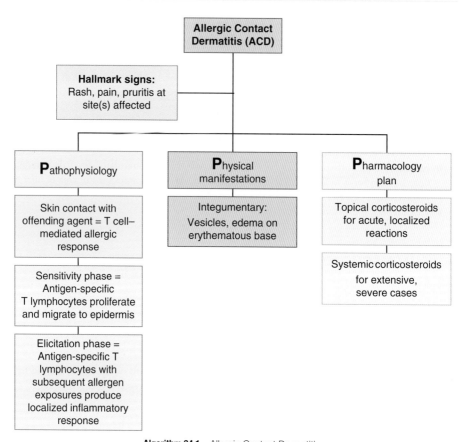

Algorithm 34.1   Allergic Contact Dermatitis

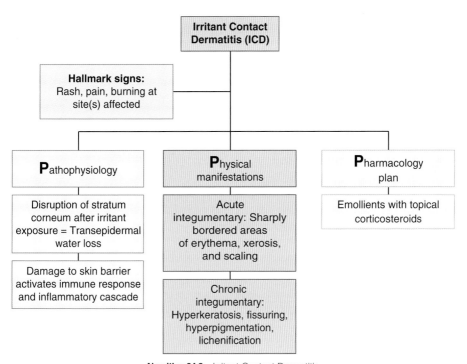

Algorithm 34.2 Irritant Contact Dermatitis

References

Bland, T. B (2020). Dermatologic disorders. In D. L. Maaks, N. Starr, M. A. Brady, N. M. Gaylord, M. Driessnack, & K. G. Duderrstadt (Eds.), *Burns' pediatric primary care* (7th ed., pp. 596–599). Elsevier.

Fonacier, L., & Feldman, E. (2020). *Contact dermatitis. Synopsis.* World Allergy Organization. https://www.worldallergy.org/component/content/article/contact-dermatitis-fonacier-l-feldman-e?catid=16&Itemid=101#:~:text=Contact%20Dermatitis:%20Synopsis&text=Contact%20dermatitis%20(CD)%20is%20a,or%20secondary%20ACD%20is%20suspected.

Fonacier, L., Bernstein, D. I., Pacheco, K., Holness, D. L., Blessing-Moore, J., Khan, D., Lang, D., Nicklas, R., Oppenheimer, J., Portnoy, J., Randolph, C., Schuller, D., Spector, S., Tilles, S., & Wallace, D. (2015). Contact dermatitis: A practice parameter—Update 2015. *Journal of Allergy and Clinical Immunology: In Practice, 3*(3), S1–S39. https://doi.org/10.1016/j.jaip.2015.02.009.

Lima, A. L., Timmermann, V., Illing, T., & Elsner, P. (2019). Contact dermatitis in the elderly: Predisposing factors, diagnosis, and management. *Drugs & Aging, 36*(5), 411–417. https://doi.org/10.1077/s40266-019-00641-4.

Nicol, N. H., & O'Haver, J (2023). Alterations of the integument in children. In J. L. Rogers (Ed.), *McCance and Huether's pathophysiology: The biologic basis for disease in adults and children* (9th ed., pp. 1543–1546). Mosby-Elsevier.

Okeke, C. V., Malik, A. M., Atwater, A. R., Powell, D. L., Czajkowski, G., Castanedo-Tardan, M. P., Montanez-Wiscovich, M., & Wu, P. A. (2022). American Contact Dermatitis Society position statement: Dermatitis and skin of color. *Dermatitis, 33*(1), 3–9. https://www.contactderm.org/UserFiles/ACDSPositionStatement-DermatitisandSkinofColor.pdf.

CHAPTER 35

Psoriasis

Jodi Allen

Psoriasis

Psoriasis is a chronic relapsing immune-mediated inflammatory disorder involving the skin of extensor areas of the body, scalp, and nails and typically demonstrates systemic comorbidities. Psoriasis occurs in approximately 0.5% to 11% of adults and is more prevalent in high-income countries and areas with older adults (Djuric & Turner, 2023). The prevalence of psoriasis in the United States is 3% (Armstrong et al., 2021). Risk is based on genetic and environmental factors, though genetics are the predominant indicator of risk. Environmental factors such as skin infection or trauma, smoking, and obesity can promote exacerbations of the condition. Psoriasis is typically diagnosed by the age of 40, though it can occur (rarely) in children (Djuric & Turner, 2023). There are multiple forms of psoriasis including plaque (the most common form), inverse, guttate, pustular, and erythrodermic, also known as exfoliative. Persons with psoriasis are at higher risk for developing psoriatic arthritis (PA) and having cardiovascular events, anxiety and depression, and multiple other comorbid conditions including uveitis, inflammatory bowel disease, and metabolic syndrome (Djuric & Turner, 2023).

Pathophysiology

Psoriasis involves a complicated inflammatory process involving macrophages, fibroblasts, dendritic cells, natural killer cells, T helper cells, and regulatory cells. These immune cells cause the secretion of multiple inflammatory mediators such as tumor necrosis factor and other cytokines that promote keratinocyte proliferation, angiogenesis, and infiltration of other immune cells into the lesions of psoriasis. One specific cytokine, IL-23, activates the T helper cell 17 pathway and is suspected to be the predominant mechanism of the condition. Both the dermis and epidermis are thickened due to cellular hyperproliferation, altered keratinocyte differentiation, and increased dermal vasculature. Epidermal shedding time becomes only 3 to 4 days versus the typical 14 to 20 days, causing cell maturation and keratinization to be bypassed and the hallmark thickening of skin with plaque formations to develop (see Algorithm 35.1). The loose cohesive keratin gives the lesion(s) a silver appearance. Capillary dilation and increased vascularization cause the presence of erythema. Psoriasis can present as mild, moderate, or severe depending on the size, distribution, and inflammation of lesions and will vacillate between remission and exacerbations (Djuric & Turner, 2023).

Physical Clinical Presentation

SUBJECTIVE

During the focused history, documentation should include the onset of symptoms; precipitating events; location, intensity, and quality of pain (if any); progression of symptoms; alleviating and aggravating factors; previous episodes; and associated symptoms. Persons will typically present

---

BOX 35.1 ■ Pediatric Considerations

Psoriasis occurs in all ages, but 30% of cases have onset in childhood. Obesity is a common comorbidity in children with psoriasis. Guttate psoriasis, which can be triggered by a streptococcal throat infection known as group A beta-hemolytic strep, is often the first sign of psoriasis in children. If a child presents with small papules on the trunk or extremities 2 to 3 weeks after diagnosis of group A beta-hemolytic strep, they should be evaluated for guttate psoriasis. Parents and the child should be informed that this subtype of psoriasis often resolves spontaneously within weeks or months of onset (Bland, 2020).

BOX 35.2 ■ Diversity Considerations

Persons of all skin colors can develop psoriasis; however, their objective presentation often differs. Fair-skinned persons typically present with erythematous or pink skin and the scales are a silvery white color. Hispanic persons are more apt to have salmon-colored psoriasis with a silvery white scale. In Black persons, the psoriasis often appears violet with gray scales. When psoriasis begins to clear on persons of color, a light or dark patch of skin where the psoriasis once was may appear, but these patches are not scars and they will resolve within 12 months. Identifying the differences in skin appearance with psoriasis in persons of color will aid in swift treatment (American Academy of Dermatology Association, 2023).

---

with concern due to pruritic, erythematous, inflamed, dry, and scaly plaques that appear to be worsening over time. The symptoms are often gradual and the plaques are found in only a few areas (such as elbows or knees); however, guttate psoriasis can also present as a rapid eruptive onset and be found in many areas. This type of rapid onset often follows a streptococcal throat infection 2 to 3 weeks prior, so asking about this in the past medical history section of the history is valuable (Box 35.1). Family history is important to ascertain, as 50% of persons diagnosed with psoriasis have an affected parent. Determine smoking status when asking social history questions, as smoking can exacerbate psoriasis (Djuric & Turner, 2023).

OBJECTIVE*

Generalized: **Fever**
  Musculoskeletal: **Arthritis mutilans with distal interphalangeal deformity** (comorbid PA)
  Integumentary: **Pitting of nails, onycholysis, subungual hyperkeratosis, nail plate dystrophy** (known as psoriatic nail disease, it can occur in all psoriasis subtypes)
  Plaque: **Well demarcated, thick, silvery, scaly, erythematous plaque surrounded by normal skin** (see Algorithm 35.1) (Box 35.2); location is typically skin of extensor areas of the body such as elbows and knees, face, and scalp (Fig. 35.1)
  Inverse: **Large, smooth, dry and deeply erythematous lesions in skinfolds**
  Guttate: **Small papules on trunk and extremities, sudden appearance**
  Pustular: **Blisters of noninfectious pus over areas of plaque psoriasis**
  Erythrodermic (exfoliative): **Widespread, erythematous, scaling lesions covering large body surface area** (Box 35.3)
  Psychiatric: Feelings of sadness related to lack of self-esteem secondary to psoriasis (Djuric & Turner, 2023)

---

*Hallmark signs bolded and <u>Red flags are bolded and underlined</u>.

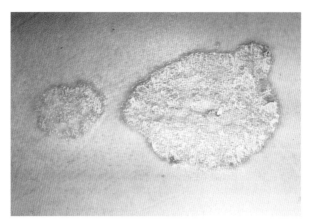

Fig. 35.1   Plaque psoriasis. Well-demarcated pink plaque with scale. (Courtesy Schaffer, J. V. (2024). Psoriasis. In J. L. Bolognia, J. V. Schaffer, & L. Cerroni (Eds.), *Dermatology* (5th ed.). Elsevier.)

BOX 35.3 ■ Acute Care Considerations

Erythrodermic (exfoliative) psoriasis is an extremely rare subtype, affecting only 2% of people living with psoriasis, but can be life-threatening. Erythrodermic psoriasis disturbs the body's normal temperature and fluid balance, leading to fluid retention, with increased risk for infection, pneumonia, and heart failure. Any person who presents with severe erythema or shedding of skin to a large area of the body (often in large sections of skin), skin that appears to be burned, elevated heart rate, severe pain/itching, and/or volatility of temperature should be evaluated in an emergency department (National Psoriasis Foundation, 2022).

Evaluation and Differential Diagnoses

DIAGNOSTICS

Laboratory, imaging, and skin biopsy are not required to diagnose psoriasis due to its distinct clinical features. Only in rare cases where determination of psoriasis subtype is needed will a skin biopsy be done. Other laboratory testing and imaging may be ordered based on diagnosis of psoriasis subtype (e.g., throat culture to rule out streptococcal throat infection and hand X-ray to rule out PA) (Djuric & Turner, 2023).

DIFFERENTIAL DIAGNOSES

- Atopic dermatitis: Poorly demarcated erythematous, dry, fine scales, commonly found on the skin of flexor surfaces of the body; also known as eczema
- Tinea corporis: Circular and clearly circumscribed mildly erythematous scaly patches with a slightly elevated ringlike border; also known as ringworm
- Seborrheic dermatitis: Lesions are pruritic erythematous plaques with greasy white or yellow scales and occur in areas rich in sebaceous glands, such as scalp, eyebrows, nasolabial folds, and axillae.

(Djuric & Turner, 2023)

Plan

Treatment of psoriasis is individualized with the goals of maintaining skin moisture, reducing epidermal cell turnover and pruritis, promoting immunomodulation, preventing and managing comorbid conditions, and supporting the person in maintaining quality of life (Djuric & Turner, 2023).

GUIDELINE RESOURCES

- Elmets, C. A., Korman, N. J., Prater, E. F., Wong, E. B., Rupani, R. N., Kivelevitch, D., Armstrong, A. W., Connor, C., Cordoro, K. M., Davis, D. M. R., Elewski, B. E., Gelfand, J. M., Gordon, G. B., Gottlieb, A. B., Kaplan, D. H., Kavanaugh, A., Kiselica, M., Kroshinsky, D., Lebwohl, M., … Mentor, A. (2021). Joint AAD–NPF guidelines of care for the management and treatment of psoriasis with topical therapy and alternative medicine modalities for psoriasis severity measures. *Journal of the American Academy of Dermatology, 84*(2), 432–470. https://doi.org/10.1016/j.jaad.2020.07.087
- Mentor, A., Gelfand, J. M., Connor, C., Armstrong, A. W., Cordoro, K. M., Davis, D. M. R., Elewski, B. E., Gordon, K. B., Gottlieb, A. B., Kaplan, D. H., Kavanaugh, A., Kiselica, M., Kivelevitch, D., Korman, N. J., Kroshinsky, D., Lebwohl, M., Leonardi, C. L., Lichten, J., Lim, H. W., … Elmets, C. A. (2020). Joint American Academy of Dermatology—National Psoriasis Foundation guidelines of care for the management of psoriasis with systemic nonbiologic therapies. *Journal of American Academy of Dermatology, 82*(6), 1445–1486. https://doi.org/10.1016/j.jaad.2020.02.044

Pharmacotherapy

- Topical corticosteroids are first-line agents (as long as less than 20% of the body is involved). Potency of the topical corticosteroid (Table 35.1) prescribed is based on psoriasis severity and location and the person's preference and age (Box 35.4). Lower-potency corticosteroids should be used on the face, intertriginous areas, and areas susceptible to steroid atrophy (e.g., forearms). Adults typically require moderate to high potency as initial therapy. Areas of thick, chronic plaques often require treatment with ultrahigh-potency corticosteroids (see Algorithm 35.1).
- Other topical options
  - Calcineurin inhibitors (tacrolimus and pimecrolimus): Can be used on face and intertriginous areas
  - Vitamin D analogue (calcipotriene): For mild to moderate plaque psoriasis
  - Combination of potent topical corticosteroids with vitamin D analogue is more effective than either agent alone; applying high-potency topical steroids in the morning and vitamin D analogue in the evening.
  - Emollient: In conjunction with topical corticosteroids can reduce itching and desquamation and prevent quick relapse when topical corticosteroids are discontinued
- Nonbiologic and biologic agents are primary options for persons with severe incapacitating psoriasis.** The most common and widely used nonbiologic is methotrexate and common biologics include etanercept and adalimumab. Prescribing these agents will be determined by a dermatologist or rheumatologist.

(Elmets et al., 2021; Mentor et al., 2020)

NONPHARMACOTHERAPY

- Educate
  - Person and family about psoriasis, treatments (including length of treatment), likely side effects of treatment (steroid atrophy), and avoidance of exacerbation triggers (e.g., skin infection, trauma, and smoking); provide support related to psychological stressors
  - Person and family about increased risk of cardiovascular comorbid conditions and encourage loss of weight as necessary to lessen risk

---

**Biologic treatment guidelines are not included in this chapter as they require specialty referral and management.

TABLE 35.1 ■ Topical Corticosteroids Potency

Ultrahigh potency	High potency
Betamethasone dipropionate, augmented 0.05%	Amcinonide 0.1%
Clobetasol propionate 0.05%	Betamethasone dipropionate 0.05%
Desoximetasone 0.25%	Betamethasone dipropionate, augmented 0.05%
Diflorasone diacetate, augmented 0.05%	Desoximetasone 0.25%, 0.05%
Fluocinonide 0.1%	Diflorasone diacetate, augmented 0.05%
Flurandrenolide 4 mcg/cm^2	Diflorasone diacetate 0.05%
Halobetasol propionate 0.05%	Fluocinonide 0.05%
	Halcinonide 0.1%
	Mometasone furoate 0.1%
	Triamcinolone acetonide 0.1%, 0.2%, 0.5%
	Betamethasone valerate 0.12%
	Fluocinolone acetonide 0.025%
	Flurandrenolide 0.5%
	Hydrocortisone valerate 0.2%
	Mometasone furoate 0.1%

Moderate potency	Low potency
Betamethasone dipropionate 0.05%	Alclometasone dipropionate 0.05%
Betamethasone valerate 0.1%	Betamethasone valerate 0.05%
Clocortolone pivalate 0.1%	Desonide 0.05%
Fluocinolone acetonide 0.01%, 0.025%	Fluocinolone acetonide 0.01%
Fluticasone propionate 0.05%	Triamcinolone acetonide 0.025%
Flurandrenolide 0.05%	Dexamethasone sodium phosphate 0.1%
Hydrocortisone butyrate 0.1%	Hydrocortisone 0.5%–2.5%
Hydrocortisone probutate 0.1%	Methylprednisolone acetate 0.25%
Hydrocortisone valerate 0.2%	
Prednicarbate 0.1%	
Triamcinolone acetonide 0.01%, 0.025%	

Adopted from Elmets, C. A., Korman, N. J., Farely Prater, E., Wong, E. B., Rupani, R. N., Kivelevitch, D., Armstrong, A. W., Connor, C., Cordoro, K. M., Davis, D. M. R., Elewski, B. E., Gelfand, J. M., Gordon, G. B., Gottlieb, A. B., Kaplan, D. H., Kavanaugh, A., Kiselica, M., Kroshinsky, D., Lebwohl, M., … Mentor, A. (2021). Joint AAD-NPF guidelines of care for the management and treatment of psoriasis with topical therapy and alternative medicine modalities for psoriasis severity measures. *Journal of American Academy of Dermatology, 84*(2), 432–470. https://doi.org/10.1016/j.jaad.2020.07.087.

BOX 35.4 ■ Older Adult Considerations

Treating older adults with psoriasis is challenging due to the prevalence of comorbid conditions, polypharmacy, and immune system impairment. Topical agents remain the first-line therapy for older adults as there are fewer systemic side effects; however, older adults are at greater risk for steroid skin atrophy due to the expected age-related changes already occurring with their skin (e.g., thinning, bruising). Considering this and evaluating the concerns of the older adult related to their psoriasis can limit unwanted and potentially harmful treatments. A thorough medication review prior to prescribing is paramount to prevent adverse drug reactions (Strong, 2021).

- Avoidance of photosensitizing medications such as tetracyclines and sulfa drugs if possible; avoidance of scratching or picking at plaques
- Controlled sun exposure can be beneficial, but sunscreen use is mandatory to prevent sunburns (which can exacerbate psoriasis).
- Seek treatment for streptococcal throat infections immediately.
- If taking methotrexate, take folic acid 5 mg by mouth weekly to prevent side effects.
- Prior to starting nonbiologic or biologic therapies, ensure that the person is up to date on vaccinations to prevent infection.

- Lifestyle
  - Smoking cessation
  - Low-fat, high-fiber diet to promote cardiovascular and immune system health
- Referral
  - Dermatology: Newly diagnosed persons who have moderate to extensive skin involvement (more than 20% of the body involved)
  - Rheumatology: Persons with PA
  - Mental health provider: For psychological evaluation and treatment as needed
  - Dietician or nutritionist: If overweight or obese to prevent complications and comorbid conditions
- Follow-up
  - Every 2 months

(Elmets et al., 2021; Mentor et al., 2020)

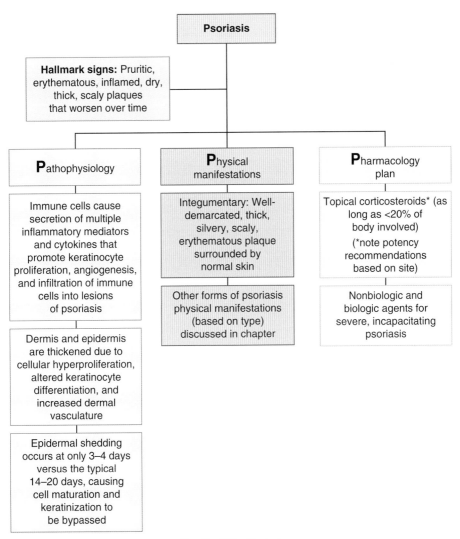

Algorithm 35.1   Psoriasis

References

American Academy of Dermatology. (2023). *Can you get psoriasis if you have skin of color?* American Academy of Dermatology. https://www.aad.org/public/diseases/psoriasis/treatment/could-have/skin-color#: ~:text=Yes.,psoriasis%20and%20silvery%2Dwhite%20scale.

Armstrong, A. W., Mehta, M. D., Schupp, C. W., Gondo, G. C., Bell, S. J., & Griffiths, C. E. (2021). Psoriasis prevalence in adults in the United States. *JAMA Dermatology, 157*(8), 1–7. https://doi.org/10.1011/jamadermatol.2021.2007.

Bland, T. B. (2020). Dermatologic disorders. In D. L. Maaks, N. Starr, M. A. Brady, N. M. Gaylord, M. Driessnack, & K. G. Duderrstadt (Eds.), *Burns' pediatric primary care* (7th ed., pp. 605–607). Elsevier.

Djuric, C. M., & Turner, K. C. (2023). Structure, function, and disorders of the integument. In J. L. Rogers (Ed.), *McCance and Huether's pathophysiology: The biologic basis for disease in adults and children* (9th ed., pp. 1516–1520). Mosby-Elsevier.

Elmets, C. A., Korman, N. J., Farely Prater, E., Wong, E. B., Rupani, R. N., Kivelevitch, D., Armstrong, A. W., Connor, C., Cordoro, K. M., Davis, D. M. R., Elewski, B. E., Gelfand, J. M., Gordon, G. B., Gottlieb, A. B., Kaplan, D. H., Kavanaugh, A., Kiselica, M., Kroshinsky, D., Lebwohl, M., ... Mentor, A. (2021). Joint AAD-NPF guidelines of care for the management and treatment of psoriasis with topical therapy and alternative medicine modalities for psoriasis severity measures. *Journal of American Academy of Dermatology, 84*(2), 432–470. https://doi.org/10.1016/j.jaad.2020.07.087.

Mentor, A., Gelfand, J. M., Connor, C., Armstrong, A. W., Cordoro, K. M., Davis, D. M. R., Elewski, B. E., Gordon, K. B., Gottlieb, A. B., Kaplan, D. H., Kavanaugh, A., Kiselica, M., Kivelevitch, D., Korman, N. J., Kroshinsky, D., Lebwohl, M., Leonardi, C. L., Lichten, J., Lim, H. W., ... Elmets, C. A. (2020). Joint American Academy of Dermatology—National Psoriasis Foundation guidelines of care for the management of psoriasis with systemic nonbiologic therapies. *Journal of American Academy of Dermatology, 82*(6), 1445–1486. https://doi.org/10.1016/j.jaad.2020.02.044.

National Psoriasis Foundation. (2022). *Erythrodermic psoriasis*. Retrieved September 6, 2024 from https://www.psoriasis.org/erythrodermic-psoriasis.

Strong, C. (2021). *Psoriasis in older adults: A treatment challenge for clinicians*. Dermatology Advisor. Retrieved September 6, 2024 from https://www.dermatologyadvisor.com/home/topics/psoriasis/discussion-of-safe-treatment-for-psoriasis-in-patients-aged-65-years-and-older.

CHAPTER 36

Malignant Skin Lesions

Jodi Allen ▪ Corrine M. Djuric

Malignant Skin Lesions

Malignant skin lesions consist of nonmelanoma skin cancers and cutaneous melanomas. Nonmelanoma skin cancers are the most prevalent form and consist of basal cell carcinoma (BCC) and squamous cell carcinoma (SCC) (Djuric & Turner, 2023). More than 5.4 million cases of nonmelanoma skin cancers have been reported in the United States, with the majority of BCC and SCC being highly curable. Malignant melanoma represents 1% of all skin cancer cases but 79% of all skin cancer deaths, making it the most serious and life-threatening malignant skin lesion (Carr et al., 2020). The overall 5-year survival rate of melanoma has risen to 93.3% in the United States; however, the survival rate for later stages, specifically stage IV, remains less than 30% (Saginala et al., 2021). Malignant skin lesions are more common in females younger than 40 years of age and in males older than 40 years of age, though risk generally increases as age progresses. Malignant skin lesions are 40 times more prevalent in White persons than in Black persons (Box 36.1) (Djuric & Turner, 2023). Risk increases with exorbitant exposure to ultraviolet (UV) radiation from the sun and/or artificial UV exposure (such as from tanning beds). Persons with a fair complexion; occupational exposures to UV rays (Box 36.2), coal tar, creosote, arsenic compounds, and radium; and a family history of skin cancer are also at increased risk (Carr et al., 2020).

Pathophysiology

Prolonged and repetitive UV exposure, especially during childhood, coupled with mutations in gene sequencing cause most malignant skin lesions. Lesions appear most frequently on sun-exposed areas of the skin such as the face, neck, arms, and hands (Djuric & Turner, 2023). BCC is a malignant growth of the surface epithelial of the skin originating in the basal layer keratinocytes (see Algorithm 36.1). Mutation of a tumor suppression gene leads to loss of keratinocyte repair functions. Tumors are slow growing and rarely metastasize, though they can be locally invasive, painful, and disfiguring (Endo, 2022). BCCs have multiple subtypes that can have different clinical presentations (Djuric & Turner, 2023). SCC originates at the keratinocyte and is a full-thickness epidermal atypia that is further classified as Bowen's disease (in situ) or invasive disease (see Algorithm 36.2). Invasive disease extends into or below the dermal layer of the skin (Djuric & Turner, 2023). Mutation of tumor suppression pathways and damaged deoxyribonucleic acid repair are the underlying pathophysiology of SCC (Endo, 2022).

Melanoma is a malignant tumor originating in the melanocyte, the cell found in the basal epidermis and hair follicles that synthesizes the pigment melanin. In the presence of UV-induced DNA damage, melanocyte-stimulating hormone is released so that the melanin pigment can shield further DNA damage (see Algorithm 36.3). Cutaneous melanoma pathophysiology is complex, but the direct transformation of normal melanocytes into neoplastic cells occurs through several mutations affecting protooncogene and tumor suppressor genes. Initially, tumors stay confined to the epidermis, but if left untreated, will spread to the subcutaneous fat and eventually to

BOX 36.1 ■ Diversity Considerations

While not common, people of color can develop malignant skin lesions. The lack of information regarding people of color and skin cancers along with the lack of dermatologic malignant skin lesion examples provided to health care providers in training have weakened the ability to identify these lesions in people of color. Unfortunately, when malignant skin lesions are identified in people of color it is often in later stages, increasing risk of disfigurement and mortality. Self-screening remains effective for all persons, but persons of color may not notice a change in skin pigmentation. If a darker than usual spot is identified, if the spot is bleeding, or if the spot has changed shape, care should be sought. If an area of skin feels rough or dry or if a dark line underneath or around a fingernail or toenail is identified, instruct persons to seek care (Shao & Feng, 2022).

BOX 36.2 ■ Older Adult Considerations

As the general population ages, the prevalence of malignant skin lesions diagnosed in older adults is increasing. Risk of skin cancer increases in older adults who have a history of working outdoors, have a previous diagnosis of any type of malignant skin lesion, and are male. Older males are found to be at the highest risk for death from melanoma. Skin examinations are not often included in the physical assessment of older adults, and health care providers may be missing suspicious lesions or mistakenly identifying benign or precancerous lesions in lieu of the proper diagnosis (Sinikumpu et al., 2022).

BOX 36.3 ■ Acute Care Considerations

Melanoma is often diagnosed in the emergency department related to complications that cause the person afflicted to seek acute care. Persons with melanoma will often present with signs and symptoms of septicemia caused by a secondary malignancy or infection. Any person with confusion or delirium, fever (or hypothermia), hypotension, rapid heart rate, and/or mottled skin should be emergently evaluated for septicemia and its underlying cause identified. Unfortunately, if melanoma is the underlying primary malignancy, this equates to a late-stage identification and prognosis is poor (Hundal et al., 2023).

regional lymph nodes. Occasionally, distant sites such as bone, lung, liver, and brain will demonstrate metastases (Box 36.3) (Djuric & Turner, 2023).

Physical Clinical Presentation

SUBJECTIVE

During the focused history, documentation should include the onset of symptoms; precipitating events; location, intensity, and quality of pain (if any); progression of symptoms; alleviating and aggravating factors; previous episodes; and associated symptoms. Persons will commonly present with a change in a nevus or a new "spot" on their skin that did not previously exist. Some pain and friability may be reported with BCC and SCC skin lesions; however, melanoma lesions can initially present as pruritic and evolve to tender lesions that bleed and ulcerate. Nonhealing ulcers may be reported as well. A personal history of being immunocompromised due to either disease or medication use as well as family history of any malignant skin lesion increases risk and is important to ascertain. Persons who have a history of repeated sunburns, particularly blistering sunburns, have an increased risk as well. Ask about social history including occupational sun or chemical exposure as these also increase the risk of malignant skin lesions. Ask about general sun exposure habits including sunscreen use on face and body (American Academy of Dermatology Association [AADA], 2023a; Djuric & Turner, 2023).

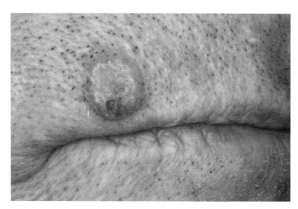

Fig. 36.1   Malignant skin lesion, basal cell carcinoma. Noduloulcerative lesion of the upper lip demonstrating telangiectasia and small ulceration. (From Allen, C. M., Damm, D. D., Chi, A. C., & Neville, B. W. (2024). *Oral and maxillofacial pathology* (5th ed.). Elsevier.)

OBJECTIVE*

Integumentary: Location typically on sun-exposed areas of the skin

BCC: **Pearl-colored nodule with fine telangiectasia over the surface and a depressed center or rolled edge** on face, ears, cheeks, nose, and neck (most common) (see Algorithm 36.1) (Fig. 36.1)

SCC: Most commonly found on lips, tips of ears, nose, cheeks, and scalp of bald males and on hands, forearms, and shins of females

- Bowen's disease: **Erythematous, well-demarcated pink or red scaly patch or plaque** (see Algorithm 36.2) (Fig. 36.2)
- Invasive disease: **Indurated, hyperkeratotic papules, plaques, or nodules 5 to 15 mm in diameter**

Malignant melanoma: **De novo lesion or increase in nevus size and change in color or shape** (Box 36.4) on the back and neck in males and legs in females (most common) (see Algorithm 36.3): **ABCDEs of melanoma** (Fig. 36.3):

A = Asymmetry
B = Border irregularity
C = Color change
D = Diameter larger than a pencil eraser (~6 mm)
E = Evolving lesion (changing over time)
(Djuric & Turner, 2023)

Evaluation and Differential Diagnoses

DIAGNOSTICS

Malignant Skin Lesions

- Skin biopsy is necessary to confirm the diagnosis of BCC, SCC, and malignant melanoma as early diagnosis and intervention is critical. BCC will rarely metastasize, so staging of lesions is not necessary. On the contrary, SCC and melanoma require staging due to their increased potential to metastasize (Djuric & Turner, 2023; Endo, 2022).

---

*Hallmark signs bolded and <u>Red flags are bolded and underlined</u>.

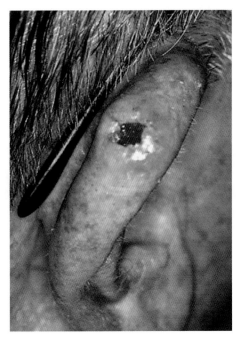

Fig. 36.2 Malignant skin lesion, squamous cell carcinoma. Notice the erythema and well-demarcated red scaly patch. (From Kenneaster, D. G. (2005). Introduction to skin cancer, *Oral and Maxillofacial Surgery Clinics of North America*, 17(2). https://doi.org/10.1016/j.coms.2005.02.001.)

BOX 36.4 ■ Pediatric Considerations

Malignant skin lesions are not common in the pediatric population, but 300 to 400 cases of melanoma are diagnosed annually. Due to the rareness of the diagnosis in children, it is often found in later stages, which increases treatment requirements, morbidity, and mortality. Signs of melanoma in children are slightly different than in adults. Melanoma is often one single color in children and may not be the typical black or brown color; also, it can be more pruritic and have increased bleeding, and the lesion is often raised (versus flat, as in adults). Educating parents and older children about melanoma and how to identify suspicious lesions is imperative to prevent later staging and improve the outcome of the diagnosis (AADA, 2023b).

DIFFERENTIAL DIAGNOSES

- Actinic keratosis: Generally considered premalignant lesions, found mainly in sun-exposed skin and present as small, 0.2- to 5-mm, flesh-colored or slightly hyperpigmented macules or plaques; surface feels rough and uneven (liken to sandpaper)
- Seborrheic keratoses: Benign lesions that are light to dark brown with soft, wartlike growths located mainly on the trunk
- Solar lentigines: Pigmented macules that appear on sun-exposed areas such as the dorsum of the hands and arms (also known as liver spots)
- Benign nevi: Round to oval with regular borders, <5 mm in diameter with evenly distributed color, do not fit into any of the ABCDEs of melanoma (also known as moles)

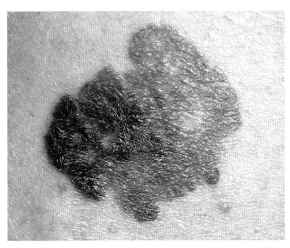

Fig. 36.3 Malignant skin lesion, melanoma. Melanoma violating the ABCDE rules. (From Habif, T. (2010). Nevi and malignant melanoma. In T. Habif (Ed.). *Clinical Dermatology* (5th ed.). St Louis, Missouri: Mosby.)

Plan

GUIDELINE RESOURCES

- Alam, M., Armstrong, A., Baum, C., Bordeaux, J. S., Brown, M., Busam, K. J., Eisen, D. B., Iyengar, V., Lober, C., Margolis, D. J., Messina, J., Miller, A., Miller, S., Mostow, E., Mowad, C., Nehal, K., Schmitt-Burr, K., Sekulic, A., Storrs, P., … Bichakjian, C. (2018). Guidelines of care for the management of cutaneous squamous cell carcinoma. *Journal of the American Academy of Dermatology, 78*(3), 560–578. https://doi.org/10.1016/j.jaad.2017.10.007
- Bichakjian, C., Armstrong, A., Baum, C., Bordeaux, J. S., Brown, M., Busam, K. J., Eisen, D. B., Iyengar, V., Lober, C., Margolis, D. J., Messina, J., Miller, A., Miller, S., Mostow, E., Mowad, C., Nehal, K., Schmitt-Burr, K., Sekulic, A., Storrs, P., … Alam, M. (2018). Guidelines of care for the management of basal cell carcinoma. *Journal of the American Academy of Dermatology, 78*(3), 540–559. https://doi.org/10.1016/j.jaad.2017.10.006
- Swetter, A. M., Tsao, H., Bichakjian, C. K., Curiel-Lewandrowski, C., Elder, D. E., Gershenwald, J. E., Guild, V., Grant-Kels, J. M., Halpern, A. C., Johnson, T. M., Sober, A. J., Thompson, J. A., Wisco, O. J., Wyatt, S., Hu, S., & Lamina, T. (2019). Guidelines of care for the management of primary cutaneous melanoma. *Journal of the American Academy of Dermatology, 80*(1), 208–250. https://doi.org/10.1016/j.jaad.2018.08.055

Pharmacotherapy

Management of nonmelanomatous and melanoma skin lesions depends on several factors and will be dictated by specialty practice. Mohs microscopic surgery is a common surgical treatment (see Algorithms 36.1, 36.2, and 36.3).

- BCC: Nonsurgical candidates or patients refusing surgical excision may be treated with topical therapies such as imiquimod, fluorouracil, cryotherapy, or photodynamic therapy. The specialist and the patient will determine which therapy suits best (Kim et al., 2018a).
- SCC: Cryotherapy, topical imiquimod, and topical fluorouracil may be options for the nonsurgical candidate (Kim et al., 2018b).
- Melanoma: Chemotherapy, radiation therapy, immunotherapy, and gene therapy are options with or without surgical intervention depending on the presentation and patient preference (Swetter et al., 2019).

NONPHARMACOTHERAPY

- Educate
  - Person and family about the diagnosis, treatment, and importance of seeing a specialist for care
  - Person and family about prevention of skin cancer, starting in early childhood if possible
  - Person and family about the ABCDE mnemonic for early detection and self-screening for melanoma
  - Survivors of any malignant skin lesion should be made aware that they are at increased risk for reoccurrence.
- Lifestyle
  - Avoid sun exposure from 11 a.m. to 4 p.m. due to intense levels of UV radiation.
  - Wear protective clothing including tight-weave fabric, long-sleeve shirt, and wide-brimmed hat.
  - Wear large-framed wraparound sunglasses with 99% to 100% UV absorption.
  - Apply sunscreen with an SPF of at least 15, even on hazy days; reapply often.
  - Avoid tanning beds.
- Referral
  - Dermatologist, even for nonmelanomatous skin lesions
  - Oncologist, if needed, is typically referred to by a dermatologist.
- Follow-up
  - Comprehensive physical assessment with skin examination every 6 to 12 months or more often if signs of new or changing skin lesions or recurring lesion at previous site of BCC, SCC, or melanoma

(Kim et al., 2018a, 2018b; Swetter et al., 2019)

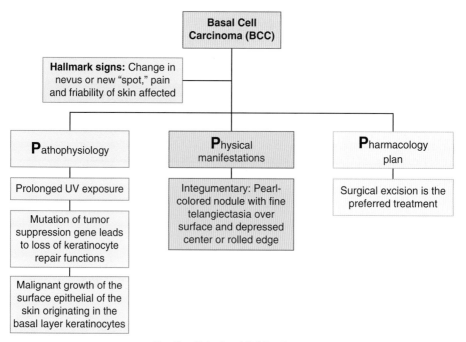

Algorithm 36.1 Basal Cell Carcinoma

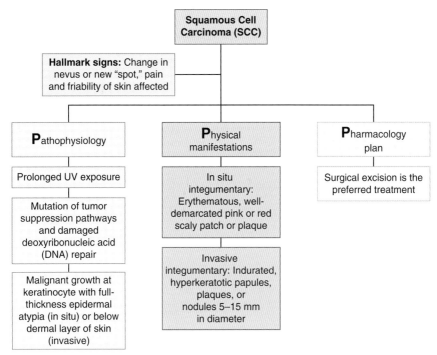

Algorithm 36.2 Squamous Cell Carcinoma

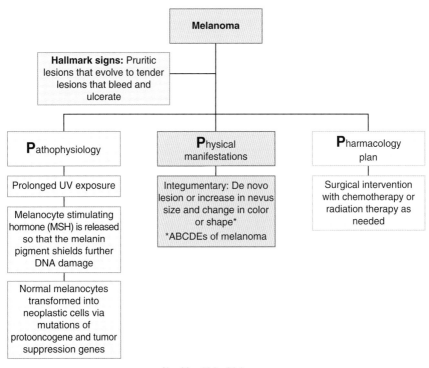

Algorithm 36.3 Melanoma

References

American Academy of Dermatology. (2023a). *Types of skin cancer*. American Academy of Dermatology. https://www.aad.org/public/diseases/skin-cancer/types/common.

American Academy of Dermatology. (2023b). *Melanoma can look different in children*. American Academy of Dermatology. https://www.aad.org/public/diseases/skin-cancer/types/common/melanoma/different-children.

Carr, S., Smith, C., & Wernber, J. (2020). Epidemiology and risk factors of melanoma. *Surgical Clinics of North America, 100*(1), 1–12. https://doi.org/10.1016/j.suc.2019.09.005.

Djuric, C. M., & Turner, K. C. (2023). Structure, function, and disorders of the integument. In J. L. Rogers (Ed.), *McCance and Huether's pathophysiology: The biologic basis for disease in adults and children* (9th ed., pp. 1527–1532). Mosby-Elsevier.

Endo, J (2022). Skin problems. In G. A. Warshaw, J. F. Potter, E. Flaherty, M. T. Heflin, M. K. McNabney, & R. J. Ham (Eds.), *Ham's primary care geriatrics* (7th ed., pp. 541–542). Elsevier.

Hundal, H., Taneja, K., Patel, K., Siegler, J. E., Thon, J., Shin, J., Hsiung, H., Diaz, M., & Toloza, E. M. (2023). Melanoma patients in the emergency department: Characteristics and outcomes. *Cancer Research, 83*(7_Supplement), 3220. https://doi.org/10.1158/1538-7445.AM2023-3220.

Kim, J. Y. S., Kozlow, J. H., Mittal, B., Moyer, J., Olencki, T., & Rodgers, P. (2018a). Guidelines of care for the management of basal cell carcinoma. *Journal of the American Academy of Dermatology, 78*(3), 540–559. https://doi.org/10.1016/j.jaad.2017.10.006.

Kim, J. Y. S., Kozlow, J. H., Mittal, B., Moyer, J., Olencki, T., & Rodgers, P. (2018b). Guidelines of care for the management of cutaneous squamous cell carcinoma. *Journal of the American Academy of Dermatology, 78*(3), 560–578. https://doi.org/10.1016/j.jaad.2017.10.007.

Saginala, K., Barsouk, A., Aluru, J. S., Rawla, P., & Barsouk, A. (2021). Epidemiology of melanoma. *Medical Sciences, 9*(4), 63. https://doi.org/10.3390/medsci9040063.

Shao, K., & Feng, H. (2022). Racial and ethnic healthcare disparities in skin cancer in the United States: A review of existing inequities, contributing factors, and potential solutions. *Journal of Clinical and Aesthetic Dermatology, 15*(7), 16–22. https://www.ncbi.nlm.nih.gov/pmc/articles/PMC9345197.

Sinikumpu, S. P., Jokelainen, J., Keinanen-Kiukaanniemi, S., & Huilaja, L. (2022). Skin cancers and their risk factors in older persons: A population-based study. *BMC Geriatrics, 22*(1), 269. https://doi.org/10.1186/s12877-022-02964-1.

Swetter, S. M., Tsao, H., Bichakjian, C. K., Curiel-Lewandrowski, C., Elder, D. E., Gershenwald, J. E., Guild, V., Grant-Kels, J. M., Halpern, A. C., Johnson, T. M., Sober, A. J., Thompson, J. A., Wisco, O. J., Wyatt, S., Hu, S., & Lamina, T. (2019). Guidelines of care for the management of primary cutaneous melanoma. *Journal of the American Academy of Dermatology, 80*(1), 208–250. https://doi.org/10.1016/j.jaad.2018.08.055.

CHAPTER 37

Integumentary Infections

Jodi Allen

Cellulitis

Cellulitis

Cellulitis is a bacterial infection of the skin involving the dermis and subcutaneous tissue often caused by group A streptococcus, streptococcus pyogenes, or staphylococcus aureus (including the methicillin-resistant strains). Cellulitis can materialize as an extension of a skin wound, as an ulcer, or from a furuncle or carbuncle. Cellulitic infections can cause systemic symptoms and can become life-threatening (Djuric & Turner, 2023). The global burden of disease for cellulitis is estimated at 43 million cases, with 14 million cases occurring in the United States annually, most often in middle-aged and older adults (Miller et al., 2022). Any break in the skin or mucus membranes is a potential portal of entry for bacterial pathogens and increases the risk of developing cellulitis. Persons with diabetes mellitus, edema, peripheral vascular disease, tinea pedis, insect bites, history of recurrent cellulitis, intravenous (IV) drug abuse, or immune suppression from disease or medication are at higher risk for developing cellulitis. Health care providers must be able to differentiate uncomplicated from severe cellulitis as well as from necrotizing fasciitis as this requires immediate acute care treatment (Box 37.1) (Djuric & Turner, 2023). Severity of cellulitis is dependent upon the virulence of the pathogen, the person's immune status, and the depth of infection (Brown & Hood Watson, 2023).

Pathophysiology

Cellulitis exhibits an acute inflammatory response secondary to cytokine and neutrophil response from bacteria breaching the epidermis. During the inflammatory process, the neutrophils along with basophils, mast cells, and platelets accumulate at the site. Necrosis of normal tissue can occur during the inflammatory process due to the proteolytic enzymes produced by the leukocytes present (see Algorithm 37.1). An increase in vascular permeability of the microcirculation of the skin allows protein-rich fluids to leak into the interstitial tissue, and vasodilation leads to bright erythema of the skin and indistinct borders, which are some of the hallmark signs of cellulitis (Brown & Hood Watson, 2023; Djuric & Turner, 2023).

Physical Clinical Presentation

SUBJECTIVE

During the focused history, documentation should include the onset of symptoms; precipitating events; location, intensity, and quality of pain; progression of symptoms; alleviating and aggravating factors; previous episodes; and associated symptoms. Typically the person with cellulitis will complain of warm, tender, and erythematous skin, noting a precipitating event that caused the site

---

BOX 37.1 ■ Acute Care Considerations

Necrotizing fasciitis is rare but is a life-threatening and "not to miss diagnosis." The hallmark of this infection is its rapid progression of tissue destruction and severity of systemic symptoms. While the progression of cellulitis is typically represented in days, necrotizing fasciitis progression is measured in hours. This infection is caused by "flesh-eating bacteria," and loss of affected limb or life is a complication. The pain at the affected site will be disproportionate to the appearance of the skin lesion, differentiating necrotizing fasciitis from cellulitis. Emergent care is needed, and swift treatment is key to a good outcome (Djuric & Turner, 2023).

BOX 37.2 ■ Pediatric Considerations

Periorbital cellulitis can be a life-threatening form of cellulitis common in young children. The typical presentation is erythema and edema over the affected periorbital area, though the edema can be so severe that the entire affected side of the face is swollen. The child may complain of pain with certain eye movements, and they may have a high fever, tachycardia, and lethargy. On exam, the child will demonstrate an inability to perform extraocular movements via cranial nerve III, IV, and VI testing. Periorbital cellulitis is an emergent condition (Bland, 2020).

---

to become "infected." Many persons presenting with cellulitis will not know what precipitated the symptoms. Persons may or may not have fatigue and fever with cellulitis. The area of involvement can vary from a few centimeters to an extremely large area of skin and is almost always unilateral if located in the extremities. Some may complain of tender and enlarged lymph nodes near the affected area (Brown & Hood Watson, 2023; Djuric & Turner, 2023). Gaining a quality history that includes recent travel and a recent injury or bite to the affected area, along with a thorough medical history, will help to determine risk of complications and severity of cellulitis. Asking pointed questions about drug use, specifically IV drug use, may identify a point of entry for the offending bacteria (Brown & Hood Watson, 2023).

OBJECTIVE*

Generalized: Malaise, **fever**
   Neurological: **Mental status changes; localized sensory loss**
   HEENT: **Periorbital edema; facial puffiness; abnormal cranial nerves III, IV, and VI** (Box 37.2)
   Cardiovascular/peripheral vascular: **Hypotension; tachycardia; diminished pulses**
   Integumentary: **Erythematous, warm, edematous area of skin with a flat, diffuse, indistinct border** (Fig. 37.1) (Box 37.3). It is beneficial for the health care provider to mark the area with a nonpermanent pen to ensure improvement or identify worsening on follow-up (see Algorithm 37.1).
   (Brown & Hood Watson, 2023; Djuric & Turner, 2023)

Evaluation and Differential Diagnoses
DIAGNOSTICS

Cellulitis is a clinical diagnosis based on presentation and history. Two of the following four criteria are required to diagnose: (1) warmth, (2) erythema, (3) edema, and (4) tenderness.

---

*Hallmark signs are bolded and <u>**Red flags are bolded and underlined**</u>.

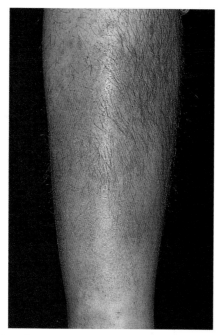

Fig. 37.1 Cellulitis, nonpurulent. Cellulitis with diffuse erythema, minimal swelling, and not well-demarcated borders. (From Habif, T. P., et al. (2011). Bacterial infections. In T. P. Habif, et al. (2012), *Skin disease* (3rd ed.). Elsevier.)

BOX 37.3 ■ Diversity Considerations

Cellulitis presents with a brightly erythematous skin color that is warm and tender to the touch in light-skinned persons; however, in darker-skinned persons, the color will present as a darker erythema. This often causes concern for a complicated cellulitic infection when it is merely representative of the amount of melanin in the skin. A complete physical assessment should be undertaken in persons of color to determine severity and comorbid conditions, which should drive the decision for inpatient versus outpatient treatment (Brown & Hood Watson, 2023).

No imaging is necessary except in persons with febrile neutropenia. Consider blood cultures only in persons who are immunocompromised, those who experienced a water-associated injury or an animal bite, and when persons have signs of systemic infection (Stevens et al., 2014).

DIFFERENTIAL DIAGNOSES

- Erysipelas: Acute, nonpurulent, superficial infection of the upper dermis and superficial lymphatics most commonly caused by beta-hemolytic streptococci. Unlike cellulitis, there is no subcutaneous layer involvement, and the affected area of skin has well-demarcated borders.
- Necrotizing fasciitis: Rare, rapidly spreading skin infection versus the somewhat slower progression of cellulitis. Greater presence of systemic symptoms, including high fever, tachycardia, hypotension, mental status changes, and pain out of proportion to the exam are emergent signs (see Box 37.1).

BOX 37.4 ■ Older Adult Considerations

Cellulitis in older adults can be frequent secondary to multiple risk factors and complicated secondary to multiple comorbid conditions. When older adults are hospitalized for cellulitis, age is an independent risk factor for an increased length of hospital stay and increased mortality, though this can be attributed to underlying comorbidities as well. Delayed administration of antibiotics can increase mortality also. Hospital readmission for cellulitis is more common in older adults, which can increase prolonged immobility, loss of independence, and poor outcomes. Careful determination of inpatient versus outpatient treatment is needed (Kumar et al., 2020).

■ Deep vein thrombosis (DVT): Typically unilateral with tenderness, erythema, warmth, and edema most commonly affecting lower extremities. History of recent surgeries, prolonged immobility, or family history of DVT increases risk. DVT rarely presents with fever. (Brown & Hood Watson, 2023; Djuric & Turner, 2023)

Plan

When developing the treatment plan for cellulitis, the severity of infection and the person's comorbid conditions should guide the need for hospitalization versus outpatient care (Box 37.4).

GUIDELINE RESOURCES

■ Stevens, D. L., Bisno, A. L., Chambers, H. F., Dellinger, E. P., Goldstein, E. J. C., Gorbach, S. L., Hirschmann, J. V., Kaplan, S. L., Montoya, J. G., Wade, J. C., & Infectious Diseases Society of America. (2014). Executive summary: Practice guidelines for the diagnosis and management of skin and soft tissue infections: 2014 update by the Infectious Diseases Society of America. *Clinical Infectious Diseases*, *59*(2), 147–159. https://doi.org/10.1093/cid/ciu444

Pharmacotherapy

Pharmacologic management presented here is specific to adults with mild to moderate cellulitis free of systemic signs of infection and can be safely treated in an outpatient setting (see Algorithm 37.1).

■ Nonpurulent cellulitis
  ▪ Cephalexin 500 mg orally every 6 hours for 5 days *OR*
  ▪ Penicillin VK 250 to 500 mg orally every 6 hours for 5 days *OR*
  ▪ Dicloxacillin 500 mg orally every 6 hours for 5 days *OR*
  ▪ Clindamycin 300 to 450 mg orally every 6 hours for 5 days
  ▪ Prednisone 40 mg orally daily for 7 days as adjunct therapy in nondiabetic persons or ibuprofen 400 mg orally 4 times daily to accelerate clinical improvement. Prednisone must *not* be used if necrotizing fasciitis is present.
■ Purulent cellulitis: Requires coverage against methicillin-resistant *Staphylococcus aureus* (MRSA)
  ▪ Trimethoprim-sulfamethoxazole 160 mg/800 mg twice daily *OR* Doxycylcine 100 mg orally BID**
  (Stevens et al., 2014)

**A longer duration of antibiotic treatment may be a consideration in a person with purulent cellulitis who shows minimal improvement with antibiotic therapy within 48 hours.

NONPHARMACOTHERAPY

- Educate
  - Person and their family about the diagnosis of cellulitis, treatments, possible side effects of treatment, importance of adherence and completion of pharmacologic therapy, and signs and symptoms that prompt immediate care (e.g., if infection worsens and if fever persists despite antibiotic use for 48 hours)
  - Elevate affected limb as often as possible.
  - Avoidance of scratching or picking at site of cellulitis
  - Wash affected area with unscented antibacterial soap and soft cloth; do not scrub. If nonpermanent pen was used to identify improvement or worsening of cellulitis, advise not to wash off. Dry well.
- Lifestyle
  - Limit sugar intake in persons with diabetes mellitus to prevent hyperglycemia, slower healing, and other complications of cellulitis.
  - Drink plenty of water, especially with antibiotic use.
- Referral
  - Emergency department: If no improvement of cellulitis after 48 to 72 hours of antibiotic therapy, worsening of cellulitis, or persistent fevers
  - Infectious disease: Likely referred via emergency department
  - Wound care: For recurring cellulitis or slow-healing cellulitis in persons with diabetes mellitus, edema, and/or peripheral vascular disease
- Follow-up
  - 48 hours after initiation of antibiotic therapy or sooner if concern. Improvement including decreased swelling, erythema, and pain to the affected area should be identified. The borders of erythema should be receding.
  - If improvement, then in 1-week increments until cellulitis is resolved.

(Brown & Hood Watson, 2023; Stevens et al., 2014)

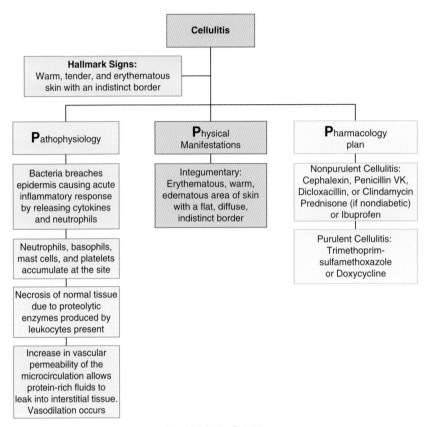

Algorithm 37.1   Cellulitis

References

Bland, T. B. (2020). Dermatologic disorders. In D. L. Maaks, N. Starr, M. A. Brady, N. M. Gaylord, M. Driessnack, & K. G. Duderrstadt (Eds.), *Burns' pediatric primary care* (7th ed., pp. 574–576). Elsevier.

Brown, B. D., & Hood Watson, K. L. (2023). Cellulitis. In: StatPearls [Internet]. https://www.ncbi.nlm.nih.
gov/books/NBK549770.

Djuric, C. M., & Turner, K. C. (2023). Structure, function, and disorders of the integument. In J. L. Rogers
(Ed.), *McCance and Huether's pathophysiology: The biologic basis for disease in adults and children* (9th ed.,
pp. 1521–1522). Mosby-Elsevier.

Kumar, M., Ngian, V. J. J., Yeong, C., Keighley, C., Nguyen, H. V., & Ong, B. S. (2020). Cellulitis in older
people over 75 years—Are there differences? *Annals of Medicine and Surgery, 49*, 37–40. https://doi.
org/10.1016/j.amsu.2019.11.012.

Miller, K. M., Lamagni, T., Hay, R., Cannon, J. W., Marks, M., Bowen, A. C., Kaslow, D., Cherian, T., Seale,
A. C., Pickering, J., Daw, J. N., Moore, H. C., Van Beneden, C., Carapetis, J. R., & Manning, L. (2022).
Standardization of epidemiological surveillance of Group A streptococcal cellulitis. *Open Forum Infectious
Disease, 9*(1_Supplement), 25–30. https://doi.org/10.1093/ofid/ofac267.

Stevens, D. L., Bisno, A. L., Chambers, H. F., Patchen Dellinger, E., Goldstein, E. J. C., Gorbach, S. L.,
Hirschmann, J. V., Kaplan, S. L., Montoya, J. G., & Wade, J. C (2014). Practice guidelines for the diag-
nosis and management of skin and soft tissue infection: 2014 update by the Infectious Disease Society of
America. *Clinical Infectious Diseases, 59*(2), 10–52. https://doi.org/10.1093/cid/ciu296.

Reproductive System

SECTION OUTLINE

38 Benign Prostatic Hypertrophy

39 Dysmenorrhea

40 Sexually Transmitted Infections

CHAPTER 38

Benign Prostatic Hypertrophy

Jodi Allen

Benign Prostatic Hypertrophy

Benign prostatic hypertrophy (BPH), also known as benign prostatic hyperplasia, is nonmalignant hyperplasia of the prostate tissue and the most common benign prostatic disease in males over age 50 (Rodway & McCance, 2023). Age is a significant predictor of the development of BPH, with 50% of males over age 50 demonstrating evidence of the disease (Box 38.1) (Rodway & McCance, 2023). The prevalence of BPH in the United States is on the rise as the population ages, with BPH present in approximately 70% of males between the ages of 60 and 69 and 80% of males over age 70 (Awedew et al., 2022). Risk factors for BPH include age, diabetes, obesity, metabolic syndrome, hypertension, diet, sex hormone levels, and family history (Boxes 38.2 and 38.3) (Granville & Suchak, 2023). Males with obesity and poor glycemic control have significantly greater lower urinary tract symptoms (LUTS), which are associated with high levels of systemic inflammation and increased levels of estrogen (Rodway & McCance, 2023). BPH is a clinical diagnosis and one of exclusion.

Pathophysiology

The cause of BPH remains fully unknown; however, the aging prostate with fluctuating levels of androgens and estrogens in addition to chronic inflammation leads to a cascade of events (Rodway & McCance, 2023). The prostate gland naturally enlarges during a male's life cycle, with the last growth phase during the fifth decade of life (Granville & Suchak, 2023). Circulating androgens disrupt the typical balance of growth factor signaling pathways, which causes growth and tissue remodeling, leading to prostate enlargement (Rodway & McCance, 2023). Chronic inflammation exacerbates growth and remodeling of the prostate tissue (see Algorithm 38.1). This growth can eventually occur in an outward fashion, leading to an enlarged prostate (Granville & Suchak, 2023). Enlargement of the prostate causes impingement on the prostatic urethra and bladder outlet while also causing tension of prostatic smooth muscle, and thus function of the muscle (Granville & Suchak, 2023). LUTS occur due to excessive growth of glandular prostate tissue that can impede or completely obstruct urinary flow (Granville & Suchak, 2023). The act of voiding is synchronized between the bladder and urethra. Stimulation of parasympathetic nerves triggers bladder muscle contraction and the action of voiding; however, stimulation of sympathetic nerves in the bladder neck and prostate causes closing of the bladder outlet, leading to voiding dysfunction (Granville & Suchak, 2023).

Physical Clinical Presentation

SUBJECTIVE

During the focused history, documentation should include the onset of symptoms; precipitating events; location, intensity, and quality of pain; progression of symptoms; alleviating and

BOX 38.1 ■ Older Adult Considerations

Benign prostatic hypertrophy (BPH) is frequently diagnosed in the fifth and sixth decades of life, in which males are considered to remain vital in all aspects of life. At this stage of life, males are often working, physically and sexually active, traveling, and carrying out activities of daily living. Lower urinary tract symptoms related to BPH range from inconvenient to severely affecting quality of life, and admitting to health care providers that these symptoms are occurring brings up a variety of anxiety-provoking feelings. In a 2019 study, males reported that identification of the disease negatively affected virility and sexual ability, increased feelings of embarrassment about the disease, and increased hesitancy to be examined. For practitioners who approach males with lower urinary tract symptoms related to BPH, respectfully educating them on what to expect during examination and treatment and how to lessen the impact of BPH on activities of daily living can aid in improved quality of life and comfort with care (Ozcan & Ozdil, 2019).

BOX 38.2 ■ Diversity Considerations

In the United States, benign prostatic hypertrophy (BPH) is disproportionately prevalent in Black males relative to the general population. The increased risk of BPH in this population is thought to be due to genetic factors and a variety of health disparities. The increased risk of prostate cancer is well known in Black males, but less research has been done on their lower urinary tract symptoms related to BPH. When caring for Black males with symptoms of BPH, it is imperative to ascertain their family history of prostate cancer and screen them appropriately. Several studies have demonstrated that vitamin D insufficiency, common in Black persons and those with higher skin melanin, exacerbates lower urinary tract symptoms (Wiedemer et al., 2021).

BOX 38.3 ■ Pediatric Considerations

Family history of prostate cancer, specifically when a brother or father is diagnosed, is known to increase the risk of prostate cancer from twofold to fourfold. What is less known is that a family history of breast cancer increases the risk for prostate cancer by 21%. When obtaining a child's history, the family history is often left out secondary to time constraints during the well child visit. Genetic red flags should be identified by practitioners, especially if multiple members of the family are affected by the same condition. Educating the child's family about heritable diagnoses during their early age can have a positive impact on disease prevention for the entire family (Barber et al., 2018).

aggravating factors; previous episodes; and associated symptoms. BPH causes LUTS related both to storage of urine (frequency, nocturia, urgency, incontinence) and voiding (slow, split, or intermittent stream; straining; hesitancy; dribbling/trickling of urine; incomplete emptying), which are frequently the first symptoms males report (Rodway & McCance, 2023). As BPH is a diagnosis of exclusion, a thorough history including past medical history as well as family and social histories should be included. Identify key inflammatory indicators that could be exacerbating LUTS, such as poorly controlled diabetes or obesity (Fig. 38.1) (Granville & Suchak, 2023). Current or former diagnoses and family history of diseases that can affect the neural control of voiding mechanisms such as cerebrovascular accident, Parkinson's disease, multiple sclerosis, and spinal cord injury should be identified (Granville & Suchak, 2023). Review medications to identify those that can affect urinary flow (e.g., anticholinergics, diuretics) and inquire about dietary habits as males who eat a diet high in red meat and low in vegetables can increase their risk of BPH (Russo et al., 2021).

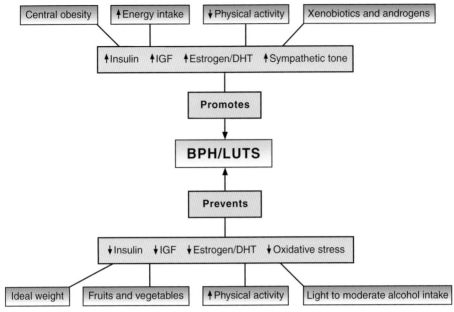

Fig. 38.1 Pathophysiologic responses that promote and strategies that prevent benign prostatic hypertrophy/lower urinary tract symptoms. *BPH*, benign prostatic hypertrophy; *LUTS*, lower urinary tract symptoms. (From Rakel, D., & Minichiello, V. J. (2023) (Eds.), *Integrative medicine* (5th ed.). Elsevier.)

BOX 38.4 ■ Acute Care Considerations

Acute urinary retention (AUR) is a significant complication of benign prostatic hypertrophy. Males will report an urgent need to urinate without the ability to do so; pain, frequently severe, to the lower abdomen; and swelling to the lower abdomen. A thorough history and physical exam including abdominal, rectal, and neurologic exams should be completed. Males with AUR will have a variety of tests done, but ultimately the urine must be drained from the bladder before damage occurs to the bladder and/or kidneys. AUR can be life threatening if left untreated; therefore swift identification and transfer to an emergency department are imperative to decrease risk of morbidity and mortality (Gelber & Singh, 2021).

OBJECTIVE*

Generalized: Fatigue

Neurological: **Decreased sensation to lower extremities, perineum, or scrotum** via light touch

Gastrointestinal: **Costovertebral angle tenderness; palpable bladder;** abdominal pain; **abdominal swelling** (Box 38.4)

Genitourinary: **Hematuria**

Reproductive: **Enlarged smooth prostate;** (see Algorithm 38.1) **firm nodular prostate** (Granville & Suchak, 2023)

---

*Hallmark signs are bolded and **Red flags are bolded and underlined**.

Evaluation and Differential Diagnoses

DIAGNOSTICS

- Measure the severity of symptoms by obtaining an American Urological Association Symptom Index (AUA-SI)/International Prostate Symptom Score (https://www.mdcalc.com/calc/10462/american-urological-association-symptom-index-aua-si).
- Urinalysis to exclude infection or hematuria
- Postvoid residual volume, if equipment readily available
- Prostate-specific antigen is optional unless family history or exam warrants. The antigen level can be elevated in both BPH and prostate cancer

(American Urological Association [AUA], 2021)

DIFFERENTIAL DIAGNOSES

- Bladder calculi: Painful urination, lower abdominal pain, and hematuria
- Prostatitis: Dysuria, fever, malaise, low back, rectal, perineal pain, and hematuria
- Prostate cancer: Often asymptomatic with symptoms similar to BPH; physical exam helpful to identify; hematuria

(Granville & Suchak, 2023)

Plan

GUIDELINE RESOURCES

- Sandhu, J. S., Bixler, B. R., Dahm, P., et al. (2023). Management of lower urinary tract symptoms attributed to benign prostatic hyperplasia (BPH): AUA Guideline amendment 2023. *Journal of Urology.* https://doi.org/10.1097/JU.0000000000003698.

Pharmacotherapy

Initiation of BPH treatment is dependent on the patient and the effects their symptoms have on their quality of life. Pharmacologic therapy is of limited benefit without concurrent initiation of nonpharmacotherapeutic interventions and lifestyle modifications (see Algorithm 38.1). A "watchful waiting" approach for males with BPH with mild symptoms and little impact on quality of life is the most appropriate form of management (AUA, 2021).

- First-line medication: Alpha blocker (e.g., alfuzosin, doxazosin, silodosin, tamsulosin, or terazosin). Base choice on age, comorbidities, and adverse effects profile.
- Second-line medication: 5a-reductase inhibitors (e.g., finasteride and dutasteride). Can be monotherapy in males with LUTS/BPH with prostatic enlargement on imaging, PSA level >1.5 ng/dL, or palpable prostate enlargement on digital rectal exam. Can be combination therapy with alpha-blocker to prevent progression of LUTS/BPH and/or decrease need for future prostate-related surgery. Educate on risks of sexual side effects, uncommon physical side effects, and low risk of prostate cancer with use.
- Phosphodiesterase-5 inhibitor: Tadalafil 5 mg daily is an option for those with lack of response with, incomplete response with, or inability to tolerate alpha-blocker and 5a-reductase inhibitor regardless of presence of comorbid erectile dysfunction.

(AUA, 2021)

NONPHARMACOTHERAPY

- Educate
  - Medication side effects
  - Optimal time to take other medication (e.g., diuretics) to decrease risk of LUTS
  - Bladder retraining
- Lifestyle
  - Avoidance of caffeine, alcohol, carbonated beverages, artificial sweeteners, and highly seasoned foods (all bladder irritants)
  - Avoid fluids 2 hours before bedtime if nocturia present
  - Weight loss if overweight or obese
  - Avoid constipation, but be mindful of need to increase water intake with increased fiber intake to prevent constipation, which can impact LUTS
- Referral
  - Urologist: Evaluate for surgical intervention in males with renal insufficiency secondary to BPH, urinary retention secondary to BPH, recurrent urinary tract infection, recurrent bladder calculi or gross hematuria, and if prostate cancer is suspected.
  - Pelvic floor therapy
- Follow-up
  - At minimum: Every 1 to 3 months to administer the American Urological Association Symptom Index/International Prostate Symptom Score and complete urodynamic testing. Digital rectal exam should be done annually.

(AUA, 2021)

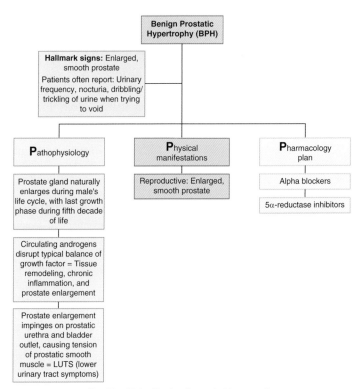

Algorithm 38.1 Benign Prostatic Hypertrophy

References

American Urological Association. (2021). *Management of lower urinary tract symptoms attributed to benign prostatic hyperplasia.* American Urological Association. https://www.auanet.org/guidelines-and-quality/guidelines/benign-prostatic-hyperplasia-(bph)-guideline.

Awedew, A. F., Han, H., Abbasi, B., Abbasi-Kangevari, M., Ahmed, M. B., Almidani, O., Amini, E., Arabloo, J., Argaw, A. M., Sthari, S. S., Atlaw, D., Banach, M., Barrow, A., Bhagavathula, A. S., Bhojaraja, V. S., Bikbov, B., Bodicha, B. B. A., Butt, N. A., Caetano dos Santos, F. L., … Dirac, M. A. (2022). The global, regional, and national burden of benign prostatic hyperplasia in 204 countries and territories from 2000 to 2019: A systematic analysis for the global burden of disease study 2019. *Lancet, 3*(11), E754–E776. https://doi.org/10.1016/S2666-7568(22)00213-6.

Barber, L., Gerke, T., Markt, S. C., Peisch, S. F., Wilson, K. M., Ahearn, T., Giovannucci, E., Parmigiani, G., & Mucci, L. A. (2018). Family history of breast and prostate cancer and prostate cancer risk. *Clinical Cancer Research, 24*(23), 5910–5917. https://doi.org/10.1158/1078-0432.CCR-18-0370.

Gelber, J., & Singh, A. (2021). Management of acute urinary retention in the emergency department. *Emergency Medicine Practice, 23*(3), 1–28. https://www.ebmedicine.net/topics/genitourinary/urinary-retention.

Granville, L. J., & Suchak, N. (2023). Benign prostate disease. In G. A. Warshaw, J. F. Potter, E. Flaherty, M. T. Heflin, M. K. McNabney, & R. J. Ham (Eds.), *Ham's primary care geriatrics: A case-based approach* (7th ed., pp. 498–506). Elsevier.

Ozcan, A., & Ozdil, K. (2019). The correlation between symptoms of benign prostatic hyperplasia and quality of life: A field study. *International Journal of Urological Nursing, 13*(1), 31–38. https://doi.org/10.1111/ijun.12180.

Rodway, G. W., & McCance, K. L. (2023). Alterations of the male reproductive system. In J. L. Rogers (Ed.), *McCance and Huether's pathophysiology: The biologic basis for disease in adults and children* (9th ed., pp. 843–844). Mosby-Elsevier.

Russo, G. I., Broggi, G., Cocci, A., Capogrosso, P., Falcone, M., Sokolakis, I., Gui, M., Caltabiano, R., & Di Mauro, M. (2021). Relationship between dietary patterns with benign prostatic hypertrophy and erectile dysfunction: A collaborative review. *Nutrients, 13*(11), 4148. https://doi.org/10.3390/nu13114148.

Wiedemer, J., McKoy, T., & Yu, M. (2021). Benign prostatic hyperplasia in African American men merits greater consideration in academic medicine. *Annals of Advanced Biomedical Sciences, 4*(2), 000164. https://doi.org.10.23880/aabsc-16000164.

CHAPTER 39

Dysmenorrhea

Jodi Allen

Dysmenorrhea

Dysmenorrhea is defined as painful menstruation, typically with absence of pain between menstrual periods. Diagnosis is further delineated as primary when there is no identifiable cause and secondary when related to organic pelvic disease (Rapkin & Gambone, 2016). Primary dysmenorrhea, the most common gynecologic condition, characteristically begins a few days prior to menstruation and persists for 48 to 72 hours. Females are more likely to report primary dysmenorrhea when they are younger than age 30, have not given birth, or have a history of sexual assault, premenstrual syndrome, or sterilization (Box 39.1) (Djuric et al., 2023). Personal history of heavy tobacco or alcohol use, a body mass index of less than 20, and family history of dysmenorrhea are risk factors as well (Djuric et al., 2023). Secondary dysmenorrhea often occurs in the later reproductive years and can occur at any time during the menstrual cycle. The most common causes of secondary dysmenorrhea are endometriosis (the foremost cause), endometritis, adenomyosis, pelvic inflammatory disease, obstructive uterine or vaginal abnormalities, uterine fibroids, polyps, tumors, ovarian cysts, pelvic congestion syndrome, and nonhormonal intrauterine devices (Djuric et al., 2023). Family history of any of these pelvic diseases can increase a female's risk for secondary dysmenorrhea. Dysmenorrhea, reportedly affecting between 45% and 95% of females, has been linked to lost work and school hours as well as a decreased quality of life for those who experience it (Box 39.2) (Ponzo et al., 2022).

Pathophysiology

Primary dysmenorrhea is caused by excessive prostaglandin synthesis of $F_2\alpha$ ($PGF_2\alpha$), which is a strong myometrial stimulant and vasoconstrictor found in secretory endometrium. This prostaglandin elevation increases myometrial contractions, constricts endometrial blood vessels, and enhances nerve hypersensitivity, leading to an increase in pain (see Algorithm 39.1). Inflammatory mediators produced in leukocytes also contribute to increased pain levels. The first 48 hours of menstruation coincide with higher prostaglandin levels, which can contribute to pain related to primary dysmenorrhea. As prostaglandins and their metabolites enter into systemic circulation, systemic symptoms (e.g., nausea, vomiting, dizziness) can occur. Anovulatory and/or thin endometrium, due to hormonal contraceptive use, decreases prostaglandin synthesis, and thus females experience little to no pain when this occurs (Djuric et al., 2023; Rapkin & Gambone, 2016).

Secondary dysmenorrhea is caused by organic pelvic condition(s) with their own individualized pathophysiology that elicit a pelvic pain response.

Physical Clinical Presentation

SUBJECTIVE

During the focused history, documentation should include the onset of symptoms; precipitating events; location, intensity, and quality of pain; progression of symptoms; alleviating and

BOX 39.1 ■ Pediatric Considerations

Ninety percent of females experience symptoms of dysmenorrhea within 2 years of menarche, making dysmenorrhea a common diagnosis in the pediatric population. In this age group, symptoms related to dysmenorrhea can increase the risk of missing school and other related activities. Appropriate treatment can be challenging, as schools often have restrictions related to medication use while attending class. Education on preferred medication use with instructions to be provided to school nurses can alleviate the discomfort of dysmenorrhea and limit school and activity time missed, improving quality of life for the young female with dysmenorrhea (Buyers & Romer, 2020).

BOX 39.2 ■ Diversity Considerations

Socioeconomic status and education are just a few of the indicators related to social determinants of health that negatively impact females with dysmenorrhea. Diets high in salt and processed sugars, which are typically less expensive than proteins, fruits, and vegetables, can increase the pain associated with dysmenorrhea. Skipping meals, particularly breakfast, and irregular eating habits also contribute to the pain intensity of dysmenorrhea. Identifying the dietary habits of females with dysmenorrhea, ensuring that they have access to appropriate foods, educating them on limiting consumption of processed foods, and encouraging them not to skip meals can decrease the severity of dysmenorrhea despite social factors (Bajalan et al., 2019).

BOX 39.3 ■ Older Adult Considerations

As females age and menopause occurs, the risk of dysmenorrhea is inherently gone due to the lack of menstruation and subsequent prostaglandin synthesis. After menopause, defined as 1 full year without menses, females should no longer experience vaginal bleeding. Bleeding after menopause is considered a red flag for endometrial and/or uterine cancer, and postmenopausal females should be educated on the importance of seeking health care if this occurs (Gambone, 2016).

aggravating factors; previous episodes; and associated symptoms. Knowing the onset of symptoms is particularly beneficial in differentiating between primary and secondary dysmenorrhea. Pain with primary dysmenorrhea typically starts within 24 hours of menses and can last for 48 to 72 hours whereas secondary dysmenorrhea may have pain 1 or more weeks prior to the start of menses and continue after the menses stops. The intensity of pain can range from uncomfortable to complete debilitation on the first day of menses or longer. Pain is frequently described as sharp, stabbing, and/or cramp-like over the lower abdominal area with radiation to the back or inner thigh(s). Persons with dysmenorrhea will commonly complain of nausea, vomiting, poor appetite, fatigue, altered bowel habits, and headache. Pain during intercourse, infertility, and abnormal uterine bleeding are more commonly reported in secondary dysmenorrhea. Personal and family histories should be ascertained to identify potential for an organic cause of dysmenorrhea. A thorough social history that includes sexual history should be obtained to identify risk for sexually transmitted infection(s) causing pelvic pain (see Chapter 40). Ask about the presence of abnormal vaginal bleeding (Box 39.3), vaginal discharge, vaginal itching, or noticeable lesions in the genital and perianal areas. Inquire about the type of birth control used, if any (Fig. 39.1).

(Djuric et al., 2023; Rapkin & Gambone, 2016)

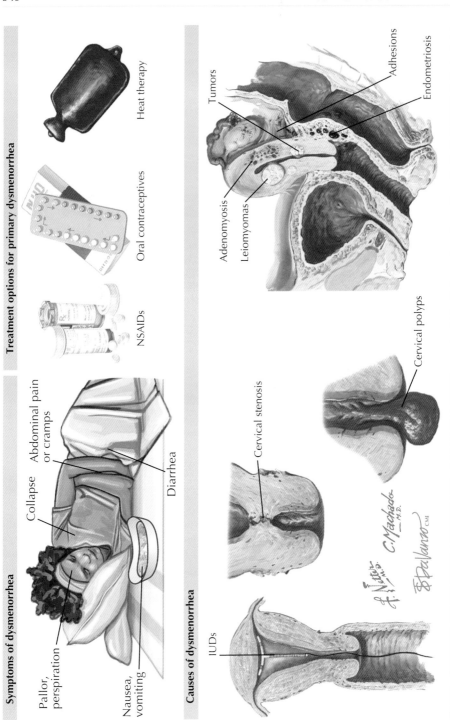

Fig. 39.1 Symptoms, possible causes, and treatment for dysmenorrhea. *NSAIDs,* nonsteroidal antiinflammatory drugs. (From Smith, R. P. (2024). *Netter's obstetrics and gynecology* (4th ed.). Elsevier.)

OBJECTIVE*

It is important to note that primary dysmenorrhea is a clinical diagnosis based on the person's menstrual history and related pain. Physical examination is often within normal limits with primary and secondary dysmenorrhea (Djuric et al., 2023).

Generalized: **Fatigue**

Gastrointestinal: **Pain to lower abdominal quadrants upon palpation**

Reproductive: Pelvic examination is essentially normal except for potential for **pain upon exam and/or identification of organic pelvic disease** (see Algorithm 39.1)

(Djuric et al., 2023; Rapkin & Gambone, 2016)

Evaluation and Differential Diagnoses

DIAGNOSTICS

Ruling out other potential causes of dysmenorrhea is the goal of diagnostics, thus diagnostics are not always required. Primary dysmenorrhea is a clinical diagnosis and does not necessarily warrant diagnostics unless an organic cause is being ruled out.

- Urine human chorionic gonadotropin or serum human chorionic gonadotropin to rule out pregnancy
- Complete blood count to rule out anemia
- Urinalysis to rule out urinary tract infection
- Gonorrhea and chlamydia via urine or culture to rule out sexually transmitted infection if risk or discharge present (see Chapter 40)
- Pelvic ultrasound to rule out organic pelvic cause

(Rapkin & Gambone, 2016)

DIFFERENTIAL DIAGNOSES

Differentiating between primary and secondary dysmenorrhea is important as each is a differential diagnosis for the other. The majority of differential diagnoses are related to organic pelvic disease causing secondary dysmenorrhea.

- Endometriosis: The most common cause of secondary dysmenorrhea; may have premenstrual spotting, fixed retroverted uterus, and/or tender pelvic nodules, particularly on the uterosacral ligaments
- Pelvic inflammatory disease: See Chapter 40
- Ovarian cyst(s): Often asymptomatic but frequent episodic pain related to menstrual cycle; often palpable on pelvic examination and visible on pelvic ultrasound (Box 39.4)

(Rapkin & Gambone, 2016)

Plan

GUIDELINE RESOURCES

- American College of Obstetricians and Gynecologists' Committee on Adolescent Health Care, Hewitt, G. D., & Gerancher, K. R. (2021). *Dysmenorrhea and endometriosis in the adolescent.* American College of Obstetricians and Gynecologists. https://www.acog.org/clinical/clinical-guidance/committee-opinion/articles/2018/12/dysmenorrhea-and-endometriosis-in-the-adolescent

---

*Hallmark signs are bolded and <u>Red flags are bolded and underlined</u>.

BOX 39.4 ■ Acute Care Considerations

Pelvic pain, frequently diagnosed as dysmenorrhea, can also be related to more acute conditions that must be ruled out to decrease morbidity. Ovarian cyst rupture, endometritis, pelvic inflammatory disease, and ectopic pregnancy can mimic dysmenorrhea in presentation depending on the stage of the condition. Appendicitis-associated pain is often thought to be related to dysmenorrhea. A thorough abdominal and pelvic assessment should be done to rule out acute alternatives to dysmenorrhea. Early diagnosis and swift treatment, often surgical, are important for safe and effective clinical management of acute pelvic pain (Rapkin & Gambone, 2016).

Pharmacotherapy

Treatment for primary and secondary dysmenorrhea is inherently the same until/if an organic pelvic cause is identified (see Algorithm 39.1). Further treatment for any organic pelvic disease will be specific to the disease identified.

- Nonsteroidal antiinflammatory drugs (NSAIDs) such as ibuprofen (800 mg once, then 400–800 mg every 8 hours as needed), naproxen sodium (440–550 mg once, then 220–550 mg every 12 hours as needed), mefenamic acid (500 mg once, then 250 mg every 6 hours as needed, not to exceed 3 days), or celecoxib (400 mg once, then 200 mg every 12 hours as needed; only in those 18 years of age and older) to be started 1 to 2 days before the onset of menses and continued through the first 2 to 3 days of bleeding
- Hormonal contraceptives such as combination oral contraceptive pills, patches, transvaginal rings, long-acting injectables, or implantable hormonal devices (if pregnancy not desired)

(American College of Obstetricians and Gynecologists [ACOG], 2021)

NONPHARMACOTHERAPY

- Educate
  - Medication side effects and importance of taking NSAIDs with food and increasing water intake to minimize side effects. Proper use of NSAIDs to limit pain in addition to maximum medication dosages and use limits should be discussed.
  - Consistent use of hormonal contraceptives can reduce risk of pregnancy and symptoms of dysmenorrhea. Hormonal contraceptives do not protect from sexually transmitted infections.
  - Use of heating pad to abdomen or hot baths to further relieve discomfort
- Lifestyle
  - Dietary changes such as caffeine and salt avoidance during first few days of menstruation
  - Increase exercise, including yoga and meditative therapies.
  - Smoking cessation
  - Acupuncture
- Referral
  - Obstetrician/gynecologist for care of organic pelvic causes of secondary dysmenorrhea or if uncontrollable symptoms of primary dysmenorrhea
  - Pelvic physical therapy
- Follow-up
  - 3 to 6 months to ensure improvement in symptoms; if no improvement, seek secondary cause and refer

(ACOG, 2021)

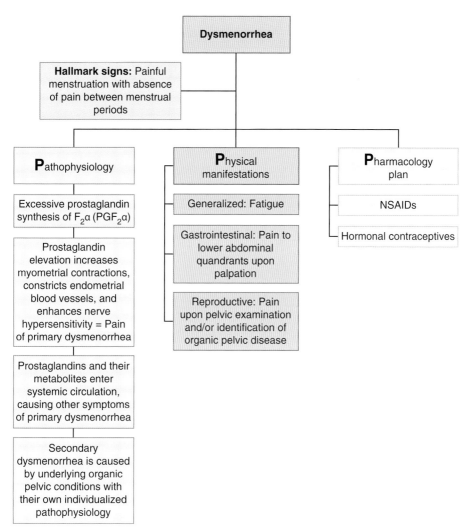

Algorithm 39.1 Dysmenorrhea

References

American College of Obstetricians and Gynecologists' Committee on Adolescent Health Care, Hewitt, G. D., & Gerancher, K. R. (2021). *Dysmenorrhea and endometriosis in the adolescent.* American College of Obstetricians and Gynecologists. https://www.acog.org/clinical/clinical-guidance/committee-opinion/articles/2018/12/dysmenorrhea-and-endometriosis-in-the-adolescent.

Bajalan, Z., Alimoradi, Z., & Moafi, F. (2019). Nutrition as a potential factor of primary dysmenorrhea: A systematic review of observational studies. *Gynecologic and Obstetric Investigation, 84*(3), 209–224. https://doi.org/10.1159/000495408.

Buyers, E., & Romer, E. (2020). Pediatric and adolescent gynecology. In D. L. Maaks, N. Starr, M. A. Brady, N. M. Gaylord, M. Driessnack, & K. G. Duderrstadt (Eds.), *Burns' pediatric primary care* (7th ed., pp. 866–867). Elsevier.

Djuric, C. M., Ruiz, S. M., & McCance, K. L. (2023). Alterations of the female reproductive system. In J. L. Rogers (Ed.), *McCance and Huether's pathophysiology: The biologic basis for disease in adults and children* (9th ed., pp. 770). Mosby-Elsevier.

Gambone, J. C. (2016). Menopause and perimenopause. In N. F. Hacker, J. C. Gambone, & C. J. Hobel (Eds.), *Hacker & Moore's essentials of obstetrics & gynecology* (6th ed., pp. 406–408). Elsevier.

Ponzo, S., Wickham, A., Bamford, R., Radovic, T., Zhaunova, L., Peven, K., Klepchukova, A., & Payne, J. L. (2022). Menstrual cycle-associated symptoms and workplace productivity in U.S. employees: A cross-sectional survey of users of the Flo mobile phone app. *Digital Health, 8*, 20552076221145852. https://doi.org/10.1177/20552076221145852.

Rapkin, A. J., & Gambone, J. C. (2016). Pelvic pain. In N. F. Hacker, J. C. Gambone, & C. J. Hobel (Eds.), *Hacker & Moore's essentials of obstetrics & gynecology* (6th ed., pp. 267–269). Elsevier.

CHAPTER 40

Sexually Transmitted Infections

Jodi Allen

Gonorrhea and Chlamydia

Sexually Transmitted Infections

Sexually transmitted infections (STIs) are the second most prevalent group of communicable diseases in the United States in both males and females (Centers for Disease Control and Prevention [CDC], 2023). Cases have been on the rise since 2020 and chlamydia infections have not returned to pre–COVID-19 pandemic levels (Boxes 40.1 and 40.2) (CDC, 2023). STIs are caused by viruses, bacteria, and parasites and infections can occur in the eyes, throat, external genitalia, vestibular glands, vagina, cervix, uterus, adnexa, and anal and perianal areas via sexual intercourse or intimate person-to-person contact (Somerall, 2023). STIs can also be transmitted from mother to child during pregnancy and birth, known as vertical transmission (Box 40.3) (Somerall, 2023). Many infected individuals are unaware of their status because symptoms are absent or minor, which increases transmission rates to others (Somerall, 2023). Risk factors for STIs are centered on behaviors such as unprotected intercourse or genital/oral contact, with multiple partners or via nonmonogamous relationships (CDC, 2023). STI transmission intensifies when the infectious agent contacts mucus membranes, specifically the mouth, oropharynx, vagina, rectum, and inner foreskin, which increases the risk for females, uncircumcised males, and males who are the receptive partner in oral or anal sex (Somerall, 2023). Broken or friable tissue increases the risk of STI transmission, and if a person has an active STI, they are at greater risk for another STI (Somerall, 2023). Untreated STIs lead to ascending infections that can affect the uterus, fallopian tubes, and ovaries in females, a serious condition known as pelvic inflammatory disease (PID) (Rimawi & Soper, 2016). Prevention, screening, and early treatment of STIs are the key to limit transmission and complications (CDC, 2023). This chapter focuses on the two most common STIs: gonorrhea and chlamydia.

Pathophysiology

Neisseria gonorrhoeae (the bacterium responsible for gonorrhea infections) is a Gram-negative diplococcus that has hairlike filaments that allow it to attach itself to host cells, predominantly epithelial cells of mucus membranes. Once the cell is invaded, the bacteria begin to damage the mucosa, causing a leukocytic response and exudate at the site of infection (see Algorithm 40.1). In females the endocervical canal is a common site of initial gonococcal infection; if untreated, the infection can ascend into the uterus and fallopian tubes where PID can develop. In males the urethra and rectum are common sites of initial infection; if untreated, the infection can cause epididymitis. Gonococci often share plasmids and DNA across species, which facilitates the transfer of antibiotic resistance, leading to multidrug-resistant gonorrhea or "super gonorrhea" (Somerall, 2023; World Health Organization, 2023).

Chlamydia trachomatis (the bacterium responsible for chlamydial infections) is a Gram-negative bacterium that is unable to reproduce without a host cell. *C. trachomatis* has a two-part growth

---

BOX 40.1 ■ Diversity Considerations

Sexually transmitted infections (STIs) are found in all populations regardless of ethnicity, socioeconomic status, or gender; however, rates are higher among some ethnic minority groups compared to the White population. These higher rates are not caused by ethnicity but rather by social conditions (social determinants of health) that are more likely to affect minority groups, such as poverty and lower socioeconomic status. Access to culturally competent care is lacking in many areas of poverty, where communities with higher rates of STIs exist. Health care providers should be culturally competent and comfortable discussing sexual health with all persons they care for to ensure risk identification for and prevention of STIs. The Centers for Disease Control and Prevention and other organizations provide culturally competent resources on their websites to assist providers (CDC, 2020).

BOX 40.2 ■ Older Adult Considerations

Sexual health is important at any age, and interest in sex does not disappear as a person ages. Older populations are not well-versed in the use of protective measures with sexual intimacy (i.e., condoms) and often lack knowledge of sexually transmitted infections (STIs) including the inherent risks they carry for themselves and their partners. These topics were not frequently discussed when they were growing up. This is reflected in the rate of STIs among those aged 55 years and older, as it has more than doubled over the past decade. Gonorrhea infections have increased from 3.5 cases per 100,000 people aged 55 years and older in 2010 to 17.2 cases per 100,000 people aged 55 years and older in 2020. Health care providers must be willing to engage in discussions about sexual health with older adults to identify risk for and prevention of STIs (Steckenrider, 2023).

BOX 40.3 ■ Pediatric Considerations

Chlamydia infection in the newborn results from perinatal exposure to a mother's infected cervix during birth. Infection to the infant's mucous membranes of the eye, oropharynx, urogenital tract, and rectum can occur. Chlamydial conjunctivitis is most frequently identified within 5 to 12 days after birth. Prophylactic use of erythromycin ointment has been found to be ineffective against chlamydial conjunctivitis versus the screening of pregnant females at risk for chlamydia and providing appropriate treatment to prevent the occurrence in the newborn. Retesting high-risk females during their third trimester and at delivery can further decrease the risk for newborns and expedite identification and treatment, if needed (CDC, 2021b).

---

cycle, the first of which consists of a small body that attaches itself to a host cell and enters it via endocytosis (see Algorithm 40.2). The second part of the cycle consists of the bacterium becoming a metabolically active parasite, reproducing up to 1000 new bodies. An inflammatory response is produced causing disruption of superficial tissues, which results in permanent scarring of affected tissues. Numerous strains of *C. trachomatis* have been identified over the years (Somerall, 2023).

The incubation period for both gonorrhea and chlamydia bacteria is 7 to 21 days, and due to the pathologic differences in how they infect cells, they can coexist and are frequently diagnosed as coinfections (Somerall, 2023).

Physical Clinical Presentation

SUBJECTIVE

According to the CDC (2023), gonorrhea and chlamydia are often asymptomatic, which requires practitioners to be astute in their history gathering to prevent worsening of infection

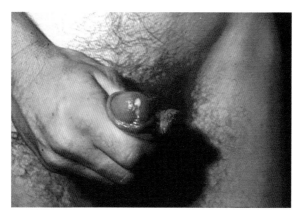

Fig. 40.1 Gonococcal urethritis. Purulent exudate common in urethritis caused by *Neisseria gonorrhoeae* bacterium. (From Centers for Disease Control and Prevention. (2020). *Sexually transmitted infections: STD clinical slides, gonorrhea.* CDC. https://www.cdc.gov/sti/hcp/clinical-slides/?CDC_AAref_Val=https://www.cdc.gov/std/training/clinicalslides/slides-dl.htm.)

and complications. Asking about the person's personal history of previous STIs and successful completion of treatment is important as often treatment is not completed and eradication of the causative bacteria is unlikely (CDC, 2021a). A thorough social history, including sexual history, is imperative for both the diagnosis of and screening for gonorrhea and chlamydia. Males may complain of dysuria, purulent penile discharge, and urethral inflammation with a gonococcal infection and females may complain of yellow or green purulent vaginal drainage, pain and/or bleeding with intercourse, and pelvic pain (Somerall, 2023). Males may complain of the same symptoms with a chlamydial infection but will often note pain or swelling of the testicles as well. Females with a chlamydial infection will report similar symptoms as gonococcal infections, making the distinction between the two bacteria challenging based on history alone. During the focused history, documentation should include the onset of symptoms; precipitating events; location, intensity, and quality of pain; progression of symptoms; alleviating and aggravating factors; previous episodes; and associated symptoms.

OBJECTIVE*

The inspection portion of the reproductive exam for suspected gonorrhea and/or chlamydia should include the external genitalia and the anal and perianal areas, urethra, and vestibular glands in females and the penis, glans, urethra, scrotum, and anal area in males.

Generalized: **Fever; chills**

HEENT: Conjunctivitis; lymphadenopathy; tonsilitis

Gastrointestinal: **Nausea; vomiting; pain to lower abdominal quadrants upon palpation**

Genitourinary: **Urethral stricture**

Reproductive: *Inspection:* **Erythema**; **inflammation** to male or female areas (noted above); **colored, purulent, odorous discharge** from vagina, vestibular glands, cervix, anus, or penis (Figs. 40.1 and 40.2). *Palpation:* **Cervical motion tenderness; adnexal tenderness; cervical or anal edema, erythema, and friability**; epididymitis; unilateral scrotal edema (see Algorithms 40.1 and 40.2)

(Somerall, 2023)

---

*Hallmark signs are bolded and Red flags are bolded and underlined.

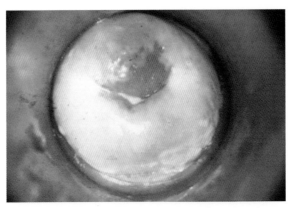

Fig. 40.2 Gonococcal cervicitis. Purulent discharge from an erythematous cervix caused by *Neisseria gonorrhoeae*. (From Centers for Disease Control and Prevention. (2020). *Sexually transmitted infections: STD clinical slides, gonorrhea*. CDC. https://www.cdc.gov/std/training/clinicalslides/slides-dl.htm.)

Evaluation and Differential Diagnoses

DIAGNOSTICS

Due to the intense similarities between the presentation of gonorrhea and chlamydia and the frequency of coinfection, they should *always* be tested for together. Note that in *all* US states, gonorrhea and chlamydia are required to be reported when identified. It can be up to the laboratory and/or health care provider to provide information such as date of diagnosis, type of treatment, pregnancy status, and partner treatment and notification.

■ Urine specimen to identify or screen for gonorrhea and chlamydia *OR* culture of discharge from cervix, urethra, rectum, oropharyngeal, or ocular sites to identify gonorrhea and chlamydia

■ Liquid-based Pap test to screen for gonorrhea and chlamydia in women (*not* as sensitive as preceding options)

■ Pregnancy test in females

■ Positive gonorrhea and chlamydia tests should lead to testing for other STIs including syphilis and HIV.

(Pagana et al., 2021)

DIFFERENTIAL DIAGNOSES

Differentiating between gonorrhea and chlamydia is important as each is a differential diagnosis for the other.

■ Trichomoniasis: Copious frothy malodorous discharge with a yellow-green to gray-green coloration; small red punctate marks called strawberry spots on vaginal walls and cervix

■ Syphilis: Chancre, a hard, firm, and painless ulcer, is visible in primary syphilis.

■ PID: Typically precipitated by gonorrhea and/or chlamydia infection in females, so similar symptoms are present. Systemic symptoms such as fever, chills, nausea, and vomiting are present with lower abdominal/pelvic pain that is often exacerbated by movement (Box 40.4).

(Somerall, 2023)

BOX 40.4 ■ Acute Care Considerations

Pelvic inflammatory disease (PID) is inflammation of the upper genital tract, uterus, fallopian tubes, and/or ovaries due to infection that sometimes requires hospitalization for treatment. Gonorrhea and chlamydia are a frequent cause of PID, especially if either of these sexually transmitted infections is left untreated or treated inappropriately. A triad of symptoms and signs are specific for PID, including pelvic pain, cervical motion and adnexal tenderness, and fever. Some females experience subtle signs of PID, making diagnosis challenging. Pelvic organ tenderness is usually present in PID and can aid in determination. Outpatient treatment for PID should include broad-spectrum coverage for a multitude of pathogens, especially gonorrhea and chlamydia, and is typically preferred over inpatient treatment. If treatment failure is occurring (i.e., no improvement with short-term treatment); treatment compliance is questionable; nausea, vomiting, and/or high fever is present; or a tubo-ovarian abscess is suspected or confirmed, inpatient care is recommended (Rimawi & Soper, 2016).

Plan

GUIDELINE RESOURCES

- Centers for Disease Control and Prevention. (2024). *Chlamydial infections—STI treatment guidelines.* CDC. https://www.cdc.gov/std/treatment-guidelines/chlamydia.htm
- Centers for Disease Control and Prevention. (2024). *Gonococcal infections among adolescents and adults—STI treatment guidelines.* CDC. https://www.cdc.gov/std/treatment-guidelines/gonorrhea-adults.htm

Pharmacotherapy

- Uncomplicated gonococcal infection of the cervix, urethra, or rectum (see Algorithm 40.1) (CDC, 2021a)
  - Ceftriaxone 500 mg IM in a single dose (for persons weighing <330 pounds [<150 kg]); ceftriaxone 1 g in a single dose (for persons weighing >330 pounds [≥150 kg])
  - If chlamydia infection has not been excluded:
    - Doxycycline 100 mg orally twice daily for 7 days
  - If cephalosporin allergy:
    - Gentamicin 240 mg IM in a single dose WITH azithromycin 2 g orally in a single dose
  - If ceftriaxone administration is not available or not feasible:
    - Cefixime 800 mg orally in a single dose with doxycycline 100 mg orally twice daily for 7 days if chlamydia infection has not been excluded
- Uncomplicated gonococcal infection of the pharynx (CDC, 2021a)
  - Ceftriaxone 500 mg IM in a single dose (for persons weighing <330 pounds [<150 kg]); ceftriaxone 1 g in a single dose (for persons weighing ≥330 pounds [≥150 kg])
  - If chlamydial infection is identified with pharyngeal gonorrhea:
    - Doxycycline 100 mg orally twice daily for 7 days
- Gonococcal conjunctivitis (CDC, 2021a)
  - Ceftriaxone 1 g IM in a single dose
- Chlamydial infection (see Algorithm 40.2) (CDC, 2021b)
  - Doxycycline 100 mg orally twice daily for 7 days
  - Alternative regimens:
    - Azithromycin 1 g orally in a single dose *OR*
    - Levofloxacin 500 mg orally daily for 7 days

- Expedited partner therapy (EPT) (CDC, 2021c)
  - An approach to treat sex partners of persons who test positive for certain STIs without previous evaluation by a health care provider. EPT is recommended for heterosexual male and female partners with gonorrhea whose prompt access to clinical evaluation and treatment is unlikely. Check your state laws to ensure that they allow EPT:
    - Cefixime 800 mg orally in a single dose
    - If chlamydia has *not* been excluded:
      - Doxycycline 100 mg orally twice daily for 7 days
      - Alternative to doxycycline → azithromycin 1 g orally in a single dose but not as efficacious

NONPHARMACOTHERAPY

- Educate
  - Medication side effects, importance of taking all medication as directed, and risk of reinfection. This education must be included with EPT as well.
  - Encouraging persons diagnosed with STIs to inform all partners and advise them to seek evaluation and treatment
  - Avoid sexual contact until treatment is complete, symptoms have resolved, and all partners have been treated. Condoms must be used if unable to abstain.
  - Signs and symptoms of PID in females; epididymitis in males
  - Importance of cervical cancer screening for females starting at age 21
  - Importance of hepatitis B vaccine and human papilloma virus vaccine (if not already received) for both males and females
- Lifestyle
  - Risk-reducing behaviors to prevent future STIs including the use of condoms with every sexual encounter and limiting number of sexual partners
- Referral
  - Obstetrician/gynecologist if pregnancy identified
  - Counseling if STI is related to trauma/nonconsensual sex
- Follow-up
  - Test to cure (i.e., repeat testing 4 weeks after therapy completion) is *not* recommended for nonpregnant persons with uncomplicated urogenital or rectal gonorrhea or chlamydia who are treated with recommended or alternative regimens unless adherence to medication is in question, symptoms persist, or reinfection is suspected.
  - Males and females should be retested 3 months after treatment of gonorrhea and chlamydia regardless.

(CDC, 2021a, 2021b)

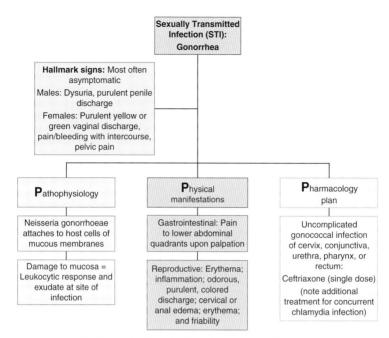

Algorithm 40.1 Sexually Transmitted Infection: Gonorrhea

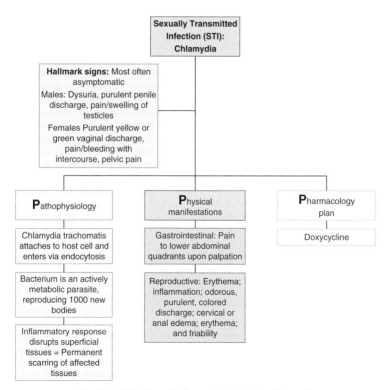

Algorithm 40.2 Sexually Transmitted Infection: Chlamydia

References

Centers for Disease Control and Prevention. (2023). *U.S. STI epidemic showed no signs of slowing in 2021—Cases continued to escalate.* Centers for Disease Control and Prevention. https://www.cdc.gov/media/releases/2023/s0411-sti.html.

Centers for Disease Control and Prevention. (2021a). *Sexually transmitted infections treatment guidelines, 2021: Gonococcal infections among adolescents and adults.* Centers for Disease Control and Prevention. https://www.cdc.gov/std/treatment-guidelines/gonorrhea-adults.htm.

Centers for Disease Control and Prevention. (2021b). *Sexually transmitted infections treatment guidelines, 2021: Chlamydial infections.* Centers for Disease Control and Prevention. https://www.cdc.gov/std/treatment-guidelines/chlamydia.htm.

Centers for Disease Control and Prevention. (2021c). *Sexually transmitted infections: Guidance on the use of expedited partner therapy in the treatment of gonorrhea.* Centers for Disease Control and Prevention. Retrieved August 17, 2023. https://www.cdc.gov/std/treatment-guidelines/clinical-EPT.htm.

Centers for Disease Control and Prevention. (2020). *Sexually transmitted infections: STD health equity.* Centers for Disease Control and Prevention. https://www.cdc.gov/std/health-disparities/default.htm.

Pagana, K. D., Pagana, T. J., & Pagana, T. N. (Eds.). (2021). *Mosby's diagnostic & laboratory test reference.* Elsevier.

Rimawi, B. H., & Soper, D. E. (2016). Infectious diseases of the female reproductive and urinary tract. In N. F. Hacker, J. C. Gambone, & C. J. Hobel (Eds.), *Hacker & Moore's essentials of obstetrics & gynecology* (6th ed., pp. 276–282). Elsevier.

Somerall, W. (2023). Sexually transmitted infections. In J. L. Rogers (Ed.), *McCance and Huether's pathophysiology: The biologic basis for disease in adults and children* (9th ed., pp. 865–884). Mosby-Elsevier.

Steckenrider, J. (2023). Sexual activity of older adults: Let's talk about it. *Lancet, 4*(3), E96–E97. https://doi.org/10.1016/S2666-7568(23)00003-X.

World Health Organization. (2023). *Multi-drug resistant gonorrhea.* World Health Organization. https://www.who.int/news-room/fact-sheets/detail/multi-drug-resistant-gonorrhoea.

INDEX

Note: Page numbers followed by "*f*" indicate figures, "*t*" indicate tables, and "*b*" indicate boxes.

A

Abdominal hernia, 251, 256*f*
  diagnosis of, 251
  evaluation of, 251
  pathophysiology, 251
  pharmacotherapy, 255
  plan for, 254
Abdominal pain, 232, 241*f*
  causes of, 238*f*
  diagnosis of, 237
  evaluation of, 237
  pharmacotherapy, 238
  plan for, 238
  sites of, 238*f*
Acanthosis nigricans, 118*f*
Acne fulminans, 306
Acne vulgaris, 304
  acute care considerations, 306*b*
  algorithm for, 309*f*
  diagnoses of, 306
  diversity considerations, 305*b*
  evaluation of, 306
  with few noninflammatory comedones, 306*f*
  hallmark signs of, 305
  nonpharmacotherapy for, 308
  older adult considerations, 305*b*
  pathophysiology, 304
  pediatric considerations, 305*b*
  pharmacotherapy for, 307
  physical clinical presentation, 304
  plan for, 307
  prevalence of, 304
Acquired hernias, 251
Actinic keratosis, 328
Acute aortic syndrome, 132*b*
Acute bacterial cystitis, 294
Acute cholecystitis, 279, 281
Acute coronary syndrome (ACS), advanced age, risk factor
    for, 132*b*, 134*b*
Acute heart failure, 154, 156*f*, 167*f*
  classification of, 157*t*–158*t*
  HFpE, pathophysiology of, 159
  medications, 159
  pathophysiology, 156*f*
  pulmonary edema, 159
  treatment of, 157*t*–158*t*
Acute pharyngitis, 222
Acute pyelonephritis, 294, 296
Acute stress disorder (ASD), 65
Acute urinary retention (AUR), 342
Adaptive immune systems, cells of, 204*f*
Adenoids, 222–223
Age
  acute coronary syndrome, risk factor of, 134*b*
  ASCVD, primary prevention strategies based on, 171*t*
  atrial fibrillation, independent risk factor as, 141*b*
Aging process, 215
Alkaline urine, 286–287
Allergic contact dermatitis, 311–312, 313*f*
  algorithm for, 316*f*
  pathophysiology, 311

Alpha-1-antitrypsin deficiency (A1ATD), 203
Alveolar abnormalities, 203
American Urological Association Symptom Index (AUA-
    SI), 343
Amiodarone, 215
Androgens, 304
Angina, 131, 138*f*
  acute care considerations, 132*b*
  diagnoses of, 135
  diversity considerations, 132*b*
  evaluation of, 135
  guideline resources, 135
  ischemia, classic finding with, 131–132
  myocardial ischemia, 131–132
  nonpharmacotherapy, 137
  older adult considerations, 134*b*
  pathophysiology, 131
  pharmacotherapy, 137
  physical clinical presentation, 133–134
  ST-segment elevation myocardial infarction, 132*b*
  unstable, 134
  vasospastic, 134
Angina pectoris, 133–134
Angiotensin-converting enzyme (ACE) inhibitors, 159, 245
Anovulatory, 346
Anxiety, 47. *See also* Generalized anxiety disorder (GAD)
Aortic aneurysm, 236*t*
Aortic dissection, 132*b*
Appendicitis-associated pain, and dysmenorrhea, 350
Arrhythmia. *See* Dysrhythmia
Arterial blood pressure (ABP), 181
Arthritis, 70
Aspiration, 195–196
Atherosclerosis, 171–172, 173*f*. *See also* Atherosclerotic
    cardiovascular disease (ASCVD)
  clinical presentation of, 172–174
  growth factors, 171–172
  inflammatory cascade, 171–172
  plaques, 171–172
  progression of, 173*f*
  T cells, 171–172
Atherosclerotic cardiovascular disease (ASCVD), 169, 172, 174
  acute care considerations, 178*b*
  age based primary prevention strategies, 171*t*
  atherosclerosis, progression of, 173*f*
  chronic kidney disease and, 176
  diagnoses of, 175
  diversity considerations, 170*b*
  drug/alcohol induced—medications, 176
  evaluation of, 175
  guideline resources, 176
  hypothyroidism, 175
  medications, and elevation of LDL, 174
  metabolic syndrome, 175
  modifiable risk factors, 169
  nonpharmacotherapy, 177
  older adult considerations, 177*b*
  onset of, 172–174
  pain/shortness of breath, 172–174
  pediatric considerations, 175*b*
  pharmacotherapy, 176

Atherosclerotic cardiovascular disease (ASCVD) *(Continued)*
  primary prevention, 169
  social determinants of health, 169
  strategies based on risk score, primary prevention, 172*t*
Atopic dermatitis, 314, 320
Atrial dysrhythmia, cardiac dysrhythmias, diagnoses in,
    142*t*–146*t*, 147*f*
Atrial fibrillation (AF), 140
  age, independent risk factor, 141*b*
  mechanisms of, 151*f*
Autoimmune diseases, 214

B
Bacterial pathogens, 224*f*
Bacterial pharyngitis, 224
Bacterial pneumonia, 196
Bacterial superinfection, 196
Basal cell carcinoma, algorithm for, 330*f*
Basophilia, 110
Benign nevi, 328
Benign prostatic hyperplasia, 340
Benign prostatic hypertrophy, 340, 341*b*, 344*f*
  acute care considerations, 342*b*
  age and, 340
  diagnoses of, 343
  diversity considerations, 341*b*
  evaluation of, 343
  hallmark signs, 342
  nonpharmacotherapy for, 344
  older adult considerations, 341*b*
  pathophysiology, 340, 342*f*
  pediatric considerations, 341*b*
  pharmacologic therapy for, 343
  pharmacotherapy for, 343
  physical clinical presentation, 340
  plan for, 343
  prevalence of, 340
  risk factors for, 340
Beta-hemolytic strep, 319
Bile stasis, 278
Biliary atresia, 278
Biliary colic, 279
Bladder calculi, 343
Blood pressure (BP)
  diversity considerations, 182*b*
  elevated, risk of HTN, 181
  factors involved in regulation of, 182*f*
  hypertensive emergency, 188*b*
  older adult considerations, 187*b*
  pediatric considerations, 187*b*
Bowel obstruction, 236*t*
Bradykinin, 223
Bronchopneumonia, 196

C
Calcineurin inhibitors, 321
Cardiac dysrhythmias, 140. *See also* Dysrhythmia
  diagnoses in
    atrial dysrhythmia, 142*t*–146*t*, 147*f*
    heart block, 142*t*–146*t*, 147*f*
    sinus dysrhythmia, 142*t*–146*t*, 147*f*
    ventricular dysrhythmia, 142*t*–146*t*, 147*f*
  electrocardiogram strip recording, 147*f*
Cauda equina syndrome (CES), 85*b*
Ceftriaxone, for gonococcal conjunctivitis, 357
Cellulitic infections, 333
Cellulitis, 333
  acute care considerations, 334*b*
  algorithm for, 337*f*

Cellulitis *(Continued)*
  criteria for, 334
  diagnoses of, 334
  with diffuse erythema, 335*f*
  diversity considerations, 335*b*
  evaluation of, 334
  hallmark signs in, 334
  nonpharmacotherapy for, 337
  nonpurulent, 335*f*
  older adult considerations, 336*b*
  pathophysiology, 333
  pediatric considerations, 334*b*
  pharmacotherapy for, 336
  physical clinical presentation, 333
  treatment plan for, 336
Centers for Disease Control and Prevention, 223
Cerebrovascular accident (CVA), 2
  acute hospital stroke management, 5*b*
  diagnoses of, 5
  evaluation of, 5
  genetics role in, 4*b*
  guideline resources, 6
  nonpharmacotherapy, 7
  pediatric considerations, 4*b*
  pharmacotherapy, 6
  physical clinical presentation, 3
Cervical spine pain, 80, 86*f*. *See also* Spine conditions
  chronicity of pain and disability, 80–81
  diagnoses of, 83
  evaluation of, 83
Charcot's triad, 278
Chest pain, 134
  cardiac causes of, 133*b*
  characteristics of, 133–134
  evaluation and diagnosis of, 136*f*
  noncardiac/cardiac causes, 133
  in pediatric patients, 133*b*
  and stable angina, 132
  and vasospastic angina, 133
Chlamydia, 353, 359*f*
  and dysmenorrhea, 349
  incubation period for, 354
Chlamydia trachomatis, 353–354
Chlamydial conjunctivitis, 354*b*
Cholecystitis, 277
Cholecystolithiasis, 277–278
Cholelithiasis, 277, 289
  acute care considerations, 281*b*
  algorithm for, 282*f*
  diagnoses of, 280
  diversity considerations, 278*b*
  evaluation of, 280
  hallmark signs of, 279
  mechanisms of, 279*f*
  nonpharmacotherapy for, 281
  older adult considerations, 281*b*
  pathophysiology, 277
  pediatric considerations, 278*b*
  pharmacotherapy for, 281
  physical clinical presentation, 278
  plan for, 280
  risk factors for, 277
Cholesterol gallstones, 277–278
Chronic autoimmune thyroiditis, 123
Chronic bronchitis, 205
Chronic gastroesophageal reflux disease, 246
Chronic heart failure, 154, 156*f*, 167*f*
Chronic obstructive pulmonary disease (COPD), 203, 208,
    210*f*

Chronic obstructive pulmonary disease (COPD) *(Continued)*
clinical presentation of, 205–206
mechanisms of, 203
pathophysiologic process of, 203
Chylomicrons, 169–170
Cluster headache, 13, 21*f*
Comedones, 304
Community-acquired pneumonia (CAP), 193, 195
Comorbidities, 209
Complete blood count (CBC), leukocytosis, diagnostics for,
112, 112*t*
Complete pulmonary function test, 216
Concussion. *See* Mild traumatic brain injury (mTBI)
Congenital hypothyroidism, 125
Congenital lobar emphysema (CLE), 206
Contact dermatitis (CD), 311
acute care considerations, 312*b*
corticosteroids for
systemic (oral), 315
topical, 315
diagnoses of, 314
diversity considerations, 314*b*
evaluation of, 314
hallmark signs of, 313
nonpharmacotherapy for, 315
older adult considerations, 312*b*
pathophysiology, 311
pediatric considerations, 312*b*
pharmacotherapy for, 315
physical clinical presentation, 312
plan for, 314
Continuous antibiotic prophylaxis, 297
Cortical spreading depression (CSD), 12
COVID-19, 196
C-reactive protein levels, 306
Crepitus, 71–72
Crohn's disease, 258–259, 260*t*
Crushing chest pain, 183
Cryotherapy, for SCC, 329
Crystal growth inhibitor deficiencies, 286–287
Cystic duct, 277–278
Cystine stone formers, 289–290
Cystitis, 294

D
Deep vein thrombosis (DVT), 336
Depression, 54. *See also* Major depressive disorder (MDD)
screening tools, 305
Diabetes mellitus type 2 (DMT2), 116, 121*f*
acute care considerations, 118*b*
ASCVD, leading cause of mortality in, 120
diagnoses of, 119
evaluation of, 119
gastrointestinal incretins, 116
guideline resources, 119
increased risk for diabetes/prediabetes, categories of, 119
insulin resistance, 116
management of, 121*b*
nonpharmacotherapy, 120
older adult considerations, 121*b*
pathophysiology, 116
pharmacotherapy, 120
physical clinical presentation, 117
proinflammatory cytokines, 116
prolonged hyperglycemia, 116
Diabetic hyperglycemic hyperosmolar state, 118*b*
Diaper dermatitis, 312, 313*f*
Diffuse recurrent muscle pain, 216
Disease-modifying antirheumatic drugs (DMARDs), 75*b*, 76

Disease progression, 214
DNA methylation patterns, 212
Doxycycline, for chlamydial infection, 357
Dysfunctional surfactant production, 213
Dysmenorrhea, 346, 351*f*
acute care considerations, 350*b*
causes for, 348*f*
diagnoses of, 349
diversity considerations, 347*b*
evaluation of, 349
nonpharmacotherapy for, 350
older adult considerations, 347*b*
pathophysiology, 346
pediatric considerations, 347*b*
persons with, 346–347
pharmacotherapy for, 350
physical clinical presentation, 346
plan for, 349
symptoms for, 348*f*
treatment for, 348*f*
Dysrhythmia, 140, 151*f*. *See also* Cardiac dysrhythmias
acute care considerations, 141*b*
atrial fibrillation, 140
categories, 140
conduction pathway defects, 140–141
diagnosis of, 142*t*–146*t*, 149
diversity considerations, 141*b*
documentation, 148
etiologies for, 140
evaluation of, 148
guideline resources, 149
nonpharmacotherapy, 150
older adult considerations, 141*b*
pathophysiology, 140
pediatric considerations, 149*b*
pharmacotherapy, 150
physical clinical presentation, 141, 148
treatment, goal in, 150

E
Ectopic pregnancy, 350
Eczematous eruption, 311
Elevated intracranial pressure (ICP), 42*b*
Emphysema, 204
Empiric pharmacotherapy, 298
Endometriosis, and dysmenorrhea, 346, 349
Endometritis, 350
Endometrium, 346
Environmental stress, 270
Environmental stresses, 214
Eosinophilia, 110
Epidermal shedding, 318
Epilepsy, 26, 33*f*. *See also* Seizure
categorizing etiology of, 26
pathophysiology, 26
Epithelial damage, 213
Erysipelas, 335
Erythrodermic (exfoliative) psoriasis, 320
Erythromycin ointment, prophylactic use of, 354*b*
Esophageal rupture, 132*b*
Exfoliative psoriasis, 318
Expedited partner therapy (EPT), 358
Extrahepatic bile duct, 277–278

F
Febrile seizures, 26, 33*f*. *See also* Seizure
clonic phase, 26–27, 28*f*
pediatric considerations, 27*b*
Flank pain, 287

"Flesh-eating bacteria," 334
Folliculitis, 307

G
Gallstones, 277
  complications, 277
GAS pharyngitis, 224–226
Gastroesophageal reflux disease (GERD), 243, 245
  diagnosis of, 246
  evaluation of, 246
  pathophysiology, 243
  pharmacotherapy, 246
  plan for, 246
Gastrointestinal
  disease, connection with IDA, 97
  incretins, in DMT2, 116
Gene polymorphisms, 215
Generalized anxiety disorder (GAD), 47, 52*f*, 65
  acute care considerations, 48*b*
  cognitive behavior therapy and, 48*b*, 51
  complication of, 47
  diagnoses of, 50
  diversity considerations, 48*b*
  evaluation of, 49
  excessive and persistent worries, 47–48
  GAD-7 scale, 49*t*
  guideline resources, 50
  health literacy, 48*b*
  nonpharmacotherapy, 51
  older adult considerations, 49*t*, 50*b*
  pathophysiology, 47, 48*b*
  pediatric considerations, 48*b*
  pharmacotherapy, 50
  physical clinical presentation, 47
  psychiatry/psych-mental health nurse practitioner, 51
Glossitis (erythema, smooth/beefy tongue), related to
    pernicious anemia (PA), 106*f*
Gonococcal cervicitis, 356*f*
Gonococcal pharyngitis, 225
Gonococcal urethritis, 355*f*
Gonorrhea, 353, 359*f*
  and dysmenorrhea, 349
  incubation period for, 354
Gram-negative bacterium, 353–354
Gram-negative diplococcus, 353
Gram-positive cocci, 294–296
Group A streptococcus (GAS), 223, 333
Guttate psoriasis, 319

H
Haemophilus influenzae, 193
Hashimoto's thyroiditis, 123
Headache syndrome, 12
Healthcare providers, 213, 233
Heart block, cardiac dysrhythmias, diagnoses in, 142*t*–146*t*, 147*f*
Heart failure (HF), 154, 167*f*
  acute care considerations, 155*b*
  acute decompensated heart failure, 155*b*
  cardinal subjective symptoms, 160
  classification of, 154, 157*t*–158*t*
  comorbid conditions and treatment, 164*t*–165*t*
  diagnoses of, 162
  diversity considerations, 155*b*
  evaluation of, 161
  guideline resources, 162
  HFrEF and HFpEF, 155
  left-sided HF, risk factors, 154
  loop diuretics, 155*b*
  nonpharmacotherapy, 165

Heart failure (HF) *(Continued)*
  older adult considerations, 160*b*
  past medical history, 160
  pathophysiology, 154, 156*f*
  pediatric considerations, 160*b*
  pharmacotherapy, 163
  physical clinical presentation, 161
  right-sided HF, risk factors, 154
  risk factors, 154
  social history, 161
  treatments, 157*t*–158*t*
Heart failure with mildly reduced ejection fraction
    (HFmEF), 154, 157*t*–158*t*
Heart failure with preserved ejection fraction (HFpEF), 154
Heart failure with reduced ejection fraction (HFrEF), 154
Helicobacter pylori infection, connection with IDA, 97
Hematuria, 287
Hemorrhagic stroke, 2
  accident, 10*f*
  acute hospital management, 5*b*
  and chronic hypertension, 2–3
Hemorrhagic strokes, 2
Hepatolithiasis, 277–278
Hernias, 252
  acquired, 251
  incisional, 251
Herpes simplex pharyngitis, 225*f*
High-density lipoprotein (HDL), 169
  contribute to hyperlipidemia, 170–171
  reverse cholesterol transport, 170–171
Hirschsprung's disease, 245
Hormonal contraceptives, for dysmenorrhea, 350
Hospital-acquired pneumonia, 194
Hospital-associated UTIs, 294–296
Hyperbilirubinemia, 278
Hypercalciuria, 286–287
Hyperchylomicronemia, 169
Hyperleukocytosis, 113*b*
Hyperlipidemia
  categorized, 169
  defined, 169
  HDL, contribute to, 170–171
  modifiable risk factors, 169
  onset of, 172–174
  pathophysiology, 169
  primary prevention, 169
Hyperoxaluria, 286–287
Hyperparathyroidism, 289
Hypertension (HTN), 181, 189*f*
  BP, factors involved in regulation of, 182*f*
  crushing chest pain and, 183
  diagnosis of, 185
  diversity considerations, 182*b*
  elevated BP and risk of, 181
  evaluation of, 184
  guideline resources, 185
  hemorrhagic stroke, primary cause of, 2–3
  natriuretic hormone, 181–183
  nonpharmacotherapy, 186*t*, 187
  obesity and, 181–183
  older adult considerations, 187*b*
  pathophysiology, 181, 182*f*
  pediatric considerations, 187*b*
  pharmacotherapy, 185, 186*t*
  physical clinical presentation, 183–184
  primary intermediaries involved, 181
Hyperuricosuria, 286–287
Hyperviscosity syndrome, 113*b*
Hypocitraturia, 286–287

Hypothyroidism, 123, 128*f*
   acute care considerations, 127*b*
   central (secondary), 124
   congenital, 125
   diagnoses of, 126
   diversity considerations, 124*b*
   evaluation of, 125
   guideline resources, 126
   laboratory testing results in euthyroid and thyroid
      disease, 126*f*
   levothyroxine (synthetic T4) as monotherapy, 126, 128*f*
   nonpharmacotherapy, 127
   older adult considerations, 125*b*
   pathophysiology, 123
   pediatric considerations, 125*b*
   pharmacotherapy, 126
   physical clinical presentation, 124
   primary, 123
Hypoxemia, 196

I
Immune-mediated inflammatory disorder, chronic relapsing, 318
Immunization, 194
Incisional hernias, 251
Inflammatory acne, 304
Inflammatory bowel disease (IBD), 258
   diagnosis of, 262
   evaluation of, 262
   pathophysiology, 258
   pharmacotherapy, 263
   plan for, 262
Initial pharmacotherapy, 270
Innate immune systems, cells of, 203–204, 204*f*
Insulin resistance, in DMT2, 116
Integumentary infections, 333
International Prostate Symptom Score, 343
Interstitial lung disease (ILD), 212–213
Intrahepatic bile duct, 277–278
Iodine deficiency, and hypothyroidism, 123
Iron deficiency anemia (IDA), 102*f*
   acute care considerations, 101*b*
   defined, 97
   diagnoses of, 100
   diversity considerations, 98*b*
   evaluation of, 99, 100*t*
   gastrointestinal disease, connection with, 97–98
   guideline resources, 100
   Koilonychia/spoon-shaped fingernails, 99*f*
   laboratory expected values and findings in adults, 100*t*
   lead poisoning, comorbid condition to, in children, 98*b*
   nonpharmacotherapy, 101
   older adult considerations, 98*b*
   pathophysiology, 97
   pediatric considerations, 98*b*
   pharmacotherapy, 100
   physical clinical presentation, 97, 99
   in pregnancy, 98*b*
   stages, 97
   symptoms and RBCs levels, 97–98
Irritable bowel syndrome, 268
   clinical presentation of, 270
   gut–brain system, 269*f*
   mechanisms of, 269*f*
   pathophysiology, 268
Irritant contact dermatitis, 311, 313*f*
   algorithm for, 317*f*
   pathophysiology, 311
Ischemic stroke, 2. *See also* cerebrovascular accidents (CVA)
   accident, 9*f*
   angina, classic finding with, 131–132

Ischemic stroke *(Continued)*
   atherosclerotic plaques, 2
   cerebral thrombosis, 2
   pathophysiology, 2
   physical clinical presentation, 3, 4*b*
   sources of embolism, 2
Isotretinoin therapy, 306

J
Jaundice, 278
Juvenile
   idiopathic arthritis, 72*b*
   pernicious anemia, 108*b*
   rheumatoid arthritis, 72*b*

K
Keloidal scarring, 305
Kidney stones, 285
Koilonychia/spoon-shaped fingernails, and iron deficiency
   anemia, condition in, 99*f*

L
Langerhans cells, 311
Lead poisoning, 98*b*
Left ventricular ejection failure (LVEF), 154
Leukocytosis, 110, 114*f*
   acute care considerations, 113*b*
   diagnoses of, 112
   diversity considerations, 111*b*
   evaluation of, 112, 112*t*, 113*f*
   guideline resources, 112
   laboratory expected values and abnormal findings, 112*t*
   nonpharmacotherapy, 113
   older adult considerations, 111*b*
   pathophysiology, 110
   pediatric considerations, 111*b*
   pharmacologic management, 114*f*
   pharmacotherapy, 113
   physical clinical presentation, 110–111
Lipids, 169–170
Liquid-based Pap test, 356
Liver disease, 236*t*
Loop diuretics, and heart failure, 155*b*
Low back pain (LBP), 80
   red flags in assessment of, 82*t*
   social determinants of health and, 81*b*
Low-density lipoprotein (LDL), 169
   enzymes reducing levels
      3-hydroxy-3-methylglutaryl coenzyme A reductase, 170
      PCSK9-inhibitors, 170
      scavenger cells, 170
      statins, 170
   macrophages transition, 170
Lower urinary tract symptoms (LUTS), 340
Lumbar spine, 83
Lung fibrosis, 213
Lymphocytosis, 110

M
Macrocytic (megaloblastic) anemia, 104
Major depressive disorder (MDD), 54, 59, 60*f*
   corticotropin-releasing hormone, overproduction of, 54
   decrease in
      norepinephrine, 54
      serotonin, 54
   diagnoses of, 58
   diversity considerations, 55*b*
   dopamine reduction and, 54
   DSM-5 criteria for, 57
   evaluation of, 57

Major depressive disorder (MDD) *(Continued)*
  guideline resources, 58
  monoamine neurotransmitter imbalance and, 54
  nonpharmacotherapy, 58
  older adult considerations, 58*b*
  pathophysiology, 54
  pediatric considerations, 55*b*
  pharmacotherapy, 58
  PHQ-9 screening tool with interpretation, 57*f*
  physical clinical presentation, 56
Malignant skin lesions, 325
  acute care considerations, 326*b*
  basal cell carcinoma, 327*f*
  diagnoses of, 327
  diversity considerations, 326*b*
  evaluation of, 327
  hallmark signs of, 327
  nonpharmacotherapy for, 330
  older adult considerations, 326*b*
  pathophysiology, 325
  pediatric considerations, 328*b*
  pharmacotherapy for, 329
  physical clinical presentation, 326
  plan for, 329
  skin biopsy, 327
  squamous cell carcinoma, 328*f*
Melanoma, 325–326, 331*f*
Metformin, 117*b*
Methicillin-resistant *Staphylococcus aureus* (MRSA), 194
Methotrexate, 215
Migraine. *See* Primary headache disorders
Mild renal tubular acidosis, 286–287
Mild traumatic brain injury (mTBI), 37, 44*f*
  contact, 37–39
  diagnosis of, 41
  evaluation of, 41
  guideline resources, 41
  nonpharmacotherapy, 42
  pathoanatomical lesions, 37–39
  pathophysiology, 37
  pediatric considerations, 39*b*
  pharmacotherapy, 42
  physical clinical presentation, 40–41
  sports-related, 38*f*
Miliary pneumonia, 196
Mohs microscopic surgery, 329
Molluscum contagiosum, 307
Monocytosis, 110
Moraxella catarrhalis, 193
Multiorgan system manifestations, 76*b*
Musculoskeletal injuries, 90*b*
Myocardial infarction (MI)
  acute care considerations, 132*b*
  diversity considerations, 132*b*
  older adult considerations, 134*b*
Myocardial ischemia, 131–132
Myxedema coma, 127*b*

N

Nasopharynx, 222–223
Natriuretic hormone, and HTNH, 181–183
Natriuretic peptides
  function, 181–183
  primary intermediaries involved BP regulation, 181
Necrosis, of normal tissue, 333
Necrotizing fasciitis, 334–335
Neisseria gonorrhoeae, 225, 353
Nephrolithiasis, 285
  acute care considerations, 289*b*

Nephrolithiasis *(Continued)*
  algorithm for, 292*f*
  diagnoses of, 288
  diversity considerations, 290*b*
  evaluation of, 288
  factors influencing, 286*f*
  hallmark signs of, 288
  nonpharmacotherapy for, 290
  older adult considerations, 287*b*
  pathophysiology, 285
  pediatric considerations, 290*b*
  pharmacotherapy for, 289
  physical clinical presentation, 287
  plan for, 289
  prevalence of, 287
Neutrophil extracellular traps, 195–196
Neutrophilia, 110, 113*f*
Newborn, physiologic jaundice of, 278
Nitrofurantoin, 215
Nodulocystic acne vulgaris, 304, 307*f*
Nonstaghorn calculi, 285–286
Nonsteroidal antiinflammatory drugs (NSAIDs), for
  dysmenorrhea, 350

O

Obesity, and HTN, 181–183
Occupational exposures, 214–215
Occupational skin disease, cases of, 311
Osteoarthritis (OA), 70, 73*f*, 78*f*
  acute care considerations, 76*b*
  diagnoses of, 74
  evaluation of, 73
  guideline resources, 74
  nonpharmacotherapy, 75
  pathophysiology, 70
  pharmacotherapy, 75
  physical clinical presentation, 71–72
Osteolytic lesions, of bone, 306
Osteoporosis, 81*b*
Ovarian cyst rupture, 350
Oxidant stress, 214
Oxidative stress, 213

P

Pain
  classification of, 235*t*
  clinical manifestations of, 236*t*
Papular lesions, 305
Parietal cells, 243
Pediatric inflammatory bowel disease, 261
Pelvic inflammatory disease (PID), 349–350, 353, 357*b*
Pelvic pain, 350
Pericarditis, 132*b*
Periorbital cellulitis, 334
Pernicious anemia (PA), 104, 108*f*
  acute care considerations, 108*b*
  diagnoses of, 107
  diversity considerations, 105*b*
  evaluation of, 106
  glossitis (erythema, smooth/beefy tongue) related to, 106*f*
  nonpharmacotherapy, 107
  older adult considerations, 105*b*
  pathophysiology, 104
  pediatric considerations, 108*b*
  pharmacotherapy, 107
  physical clinical presentation, 104–105
Pharyngitis, 229*f*
Pharynx, uncomplicated gonococcal infection of, 357
Phosphodiesterase-5 inhibitor, 343

Plaque psoriasis, 320*f*
Pneumonia, 195–196
Posttraumatic stress disorder (PTSD), 62, 67*f*
  acute care considerations, 65*b*
  behavioral symptom diagnostic clusters, 62–64, 64*f*
  diagnoses of, 65
  diversity considerations, 63*b*
  dopamine influence, 62
  evaluation of, 64
  guidelines for, 65
  nonpharmacotherapy, 65
  older adult considerations, 63*b*
  pathophysiology, 62
  pharmacotherapy, 65
  prevalence of, 62
Postvoid residual volume, 343
Prazosin, 65
Primary dysmenorrhea, 346
Primary headache disorders, 12
  cluster, 13*f*, 13
  criteria for, 15*t*
  diagnoses of, 16
  diversity considerations, 14*b*
  evaluation of, 16
  guideline resources, 17
  migraine, 12, 13*f*
  nonpharmacotherapy, 18
  pathophysiology, 12, 13*f*
  pediatric considerations, 17*b*
  pharmacotherapy, 18
  prophylactic treatment, 18
  tension and, 18, 22*f*
Proinflammatory cytokines, in DMT2, 116
Prolonged hyperglycemia, in DMT2, 116
Proprotein convertase subtilisin/kexin type 9 (PCSK9), 170
Prostaglandin synthesis, 346
Prostate cancer, 343
Prostate-specific antigen, 343
Prostatitis, 343
Protective barrier ointments, 312
Protein-rich hyaline membranes, 196
Psoriasis, 314, 318
  acute care considerations, 320*b*
  algorithm for, 323*f*
  diagnoses of, 320
  diversity considerations, 319*b*
  evaluation of, 320
  hallmark signs of, 319
  nonpharmacotherapy for, 321
  older adult considerations, 322*b*
  pathophysiology, 318
  pediatric considerations, 319*b*
  pharmacotherapy for, 321
  physical clinical presentation, 318
  topical corticosteroids potency, 322*t*
  treatment plan for, 320
Psoriatic arthritis, 318
Pulmonary emboli, 132*b*
Pulmonary fibrosis, 212, 215, 219*f*
Pyelonephritis, 294

R
Raynaud's phenomenon, 216
Reactive oxygen species (ROS), 203–204
Red blood cells (RBCs), and IDA, relation with, 97
Referred pain, 233
Renal calculi, 285
Renal colic, 287
Renin-angiotensin-aldosterone system (RAAS), 154–155
  overactivity, 181–183
  primary intermediaries involved BP regulation, 181

Respiratory syncytial virus (RSV), 194
Respiratory viruses, 196
Reverse cholesterol transport, 170–171
Review of systems (ROS), 233
Reye's syndrome, 223
Rheumatic heart disease (RHD), 224
Rheumatoid arthritis (RA), 70, 74*f*, 77*f*, 214
  acute care considerations, 76*b*
  diagnoses of, 74
  evaluation of, 74
  guideline resources, 74
  nonpharmacotherapy, 76
  older adults, treatment in, 75*b*
  pathophysiology, 71
  pharmacotherapy, 75
  physical clinical presentation, 71–72
Rosacea, 307
Rust-colored sputum, 197

S
Saddle anesthesia/paresthesia, 85*b*
Scabies, 314
Scleroderma, 214
Seborrheic dermatitis, 320
Seborrheic keratoses, 328
Secondary dysmenorrhea, 346
Seizure, 26. *See also* Epilepsy
  acute care considerations, 31*b*
  clonic phase, 26–27, 28*f*
  complementary treatment, 32
  diagnoses of, 30
  diversity considerations, 27*b*
  evaluation of, 29
  guideline resources, 30
  lifestyle and behavioral modifications, 32
  medications, 30, 35*f*
  nonpharmacotherapy, 30
  older adult considerations, 31*b*
  oxygen consumption, concern about, 27
  pediatric considerations, 27*b*
  pharmacotherapy, 30
  physical clinical presentation, 28
  tonic-clonic seizure activity, 28*f*
Selective serotonin reuptake inhibitors (SSRIs), 59*b*, 65
Serotonin
  and norepinephrine reuptake inhibitors, 65
  syndrome, 59*b*
Serum human chorionic gonadotropin, for dysmenorrhea, 349
Sexually transmitted infections (STIs), 353
  acute care considerations, 357*b*
  chlamydia
    diagnoses of, 356
    evaluation of, 356
    nonpharmacotherapy for, 358
    pathophysiology, 353
    pharmacotherapy for, 357
    physical clinical presentation, 354
  diversity considerations, 354*b*
  gonorrhea
    diagnoses of, 356
    evaluation of, 356
    nonpharmacotherapy for, 358
    pathophysiology, 353
    pharmacotherapy for, 357
    physical clinical presentation, 354
  older adult considerations, 354*b*
  pediatric considerations, 354*b*
Sexually transmitted pharyngitis, 225
Single broad-spectrum antibiotic, 281
Sinus dysrhythmia, cardiac dysrhythmias, diagnoses in, 142*t*–146*t*, 147*f*

Sjogren's syndrome, 214
Skin pigmentation, 207
Smoking cessation, 290
Social determinants of health (SDoH), 169
Soft tissue disorders, 89, 94*f. See also* Sprains/Strains
Solar lentigines, 328
Somatic pain, 232–233
Spine conditions, 80, 87*f*
  cervical pain, 80
  diagnoses of, 83
  diversity considerations, 81*b*
  evaluation of, 83
  guideline resources, 84
  neck pain, red flags in assessment of, 82*t*
  nonpharmacotherapy, 84
  older adult considerations, 81*b*
  pathophysiology, 80
  pediatric considerations, 82*b*
  pharmacotherapy, 84
  physical clinical presentation, 81
Spirometry postbronchodilator, 206–207
Sprains/strains, 89, 94*f*
  diagnoses of, 92
  diversity considerations, 90*b*
  evaluation of, 92
  guideline resources, 93
  musculoskeletal injuries, 90*b*
  nonpharmacologic therapy, 93
  older adult considerations, 91*b*
  pathophysiology, 89
  pediatric considerations, 90*b*
  pharmacotherapy, 93
  physical clinical presentation, 89, 91
  workplace injuries, 90
Squamous cell carcinoma, algorithm for, 331*f*
Stable angina
  and chest pain, 132
  pathophysiology, 132
  potential condition, 132–133
Staghorn calculi, 285–286
Staghorn configuration, 286–287
Staphylococcus aureus, 333
Staphylococcus saprophyticus, 294–296
Statins, 170
Stone composition analysis, 288
Stone inhibitors, 285
Stopping Elderly Accidents, Deaths, and Injuries
  (STEADI), 39*b*
Streptococcal toxic shock syndrome, 223
Streptococcus pharyngitis, 224*f*, 227
Streptococcus pyogenes, 333
Stroke, 2. *See also* Cerebrovascular accident (CVA),
  Ischemic stroke; Hemorrhagic stroke
Struvite stones, 286–287
Substance-induced anxiety, 65
"Super gonorrhea," 353
Supersaturation, 277–278, 285
Sympathetic nervous system (SNS), primary intermediaries
  involved BP regulation, 181
Syphilis, 356

T
T cell–mediated allergic response, 311
Tamm-Horsfall protein, 285
Tension-type headaches, 14, 17*b*, 21*f. See also* Primary
  headache disorders
Thyroid-stimulating hormone (TSH), 123
Thyrotropin-releasing hormone (TRH), 123
Tinea corporis, 320

TNF alpha and interleukin-1, 195
Tonsils, 222–223
Toxic shock syndrome toxin-1, 195
Transcriptional abnormalities, 215
Traumatic brain injury (TBI), 37, 39*b. See also* Mild
  traumatic brain injury (mTBI)
  acute care considerations, 42*b*
  diversity considerations, 40*b*
  and unintentional falls, 39*b*
Trichomoniasis, 356

U
Ulcerative colitis, 258–259, 260*t*
Umbilical hernia, 253*f*
Uncomplicated urinary tract infections, 294
Unscheduled return visits with admission, 239
Unstable angina, 134
  pathophysiology, 133
  pressure/pain, radiating to left side of neck, jaws, and
    arms, 134
  rest, pain occurrence, 133
Ureteral stones, obstructing, 289
Urinary tract infections (UTIs), 294
  acute care considerations, 296*b*
  algorithm for, 300*f*
  classification of, 294
  diagnoses of, 297
  diversity considerations, 296*b*
  evaluation of, 297
  hallmark signs of, 297
  nonpharmacotherapy for, 299
  older adult considerations, 296*b*
  pathogenesis and mechanisms of, 295*f*
  pathophysiology, 294
  pediatric considerations, 297*b*
  pharmacotherapy for, 298
  physical assessment, 296
  plan for, 298
  risk factors, 294–296
Urinary tract obstruction, 286
Urine human chorionic gonadotropin, for dysmenorrhea, 349
Urolithiasis, 285, 298

V
Vasospastic angina, 134
  and chest pain, 133
  pain at rest, 134
  pathophysiology, 133
Ventricular dysrhythmia, cardiac dysrhythmias, diagnoses
  in, 142*t*–146*t*, 147*f*
Vertical transmission, 353
Very-low-density lipoprotein (VLDL), 169–171
Viral lung infections, 193
Viral pathogens, 224*f*
Viral pharyngitis, 223*f*, 224
Viral pneumonia, 196
Visceral hypersensitivity, 268
Vitamin B12 deficiency, 104. *See also* Pernicious anemia (PA)

W
Wheezing, 194
White blood cells (WBCs)
  elevated count and risk of infection, 112
  and leukocyte function, 110
Whooping cough (pertussis), 194
Workplace injuries, 90

X
Xanthine, 285–286